# AUTOHEMOTHERAPY REFERENCE MANUAL

### \*\*\*

## AUTOBLOOD – THE MAGIC SHOT
## DEFINITIVE GUIDE & HISTORICAL REVIEW
## FROM BLOODLETTING TO STEM CELLS

By

# S. Hale Shakman
## INSTITUTE OF SCIENCE
*www.InstituteOfScience.com*

Warning and Disclaimer:  Although every possible effort has been
made to assure the accuracy and correctness of information
herein, the publisher hereby: apologizes and disclaims liability
for any errors which have escaped editing; and disclaims any and
all dental, medical or legal liability in the event the contents
of this book are utilized as a direct or indirect source of any
dental or medical advice.  The reader is encouraged to access
original works discussed herein to assure accuracy of
information, particularly on such critical matters as vaccine
preparation, etc., and to refer any medical questions concerning
discussions herein and related dental or medical treatment to
appropriate professionals.  A proper professional assessment of
all of a person's medical conditions must always be taken into
account prior to development of a treatment plan.  In this
regard, as differing professional opinions abound, "second (or
more) opinions" are highly recommended.

The AUTOMED Project:
- **AUTOHEMOTHERAPY REFERENCE MANUAL**
- *REFERENCE MANUAL ROSENOW ET AL*
- *MEDICINE'S GRANDEST FRAUD PHD*

AUTOHEMOTHERAPY REFERENCE MANUAL

TABLE OF CONTENTS

## AUTHOR BIOGRAPHICAL SKETCH

S. Hale Shakman has been involved with analysis of health and related programs since 1966-9, when he served with the U.S. State Department's Agency for International Development (A.I.D.) in Washington, D.C. As Program Officer for the Vietnam Program's Public Health Sector, he participated in the overall planning, development and coordination of both direct assistance and training efforts, including oversight of American Medical Association and American Dental Association education contracts, assessments of health facility and construction needs, and coordination with U.S. military and other free world contributors. This included two temporary assignments to Vietnam totaling 5 months, and a Meritorious Service award. He subsequently served in a program management capacity at the Office of Economic Opportunity in Washington, D.C.

Shakman left government service to accept the position of Deputy Director of International Programs (Operations) for the Pathfinder Fund, a private non profit population and health service organization. Later, as an independent consultant and writer, he assisted Maryland, Washington State and Alaska in developing Administration on Aging sponsored nutrition programs; researched, designed and wrote the Planning and Operations Guide for the National Summer Youth Sports Program (sponsored by the President's Council on Physical Fitness and the N.C.A.A.); designed an information system to serve disabled children in the Headstart Program; and compiled and edited THE BLACK PAGES Directory and Resource Guide for People of Color Publications of San Francisco. Additional publications include articles in USA TODAY and the British journal Nature.

Following graduation from Northwestern University (BA), Shakman was accepted into Georgetown University Graduate School's direct to PhD program in History of Political Thought, earning honors and election to Pi Sigma Alpha honor society. He withdrew with permission from Georgetown to accept temporary assignment to Vietnam for the U.S. Department of State. He was subsequently a participant in the Scholars' Colloquium at the Library of Congress, and resumed and completed his Ph.D. program requirements in History of Dentistry by special petition through the American Academy of Biological Dentistry. His PhD dissertation is published under the title, MEDICINE'S GRANDEST FRAUD PHD.

This "AUTOMED" project resulted from the serendipitous set of circumstances discussed below in the "Preface".

PREFACE TO THE SECOND EDITION – 2016: CASE STUDIES

This volume has been augmented with a "Preface to the Second Edition" which has been reissued in a more conventional 6 x 9 inch format as "*Autoblood: The Magic Shot*" (alternate title as per publisher requirement).  Other than this title change, the contents of the larger-print original publication are being fully retained as they are not otherwise available through Medline, etc.

We are reminded of:
- autohemotherapy's history in a range of diseases (as documented herein);
- its tradition as a "treatment of last resort" in otherwise hopeless cases;
- its potential for service against AIDS, ebola, dengue fever, Zika, etc.;
- its logical use for sepsis, which by definition involves antigen in blood;
- its role in immunotherapy vis a vis blocking metastasis of carcinoma;
- and its no-brainer potential as a tool to be integrated into basic first aid.

Beyond re-emphasis on the continuing value of this publication, this "Preface to the Second Edition" highlights notable recent developments:
(1) the growth in popularity of autohemotherapy in Latin America;
(2) alternate modern "guises" of autohemotherapy;
(3) growing use of stem cells from blood rather than from bone marrow; and
(4) the continuing association of autologous methods with cancer;

plus:
  --- Remembering "Autohemotherapist" Sam Tasker (1907-1999) ---

------------------------------------------

(1)  Popularity of autohemotherapy in Latin America.
Searching Google for alternate terms, the dominance of "autohemoterapia" vs "autohemotherapy" – seemingly reflects the particular interest in autoblood therapy in Latin America, e.g., Brazil, as well as in Mexico.

| Google Search Alternate Terms - 1 July 2016 | | | |
|---|---|---|---|
| | Total | Mexico | Brazil | Brasil |
| Autohemotherapy | 113,000 | 33,800 | 19,500 | 8,460 |
| Autohemoterapia | 359,000 | 56,600 | 126,000 | 101,000 |
| Autohemo-terapia | 221,000 | 2,070 | 116,000 | 3,810 |
| Auto-hemoterapia | 252,000 | 80,400 | 22,400 | 115,00 |

Particularly well known in Brazil is the "crusading" work of Dr. Luiz Moura, who has been practicing autohemotherapy since the 1940s, taking the mantle from his father who was also a doctor. Dr. Moura and associates have been engaged in controversy with governmental and medical authorities, who have sought to outlaw the practice.  Advocates have organized with the "Campanha Nacional Em Defesa Da Auto-Hemoterapia" which seems to have been effective to date in keeping the practice available..  Dr. Moura in particular has been very active in promoting awareness of autohemotherapy through a series of youtube.com videos.  See youtube.com.

(2)  Alternate "guises" of autohemotherapy.
  Over the years many, if not most, therapies that have involved extravascular reinjection of autologous blood or serum seemingly have **not** been generally categorized as "autohemotherapy" as such.
  Nonetheless the same or associated underlying physiologic processes seemingly are involved.
  Some prominent modern methods that have received popular attention:
      (a) autologous (whole) blood injection (so-called ABI), alone or with "dry needling" (introduction of a fine needle), usually to treat injured tendons; and
      (b) other methods that involve centrifuging the blood, which separates out a concentrated mix of plasma, etc., which then is injected into injured tissues in various conditions: Autologous Conditioned Plasma (ACP) for tendons; Platelet Rich Plasma (PRP) to treat "tennis elbow"; Blood-spinning, used by professional athletes in a number of sports, i.e., tennis, golf, football, soccer.
      But to date there is no indication that any of these more complex methods is preferable to ABI.  On the contrary, ABI seems to be better, or results are arguably mixed or inconclusive.  And ABI is … autohemotherapy!

(3) Therapy with stem cells from blood rather than bone marrow.
      The field of stem cell therapy had already become prominent as the cutting edge of medical science in the early years of the new millennium (as seen in trends within Medline & Google).
      The past decade has seen further acceleration of the replacement of bone-marrow transplantation (BMT) with stem-cell transplantation (SCT).
      The numbers of SCT articles listed in MEDLINE between 2006 and 2016 are nearly four times greater than the number of BMT articles (60,360 versus 15,812).  This is a dramatic departure from historical trends prior to the past decade, when articles on BMT out-numbered SCT articles two to one (63,632 to 32,158).  As noted in the case of non-Hodgkin's Lymphoma, "marrow collections have largely been abandoned in favour of this safer and better procedure [i.e., "peripheral blood stem cell harvest"] nhlcyberfamily.org/treatments/collection.htm).

| MEDLINE: | BMT | SCT |
|---|---|---|
| Prior to 2006 | 63632 | 32158 |
| 2006 – 2016 | 15812 | 60360 |
| Total all years | 79444 | 92518 |

  Thus stem cell therapy, which predominately uses stem cells from blood, has fundamentally become a form of autohemotherapy.

(4) the continuing association of autologous methods with cancer.

It is striking that the vast majority of autologous immunization methods in MEDLINE, both active and passive respectively, are involved with cancer. This is of course a grand endorsement of the use of autologous (or "personalized") methods in the treatment of cancer.

| MEDLINE a/o 1 July 2016 | | |
|---|---|---|
| Active immunization 142,384 | | |
| + autologous | 1,699 | |
| + cancer | 1,256 | 74% |
| Vaccine therapy | 100,129 | |
| + autologous | 1,773 | |
| + cancer | 1,510 | 85% |
| Passive Immunization 33,884 | | |
| + autologous | 1,566 | |
| + cancer | 1,239 | 79% |
| Serotherapy | 34,016 | |
| + autologous | 1,572 | |
| + cancer | 1,245 | 79% |
| Serum therapy | 230,626 | |
| + autologous | 3,821 | |
| + cancer | 2,205 | 58% |

At the same time, the confusion over the meaning of "active" versus "passive" Immunization continues, as discussed in detail in Chapter 7, "Theoretical Considerations". Sir Almroth Wright had argued that "passive immunization" was actually "active immunization", as clearly evidenced by the observation that, when effective, so-called "serum therapy" involved the application of increasing doses in a similar fashion as with "vaccine-therapy". To this we might well add the success in general of autologous methods against cancer, however they may be labeled. If is autologous, by definition it comprises a self-generated vaccine against one's own cancer, providing additional support for the Wright contention that so-called "passive immunization" is indeed a form of "active immunization", as discussed in Chapters 1, 2 and 5.

## -- Remembering "Autohemotherapist" Sam Tasker (1907-1999) --

When I attempted to find a practitioner in Los Angeles in the early 1990's, I was able to make contact with a dermatologist, Sam Tasker MD. Dr. Tasker had been using autohemotherapy in his dermatology practice for years, albeit on difficult cases. He clearly characterized it as a "treatment of last resort" - if nothing else worked, he would try autohemotherapy. Dr. Tasker used a method he described as "the Russian method". This was comprised of 3 cc of freshly drawn blood, with a small amount residual air in the syringe, which was then briefly shaken to more thoroughly mix the oxygen, and then nearly immediately re-injected into the muscle in the upper-arm / shoulder. He did not change the needle in the process, using the same size needle, 25 x 5/8, for both withdrawing and re-injection. His practice was to repeat the treatment as needed bi-weekly or weekly.

Dr. Tasker closed his practice in the 1990s and is longer with us. Fortunately Dr. Tasker had consented to a lengthy interview before his passing, available on YouTube, accessible through instituteofscience.com or youtube.com (s h shakman). https://www.youtube.com/watch?v=K29GXlFiOCs&feature=related https://www.youtube.com/watch?v=4cwjdL2-5ys

# CASE STUDIES

CROHN'S DISEASE

-- 10cc weekly IM for 3 months, 1 month break, + 3 added months --

Result:  Total healing of the ulcers and clearing of the polyps, proven via colonoscopy; improvement of  functioning of the intestine, weight gain, and general condition; the difference in the condition of the skin is enormous.

**BEFORE** (15 January 2007)      **AFTER** (13 October 2008)

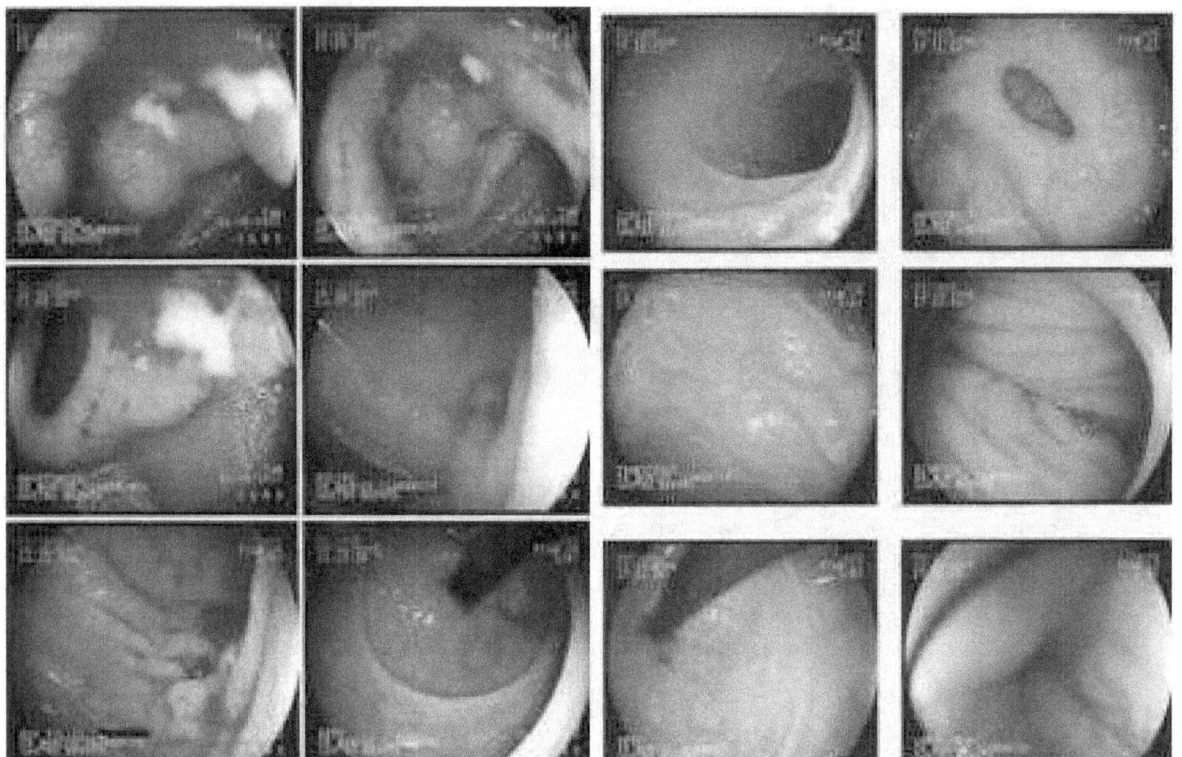

ITAIGARA MEMORIAL HOSPITAL - GASTRO-HEPATO
Information: fetha@ ibest.com.br or Jose Dutra Luiz:
dutrajl@ ig.com.br;  http://inforum.insite.com.br/39550/

## SCLERODERMA

### -- 21 Treatments between 9/08/2006 and 12/20/2006 --

Patient ADB was aged 48 years, white, lived at home and was diagnosed with auto-immune scleroderma; she had extensive wounds with prominent necrosis on the right breast and on the legs below the knees.   The patient had only autohaemotherapy during a 4-month period, and the wounds were cleaned with magnesium isotonic chloride solution 10%. As result of this treatment, we saw a marked improvement in the clinical picture and the lesions, with granulation of 70% of the areas affected in the lower limbs and healing of the breast wounds, confirmed by the photographic evidence.

Telma Geovanini, Manoel Mozart Corrêa Norberto, REFERENCIA, Coimbra U.Portugal  -- Última Edição da Revista Referência – II Série n°9 Março de 2009

**BEFORE**                                      **AFTER**

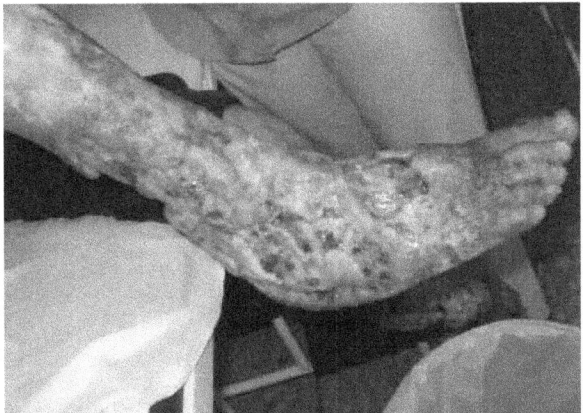

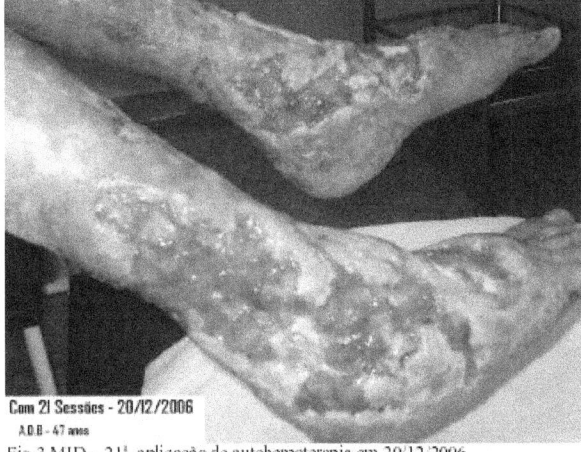

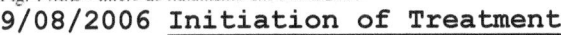
Fig. 1 MID - Início do tratamento em 09/08/2006

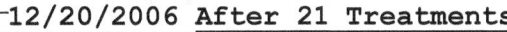
Fig 3 MID – 21ª. aplicação de autohemoterapia em 20/12/2006

**9/08/2006 Initiation of Treatment** ——**12/20/2006 After 21 Treatments**

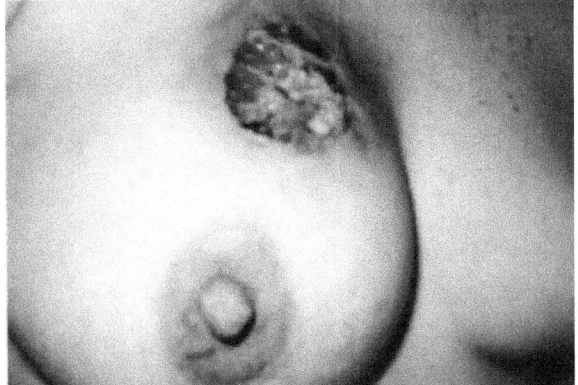

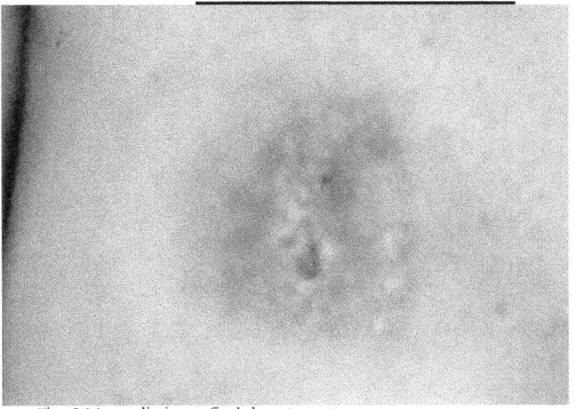

Fig. 4 Mama direita no início do tratamento            Fig. 5 Mama direita ao final do tratamento

## GOATS WITH CONTAGIOUS ECZEMA

IM injection of 5 ml every 7 days over 28 days; cured in 15 days

**BEFORE**

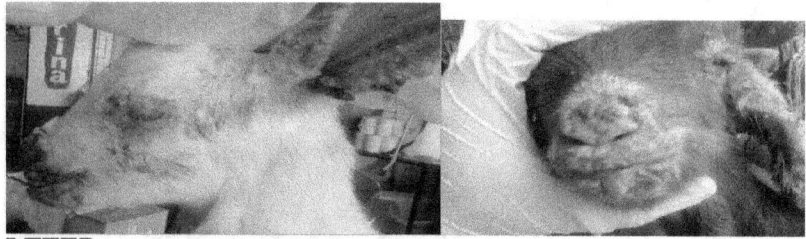

**AFTER**

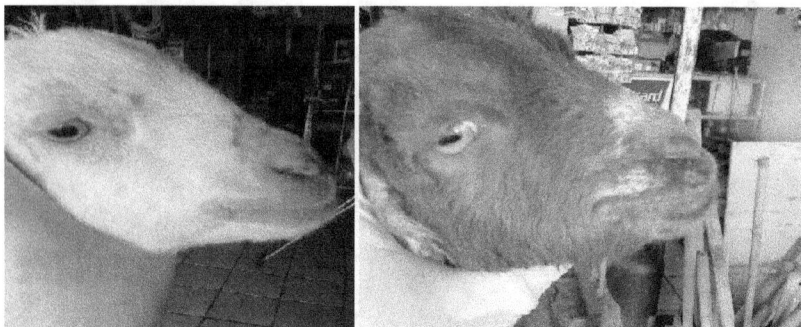

José Honorato de França Neto1  et al., [Primeiro Autor é Graduando do Curso de Medicina Veterinária, Bolsista de extensão, Universidade Federal Rural de Pernambuco, Av. Dom Manoel ds Irmãos, Recife, PE, CEP 52171-900.]

---------------------------

## SKIN DISEASE IN AKITA INU DOG

15 injections - autologous blood -- 10ml - every 15 day

**BEFORE ---** 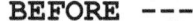                    **AFTER ---**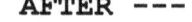

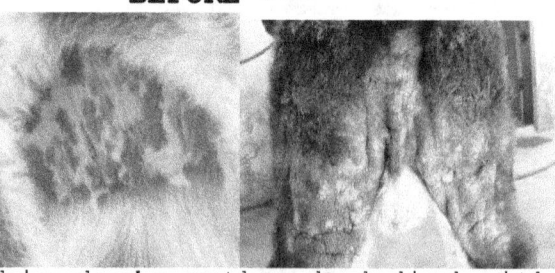          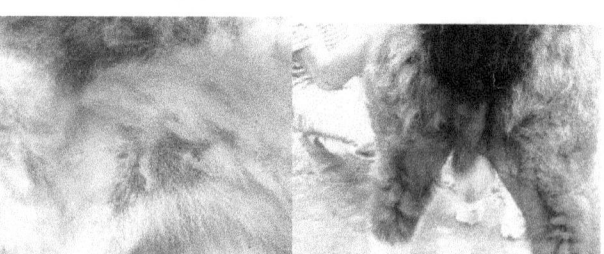

This dog's mother had died without a single hair, with many wounds all over its body, and in indescribable suffering.

**Telma Geovanini** -- Nursing Master Degree -- Auto-hemotherapy Researcher

https://www.youtube.com/watch?v=XgFB368utTY
https://www.youtube.com/watch?v=LXTONbeaiTI

PREFACE TO THE FIRST EDITION

## SOME NOVEL TWISTS & TURNS ALONG THE RESEARCH HIGHWAY

A. GENESIS: STRANDED IN THE JUNGLE
San Francisco, California, Dec. 1987:
   Upon learning of the writer's interest in science, San
Francisco restaurateur Roberto Cuyugan began vividly talking
about the Japanese invasion of the Philippines in 1941, and how
it had caused the male residents of Angeles (site of Clark AFB)
to seek refuge in the nearby mountains of Pampanga Province.  At
the time Mr. Cuyugan was 14 years-of-age, and was with his 65-
year-old father, Dr. Eutiquiano Cuyugan.
   After two months and in the height of the malaria season, Dr.
Cuyugan ran out of quinine, and he immediately engaged his son's
assistance in "drawing blood".  About 10cc of blood was drawn
from each patient, swirled around in a culture dish, and then
reinjected intramuscularly into the same person.
   Mr. Cuyugan suggested that this treatment must have somehow
immobilized the malaria parasite so that the body was able to
identify it and mount a defense; and that, because the AIDS
"virus" is carried in the blood, the treatment might similarly
work with AIDS.  This project originated in Mr. Cuyugan's
suggestions and his request to help publicize this treatment.
   Biographical Sketch:  Eutiquiano Cuyugan was a rather well-
and broadly-educated physician of his time: Born in 1876 to a
wealthy Filipino family, he was educated at the U. of St. Tomas
in Manila, and subsequently studied plastic surgery in Germany;
mental telepathy and the power of the brain in England; and other
subjects in Spain.  He died in 1958 at the age of 82, of a
cerebral hemorrhage, on the Isle of Cebu.

B. THESIS:  WRIGHT?
   The subject was put to friends who were more knowledgeable of
medical matters, who offered that it makes logical sense - it
might make the foreign organism more visible; however, as far as
they knew, there was no history of its use or its safety.
   The local library wasn't much help regarding the history of
blood injections except for a couple of disgusting stories about
fools who injected others' infected blood; however, there <u>was</u>
some mention of vaccine-therapy and the autogenously vaccines of
Sir Almroth Wright which seemed to relate.  And it <u>was</u> possible
to piece together a plausible connect-a-dot explanation as to how
such a method might work for AIDS, incorporating Wright's work to
explain how one's own blood might serve as a vaccine when
reinjected intramuscularly.
   A science convention was coming up in Corvallis, Oregon; the
story was put into proper 5-inch-square "abstract" form for
publication and for use as an outline for a June 20 oral
presentation in Corvallis.  Coincidentally, earlier that week <u>USA
TODAY</u> (6-15-88) had run a story on reinjecting heated blood along

with an anti-cancer drug to treat melanoma, and in a discussion following the Corvallis presentation someone noted that a friend had recently had his blood reinjected to treat allergies.  [See below "Abstract of Presentation" and "Transcript of Discussion".]

## C.  ANTITHESIS: NOT EXACTLY WRIGHT

Following the convention, Dr. Cuyugan's method was described to a dermatologist who immediately identified it as "autohemotherapy".  He personally had used it only once in a stubborn case of lichen planus (successfully).

A medical-library search located the term "autohemotherapy", not as a distinct category on its own, but rather within the subject area "serum therapy".  Over the years, mostly from the 1920s through the early 1940s, several hundred autohemotherapy articles were found so tucked away.  Now things started getting confusing, because "vaccine therapy" and "serum therapy" are thought to involve different immune mechanisms.  Serum therapy is generally thought to involve the transfer of immunity, via the serum, from a previously infected and immunized person or animal ("passive immunization"); obviously no such transfer of immunity is involved in autohemotherapy.

At this point the writer was inclined to favorably consider Sir Almroth Wright's assertion that serum therapy may actually be a form of vaccine-therapy, which would allow for wrapping autohemotherapy and autogenous vaccine therapy into a nice little package with Sir A.E. Wright as theoretician.  But the question of so dispensing with the whole of "serum therapy" was contemplated with no small measure of trepidation.  After all, the National Institute of Health's MEDLINE computer index continues to treat "serum therapy" as virtually synonymous with "passive immunization", in contrast to "active immunization", the principle thought to underlie vaccine-therapy.

Then a new wrinkle appeared, compelling further inquiry.

## D.  SYNTHESIS:  ROSENOW'S REVOLUTION

A 1915 article by C.H. Pierce on autogenous vaccine therapy lavishly praised an E. C. Rosenow, and totally ignored vaccine-therapy founder and prime guru Sir Almroth Wright.  Who was this Dr. Rosenow?  This question opened a Pandora's vault.

By the end of 1915 Dr. Rosenow had already published more than 70 articles including a landmark 1915 JAMA summary article which showed how bacteria from humans with various diseases (e.g. arthritis, appendicitis, stomach ulcers, etc.) would "electively locate" in corresponding organs of laboratory animals.  Dr. Rosenow solidified and expanded on this work over the next four decades, mostly as the Mayo Clinic's Head of Experimental Bacteriology.  This work identified blood-borne agents from oral infections as the cause of many such diseases in "constitutionally-predisposed persons", including even such still-mysterious conditions as schizophrenia; thus (1) the very presence in the blood of causative agents also explains autohemotherapy's reported successes in such conditions; and (2)

Beyond this, Dr. Rosenow seems to have found what modern science continues to search for - an environmental (bacterial) cause for many of these same diseases in "genetically-predisposed persons".

E.  ASYNTHESIS:  HOLMAN'S DECEPTION
  A review of literature critical of Dr. Rosenow's work, and underlying references, was undertaken in an attempt to determine what had happened to him; this review disclosed common and indispensable reference to a 1928 article by W. Holman, which had portrayed Dr. Rosenow's 1915 data as inconclusive.  On examination, it was found that Holman had perpetrated a clever but nonetheless blatant deception - one that has successfully deflected generations of doctors and patients, up to the present time, from essential facts concerning the nature of a wide range of diseases.

F.  SUPERSYNTHESIS:
  AUTOMED AS UNIMED - AN HYPOTHESIS
  This work seeks to integrate within a cohesive framework the subjects of autohemotherapy, autovaccine therapy, and Dr. Rosenow's bacteriology; and to flag and assess the conceptual significance of this framework within the history and future of medicine.
  The work is being presented in a series of three reports including: (1) this volume, *AUTOHEMOTHERAPY REFERENCE MANUAL*; (2) *REFERENCE MANUAL ROSENOW ET AL;* and (3) *MEDICINE'S GRANDEST FRAUD PHD*.  These may be followed by other reports as required on cross-cutting general and disease-specific considerations, and other relevant subjects.
  Table i-1, "Autologous Inoculation Therapy Trends", lists numbers of citations in the INDEX MEDICUS and other relevant sources for each of: autohemotherapy, auto-vaccine, E.C. Rosenow; these have compiled and indexed .  (A comprehensive listing of these autohemotherapy and auto-vaccine citations is included herein.  See *REFERENCE MANUAL ROSENOW ET AL* for Rosenow's bibliography.

  The term "AUTOMED" has been chosen as designation for this overall project for want of another term which would encompass both therapeutic and causative disease-related factors from an "autogenous" (or "autologous") perspective.
  This current volume, *AUTOHEMOTHERAPY REFERENCE MANUAL,* is particularly concerned with the therapeutic side.  Although the scope is broader than "autohemotherapy" per se, the primary focus is "hemo"(blood)-related - including reference to bone-marrow transplantation and venesection (bloodletting).  At the same time it is recognized that autohemotherapy might as well be viewed as a form of either of two other entities presented herein as sub-categories - autovaccinetherapy and autotherapy.
  For discussions of the causation of systemic disease and a comprehensive overview and index to the works of Dr. Rosenow, including reference to therapeutic vaccine and antibody, please

refer to *REFERENCE MANUAL ROSENOW ET AL.* For discussion of key factors contributing to the suppression of E. C. Rosenow's work and the focal infection concept in general, please see *MEDICINE'S GRANDEST FRAUD PHD.*

ABSTRACT OF PRESENTATION (6-20-88): Cuyugan's Malaria Treatment - Aid vs. AIDS?
[Shakman SH, Proc.Pac.Div. AAAS 7, 1988, 42]
In 1941 Filipino Dr. Eutiquiano Cuyugan treated approx. 40 malaria patients as follows: Blood (10 cc) was drawn from the arm, put in a culture dish for 2-3 mins. (swirled a bit to keep coagulation even), & injected into the same patient's buttock muscle. After 8-10 hours the site of injection became red. After 1 day chills would cease but fever remained. Over 2-3 days, fever would diminish and then disappear. By the 4th day patients could generally resume normal activity. A dose of about 3cc was not effective for a 10-year-old but a subsequent dose of about 5cc was. Cuyugan's son Roberto performed the procedure on others and self and believes it safe, suggesting possible use against AIDS.* Cuyugan's (anti-protozoa) method may be viewed as a synthesis of Sir Almroth Wright's studies**: (a) "auto-inoculation"{350-1} of blood undergoing (b) coagulation [as may be related to blood's "antibacterial power"{301}] into (c) the tissues where "bacteriotropic substances are manufactured"{353} [incl. (d) "opsonins"{83}]; comprising (e) "vaccine-therapy" with preferred "vaccines prepared from the original patient"{375}. Antibody known to opsonize bacteria (e.g. IgG & IgM)*** may also relate to viruses: IgG may neutralize (polio) virus in bloodstream***; and a deficient IgM response is associated with AIDS ****.

*Interviews with R. Cuyugan, San Francisco, USA, Jan.,1988.
**WRIGHT, A.E., Studies on Immunization (1909). ***CLARK, W.R., Experimental Foundations of Modern Immuniz. (1986), 416.
****FAUCI, A.S., Science 239 (5 Feb. 1988), 620.

DISCUSSION FOLLOWING PRESENTATION
Q1: I have an observation. I had a friend who was undergoing that treatment for allergies. I have allergies. I had never heard of the treatment and I thought to myself, "That's too good to be true. The guy must be a quack." On the other hand, if it works... And the variable is simply what you do with the blood between the time you take it out and put it back in.
A: Cuyugan just had it out for 2-3 minutes, until it started to coagulate. That seemed to Roberto Cuyugan to be very important, very significant. He swirled it around so that the serum would not separate out, and then injected it whole.
Q1: As a practical matter it would be fascinating to test it, since they're taking blood out, adding to it and then re-entering it. [melanoma doctors, as per USA TODAY 6-15-88]
A: Precisely. Maybe this article enhances prospects for a test.

Q2: Does this rise to the dignity of science?  In other words, is it science when you can't tell why something occurs?

A: The theories of Wright may explain why it occurs, or at least provide a possible explanation if in fact it does work.

Q2: Then it could be subject to experimentation, couldn't it?

A: One would think so.  There's a lot we don't know.  Science attempts to separate out what we know from what we don't.   ###

Table i-1:  AUTO-INOCULATION THERAPY TRENDS
- Numbers of articles by type, year, source:
IM=Index Medicus QCIM=Quarterly Cum.IM CL=Current List CIM=Cum.IM

| | AUTOHEMOTHERAPY/AUTOSEROTHERAPY | | | | AUTOVACCINOTHERAPY | | | | ROSENOW [TOT] |
|---|---|---|---|---|---|---|---|---|---|
| source> | IM | QCIM | CL | CIM | IM | QCIM | CL | CIM | VARIOUS |
| 1902 | | | | | | | | | 1 |
| 1903 | | | | | | | | | 2 |
| 1904 | | | | | | | | | 2 |
| 1905 | 1 | | | | | | | | 1 |
| 1906 | 2 | | | | | | | | 1 |
| 1907 | | | | | | | | | 2 |
| 1908 | | | | | | | | | 2 |
| 1909 | 1 | | | | 1 | | | | 9 |
| 1910 | 3 | | | | 3 | | | | 4 |
| 1911 | 10 | | | | 4 | | | | 3 |
| 1912 | 9 | | | | 3 | | | | 12 |
| 1913 | 11 | | | | 2 | | | | 8 |
| 1914 | 6 | | | | 3 | | | | 13 |
| 1915 | 8 | | | | 3 | | | | 11 |
| 1916 | 4 | 2 | | | 1 | 2 | | | 8 |
| 1917 | 4 | 1 | | | 2 | 2 | | | 7 |
| 1918 | 6 | | | | 1 | 4 | | | 9 |
| 1919 | 2 | | | | 2 | 2 | | | 7 |
| 1920 | 1 | 1 | | | 5 | | | | 2 |
| 1921 | 5 | 4 | | | 5 | 2 | | | 7 |
| 1922 | | 2 | | | 2 | 2 | | | 5 |
| 1923 | 10 | 9 | | | 2 | 1 | | | 10 |
| 1924 | 12 | 10 | | | 3 | 5 | | | 8 |
| 1925 | 12 | 27 | | | 1 | 14 | | | 2 |
| 1926 | 9 | 25 | | | 3 | 15 | | | 9 |
| 1927 | | 50 | | | | 35 | | | 9 |
| 1928 | | 41 | | | | 24 | | | 9 |
| 1929 | | 37 | | | | 22 | | | 4 |
| 1930 | | 35 | | | | 19 | | | 12 |
| 1931 | | 37 | | | | 10 | | | 6 |
| 1932 | | 29 | | | | 12 | | | 9 |
| 1933 | | 41 | | | | 14 | | | 9 |
| 1934 | | 38 | | | | 24 | | | 6 |
| 1935 | | 47 | | | | 21 | | | 6 |
| 1936 | | 24 | | | | 20 | | | 4 |
| 1937 | | 52 | | | | 8 | | | 4 |
| 1938 | | 33 | | | | 16 | | | 5 |
| 1939 | | 20 | | | | 11 | | | 5 |
| 1940 | | 23 | | | | 8 | | | 3 |
| 1941 | | 24 | 1 | | | 7 | | | 2 |
| 1942 | | 7 | | | | 4 | | | 6 |
| 1943 | | 8 | | | | 2 | 2 | | 6 |
| 1944 | | 10 | | | | 2 | | | 10 |
| 1945 | | 3 | 2 | | | 3 | | | 7 |
| 1946 | | 7 | 1 | | | 1 | | | |
| 1947 | | 7 | 1 | | | 5 | | | 2 |
| 1948 | | 5 | 1 | | | 5 | 1 | | 5 |

| Year | | | | | | | | | | | |
|---|---|---|---|---|---|---|---|---|---|---|---|
| 1949 | | 5 | 2 | | | 3 | 1 | | | 1 | |
| 1950 | | 6 | 2 | | | 4 | 2 | | | 3 | |
| 1951 | | 3 | 11 | | | 1 | 1 | | | 5 | |
| 1952 | | 3 | 4 | | | 4 | 3 | | | 3 | |
| 1953 | | 8 | 7 | | | 3 | 4 | | | 2 | |
| 1954 | | 2 | 10 | | | 2 | 5 | | | 1 | |
| 1955 | | 3 | 6 | | | 4 | 5 | | | 2 | |
| 1956 | | 1 | 7 | | | 2 | 2 | | | | |
| 1957 | | | 7 | | | | 3 | | | 1 | |
| 1958 | | | 4 | | | | 3 | | | 1 | |
| 1959 | | | 3 | | | | 6 | | | | |
| 1960 | | | | 1 | | | | | 2 | | |
| 1961 | | | | 2 | | | | | 3 | | |
| 1962 | | | | 1 | | | | | 3 | | |
| 1963 | | | | 2 | | | | | 4 | | |
| 1964 | | | | 2 | | | | | 6 | | |
| 1965 | | | | 4 | | | | | 1 | | |
| 1966 | | | | 3 | | | | | 1 | | |
| 1967 | | | | – | | | | | 2 | | |
| 1968 | | | | 3 | | | | | 2 | | |
| 1969 | | | | 1 | | | | | 4 | | |
| 1970 | | | | 2 | | | | | 2 | | |
| 1971 | | | | 1 | | | | | 1 | | |
| 1972 | | | | 3 | | | | | 5 | | |
| 1973 | | | | 1 | | | | | 5 | | |
| 1974 | | | | 1 | | | | | 2 | | |
| 1975 | | | | 1 | | | | | 3 | | |
| 1976 | | | | – | | | | | 2 | | |
| 1977 | | | | – | | | | | 2 | | |
| 1978 | | | | – | | | | | 2 | | |
| 1979 | | | | – | | | | | 1 | | |
| 1980 | | | | 1 | | | | | 1 | | |
| 1981 | | | | 2 | | | | | 1 | | |
| 1982 | | | | – | | | | | 2 | | |
| TOTALS | 126 | 690 | 69 | 31 | [916] | 46 | 345 | 38 | 57 | 293 | [774] |

## Chapter 1: INTRODUCTION

Life as we comprise it certainly could not have evolved, were it not for the ability, even tendency, of living things to recover from injury and disease. Somehow, even though the first lines of bodily defense may be breached by some foreign agent, the invader tends to be identified, isolated, resisted, repelled and/or conquered, or at least sufficiently restrained. However, when this does not occur, the living being may be doomed, consumed by the microbial enemy within. During the first half of the 20th century, two major types of therapies were developed which encompassed removing an invader from a "safe-haven" within the being and reinjecting it into tissues where an adequate response may be elicited - autohemotherapy and autogenous vaccines.

From the early 20th century, both autohemotherapy and autogenous vaccine therapy (the latter often in association with removal of infected oral foci) have been reported as useful in a wide and common range of disease conditions. About midway through the 20th century, largely in the wake of the medical-drug-craze era that followed World War II, both fell somewhat out of vogue, although essential elements of both are found in continuing medical practices. And as the 20th century draws to a close, a growing recognition of the limits of contemporary technology has prompted explicit calls in medical journals for revival of interest in both types of therapy. [see MEDLINE UPDATES] Both, in some fashion, have already been proposed for AIDS. [see AIDS]

Autohemotherapy consists of the simple reinjection of one's own blood, usually <u>intramuscularly or subcutaneously</u>. The procedure evolved in part from the "serum therapy" tradition of Kitasato and von Behring, which had involved <u>intravenously</u> injected "immunized" serum and a presumed passive transfer of immunity to the patient. Along the way, someone tried a mother's serum, and others, including Spiethoff, used the patient's own serum. Thus while autohemotherapy has from its inception been grouped with "serum-therapy", as early as 1917, Spiethoff noted: "The benefit [of autohemotherapy] does not depend on supplying certain lacking elements but on a broader principle which includes the individual's own serum." (17A1 in Appendix C of this volume, "Autohemotherapy Bibliography".) Such a "broader principle" might logically encompass that which underlies autogenous vaccine-therapy's action.

While autohemotherapy as a distinct entity enjoyed a well-documented period of popularity during the first half of the 20th century, which period is particularly emphasized herein, it also represents the culmination of a fundamental thread weaving through the healing arts for at least a few millennia. Such diverse traditional practices as bloodletting, acupuncture, coining and moxibustion, and modern-day plasmapheresis, innovations in bone marrow transplantation (use of autologous marrow and use of stem cells from blood in place of marrow), and to some extent even autotransfusions - all may involve the manipulation of one's own blood or blood-components and the possibility that benefits may at least in part be due to a forced defensive response within the body's tissues against harmful substances in the blood, like a vaccine. In this light, autohemotherapy may be viewed as simply the direct application of such a process.

Autogenous vaccine therapy involves the extraction, culturing, inactivation and reinjection of a presumed responsible disease-causing organism, and rests on the theoretical foundations of Louis Pasteur and Sir Almroth Wright. Pasteur (1822-1895) had discovered that injecting "attenuated" microbes may protect animals from future exposures to virulent ones, and Wright extended this to therapy with autogenous (self-generated) vaccines. As compared to autohemotherapy, autogenous vaccines allow particularly for greater control of dosage; however, making a vaccine involves much more time and expense, along with the risk of inadvertently excluding or altering the disease-causing agent(s). If such an agent is in one's blood, autohemotherapy ensures its inclusion.

Although Sir Almroth Wright does not appear to have directly addressed autohemotherapy, we may safely assume he would have considered it a form of vaccine-therapy. Wright had asserted that the overall concept of serum therapy rests on a "foundation of sand" and "many of the successful results which have been achieved by serum therapy would find their simplest explanation in the assumption that the sera ... operated as bacterial vaccines." Even without invoking Wright, autohemotherapy clearly defies ready classification as "passive immunization" in that the blood is coming not from an immunized other but from the same individual!

On the other hand, convincing arguments against the extreme Wright position come from a most prominent protege of Wright on the subject of autogenous vaccine therapy, Dr. Edward C. Rosenow, with whom we shall spend considerable time with reference to his own accomplishments. Dr. Rosenow extravascularly (intramuscularly or subcutaneously) administered both "antigen" and "antibody" (presumed agents of active and passive immunization respectively), and his specific and separate skin-test results with these substances might also be invoked to support the suggestion that autohemotherapy's action may in part be attributed to the presence and distinct action of both antigen and antibody.

Thanks primarily to the legendary works of Dr. Rosenow, who served as head of Experimental Bacteriology for the Mayo Clinic from 1915-1944, it is possible, today, to produce proper autogenous vaccines and antibody even in the case of many diseases for which causes are generally considered unknown.  The "secret" to Dr. Rosenow's successes involved the use of culture mediums that recreated conditions that exist within the human body, particularly with respect to the use of reduced oxygen gradients.  In so doing, Dr. Rosenow definitively identified causative organisms for a wide range of diseases (e.g., arthritis, diabetes, epilepsy, MS, myasthenia gravis, schizophrenia, stomach ulcers and many more), traced them to their source in oral foci (primarily diseased teeth and/or tonsils), and reproduced corresponding symptoms in laboratory animals.  Dr. Rosenow's confirmation of these results with a battery of independent tests clearly exceeded merely fulfilling the Henle/Koch postulates of causation.  (see *MEDICINE'S GRANDEST FRAUD PHD*).

    The bodies of work integrated within the AUTOMED concept are not correctly categorized as "alternative" approaches, but rather are clearly in the mainstream of medical history; e.g., some 29 autohemotherapy and 42 Rosenow items were published in J.A.M.A. Moreover, many disease conditions are common to all three categories, as shown in Table 1-1.

Table 1-1: Diseases addressed in literature of: autohemotherapy (H); autovaccine (V); Rosenow (R)

| | | | |
|---|---|---|---|
| Abscesses | HV | Migraine | H R |
| Acne | HV | Mouth Infect. | H R |
| Alcoholism | H R | Multiple Sclerosis | H R |
| Allergies | HVR | Nasal Infection etc | HV |
| Anemia | H R | Nephritis | VR |
| Angina | H R | Nervous System Dis. | H R |
| Appendicitis | H R | Ozena | HV |
| Arthritis | HVR | Pancreatic Disease | H R |
| Bacterial Infection | HV | Pemphigus | HVR |
| Boils | HV | Pneumonia | HVR |
| Bronchitis | HVR | Poliomyelitis | H R |
| Cancer | HVR | Prostatitis | VR |
| Chorea | H R | Psoriasis | HV |
| Colitis, Ulcerative | HVR | Puerperal Infection | VR |
| Common cold | VR | Pulmonary Diseases | VR |
| Diabetes | H R | Pyelonephritis | VR |
| Encephalitis | H R | Pyogenic Infection | HV |
| Endocarditis | VR | Respiratory Infect. | VR |
| Epilepsy | H R | Rheumatism | HVR |
| Erythema | H R | Rhinitis | HV |
| Eye Diseases | H R | Scarlet Fever | VR |
| Furuncles | HV | Septicemia | HV |
| Glaucoma | H R | Stomach Ulcer | H R |
| Gonorrhea | HV | Streptococcal Inf. | VR |
| Hayfever | HVR | Typhoid | HV |
| Headache | H R | Urethritis | HV |
| Herpes simplex | H R | Verucca | HV |
| Herpes Zoster | H R | Virus Diseases | HVR |
| Hypertension | H R | Whooping Cough | HV |
| Inflammatory Inf. | HV | | |
| Influenza | HVR | | |
| Iridocyclitis | H R | | |
| Leprosy | HV | | |
| Leukemia | H R | | |
| Lung Disease | H R | | |
| Meningitis | VR | | |
| Mental Illness | H R | | |

RECOMMENDATIONS FOR IMMEDIATE ACTION


  At the outset and in summation, the following recommendations
come to mind most prominently, as appears indicated by the study
of materials in this compilation:


  WAR ON DISEASE: MOVE AUTOHEMOTHERAPY TO FRONT LINES
  Autohemotherapy would well be incorporated into all first-aid
classes, scout training programs, survival training, etc., and
adopted as a universal treatment of first resort.  Once so
adopted, the patient of any systemic disease may be placed
immediately on the road to recovery or at least effective
defense, while medical help is sought and while that medical help
is trying to figure out what's wrong and how to fix it.
Autohemotherapy is the ideal immediate response in so many
diseases:  Insofar as modern medical practice involves the
withdrawing and testing of blood samples in order to determine
the nature of diseases, it would be both easy and prudent, as a
general practice, to draw out 3-10 cc more than is needed for
testing, and reinject that amount of blood subcutaneously or
intramuscularly.  Thus the patient would be in an enhanced
position for getting better even if the doctor never figures out
what's wrong.  And in this fashion, the "getting better" costs
nothing, in contrast to the blood tests themselves which may be
very time-consuming, costly, and not always conclusive.

  It might also be suggested that consideration of Dr. Rosenow's
work be incorporated into the blood testing process itself; e.g.
for discussion of Rosenow's blood culture methodology, please see
*Postgrad. Med.* 124-136, Feb. 1948.


  High on the priority list for autohemotherapy applications is
malaria.  To our dear friends at the U.S. Agency for
International Development, a recommended first step would involve
the testing of Cuyugan's method (a single shot of blood nearing
the coagulation point) as compared with that of Padoan and
Frizzerio (30B13), involving series of injections of freshly
drawn autoblood); and the training of indigenous personnel in the
administration of autohemotherapy.  The beauty of
autohemotherapy, beyond its unrivaled specificity and safety, is
simplicity.  Operators need not be trained in other areas, and
extensive programs can be undertaken by "armies" of indigenous
workers in rural or otherwise remote areas.  If this program is
followed, malaria, which now infects hundreds of millions and
kills millions each year, may be rendered impotent in a
ridiculously short period of time.

  This prescription would also seem appropriate for other insect-
vector diseases, and the likes of insidious mysterious emerging
conditions, e.g. ebola.

ON MALARIA AND OTHER ACUTE DISEASES; THERAPEUTIC REGIMENS

It may be worthwhile to note apparent similarities between Dr. Cuyugan's reported successful therapeutic methodology in the case of acute malaria attacks and Dr. Rosenow's evolved and reported successful method in treating acute poliomyelitis.  Dr. Cuyugan's method involved bringing blood to near-coagulation and thus the formation of substances which may relate to antibody [see THEORETICAL CONSIDERATIONS]; Dr. Rosenow's last-reported and spectacularly successful method in the case of polio involved single subcutaneous or intramuscular injections of massive amounts of so-called "thermal" antibody derived from antigen [see Chapter 6. Poliomyelitis, in *REFERENCE MANUAL ROSENOW ET AL*]. The question of whether the action of such substances, administered extravascularly, is properly characterized as "active" or "passive" immunization will be revisited herein, but not definitively resolved.  [see particularly THEORETICAL CONSIDERATIONS]

And for what it's worth, on the subject of acute afflictions, both Hippocrates and the 12th Century's "code of health" had called for bloodletting. [see BLOODLETTING]


ON THE NEED TO ERADICATE ORAL FOCI, INCLUDING PULPLESS TEETH

Often-symptomless foci, including inconspicuous tonsils and diseased teeth or gums, particularly including devitalized teeth, have been conclusively implicated in a wide range of systemic disease conditions, as per the works of Rosenow, Price, Haden, Billings, C.Mayo, and others.  Accordingly, so-called root-canal-"therapy" must be abandoned, until such a time as such resulting "locations of least resistance" may be rendered permanently sterile, which time has not yet arrived (this according to Dr. S. Seltzer, Head of Endodontics Section, Oral Pathology ...).

Surgical correction of residual bone infections may also be indicated. (see *REFERENCE MANUAL ROSENOW ET AL*).


AIDS AND OTHER STILL-MYSTERIOUS, SYSTEMIC CHRONIC DISEASES

Regarding the disease phenomenon known as AIDS and other still-mysterious systemic diseases as well as yet-to-emerge diseases, a three-step programme appears to be merit serious consideration:

1.  Autohemotherapy:  A therapy is immediately available that will unquestionably cause no aggravation of conditions in victims, but rather will undoubtedly provide some measure of assistance in forestalling the disease process - autohemotherapy.  It makes no difference what the causative agent really is, or where it comes from, as long as it's in the blood.  In order to provide continuous coverage, in that antibodies are produced for 3-4 days in the reticulo-endothelial system (as discussed by Florence Sabin 1939 and others), extravascular autohemotherapy

might be performed at intervals of 2-3 days.  To assure
compliance with this schedule, patients (or responsible family
members) might be instructed in self-administration as is
currently done in the cases of self-administered therapies for
the likes of diabetes and migraine.  Assuming there is no
persistent focus in the host that is continuing to feed pathogens
or their derivative forms into the bloodstream, autohemotherapy
might hopefully be curative.  However, in the continued presence
of such a focus, continued therapy would be indicated at least
until the focus is fully removed.

   2.  Autovaccine:  Insofar as:  (a) tonsils and teeth are known
"reservoirs" for HIV (the entity commonly associated with AIDS),
(b) these are by definition infected oral foci.  (c) Dr. Rosenow
and others have conclusively demonstrated a causative relation
between oral foci and a wide range of human diseases of "unknown"
or hypothesized "autoimmune" etiology.  This and many other
similarities between AIDS and MS, for example, coupled with Dr.
Rosenow's definitive showing of a causal relation between oral
foci and MS, certainly suggests that such a relation might apply
in the case of AIDS.  This, coupled with the finding of HIV in
oral foci suggests the possibility that HIV is a simple
degenerative form or other phase of the true causative organism
of the disease syndrome associated with AIDS, which degenerative
phase results from removal of the causative organism from its
natural in-vivo environment (for further discussions, see AIDS
Chapter in *REFERENCE MANUAL ROSENOW ET AL.*

   Thus it is time to put two-plus-two together, use Rosenow's
methods to culture the streptococcal form of the organism that is
growing in oral foci and probably causing the range of diseases
known as AIDS, and make autogenous therapeutic vaccines and
antibody in accord with Rosenow's instructions.  Once available
these autogenous inoculums can comprise the most specific and
powerful therapy possible, as demonstrated effective by Dr.
Rosenow for M.S. and other diseases.  These could theoretically
also provide prophylactic cover possible against septicemia
resulting from the necessary surgical procedure in step 3, below.
 Meanwhile, use autohemotherapy on a regular basis.

   3.  Remove the focus:  The body must be cleansed of the nests
in which the organism replicates; while achieving the necessary
goal of full general acceptance of this hypothesis may be "like
pulling teeth", for AIDS as well as for other chronic-systemic
mysterious or otherwise-still-vital diseases, acceptance is
inevitable and will in fact require just that - pulling teeth -
all non-vital teeth; other infected teeth wherein infection has
accessed the interior; infected areas about these teeth; and as
required other residually-infected oral foci, e.g. tonsils.
Concurrent with and following the removal of infected oral foci,
autogenous vaccine and antibody is to be continued so long as it
is determined that secondary foci elsewhere within the body may
be self-sustaining and/or continue to feed the bloodstream with

infection.

4.   Overall the works of Dr. Rosenow merit particularly thorough review and consideration as a standard and base against which on-going and future work on bacteriology/ virology may be judged and progress; to not do so seems irresponsible and even foolhardy.


In a somewhat roundabout manner, Mr. Cuyugan's proposal of reinjecting one's blood for AIDS has led to an investigation of the history of autogenous vaccines, then to the discovery of the "lost" archives of autohemotherapy, then into the nature and scope of oral-focal-related diseases, and then to the hypothesis that AIDS is indeed one of these; and along the way to an impressive body of clinical and theoretical argument that autohemotherapy may usefully and immediately be employed against AIDS and other blood-borne diseases pending the identification and removal of primary (and any now-established secondary, if possible) foci.

At least that's the way it looks from here.

Chapter 2: AUTOHEMOTHERAPY OVERVIEW (THE MAGIC SHOT)

Enabling technological advance:
The Hypodermic Needle

OVERVIEW, ACTION, SCOPE, FREQUENCY

The ability of the living body to combat infection is itself truly magical. Autohemotherapy may uniquely help the body perform this magic, by facilitating the identification of infective organisms in the bloodstream, and enabling the launching of a counterattack.

Autohemotherapy, defined herein (and commonly but not exclusively in the historical literature) as the immediate intramuscular or subcutaneous reinjection of one's own blood, appears to comprise a compelling therapy option in the absence of others, one that may also merit replacing other (experimental and often risky) attempts at therapy currently in vogue. Since the introduction of this method by Ravaut in 1913 [*1], autohemotherapy has been employed in a wide range of disease conditions. Several hundred articles on the subject have been published in mainstream medical journals mostly from the early 1920s through the early 1940s, as listed in the various Index Medicus volumes (generally under the subject category "serum therapy"). Additionally, the subcutaneous or intramuscular reinjection of autologous blood or components is often discussed in the literature without specific reference to the term "autohemotherapy", as may be noted in a number of contemporary examples [*2].

Autohemotherapy is not "alternative therapy". Numerous items on the subject which have been published in the authoritative Journal of the American Medical Association, including a 1938 editor's endorsement of autohemotherapy against psoriasis [*3] and referral to its use against other diseases, often with "spectacular" results [*4]. Autohemotherapy has also been proposed as a preventive measure. For example, a 1935 report of favorable results against cerebral hemorrhage asserted that autohemotherapy is absolutely indicated as preventive treatment in cases of established hereditary disposition to high blood pressure[*5].

The reported beneficial action of autohemotherapy has been attributed to the presence of antigens in the blood [*6] which stimulate the production of antibodies when injected into the tissues. This explanation finds support in the work of Dr. E. C.

Rosenow (Mayo Foundation, 1915-44), which established the presence of a causative organism or antigen in the blood [*7] during active stages of many diseases.  Thus might the action of autohemotherapy be likened to that of an autogenous vaccine.


The safety and utility of a twice-weekly schedule for autohemotherapy has been demonstrated in the historical literature [*8], which schedule is in concert with Dr. Rosenow's twice-weekly administration of antigen and antibody for chronic diseases such as MS.  As advocated by Dr. Rosenow in the case of MS, a responsible family member might be instructed in administering the therapy, insofar as it may have to be continued indefinitely.  As Dr. Rosenow has emphasized, the continued presence of primary oral foci, undetected symptomless oral foci or inaccessible secondary foci would serve to ensure the continued presence of causative pathogens in the circulation. Under such circumstances, neither the vaccines of Dr. Rosenow nor autohemotherapy would be expected to effect elimination of the causative organism (which elimination might be equated to a "cure"), hence the indicated need for the continuation of therapy over an indefinite period of time.


Autohemotherapy's attributes of safety, low cost, and immediate availability suggest continuing potential utility against a broad spectrum of diseases in which a causative organism disseminates through the bloodstream, regardless of the source or identity of the causative organism - including the likes of malaria, ebola and AIDS.  Autohemotherapy, as reportedly successfully used against malaria, has been proposed for AIDS in 1988 [*9] (an experimental intravenous form has also been proposed, in 1992). [*10]  In cases where a persistent focus of infection does not exist (or may be eradicated), autohemotherapy may indeed be sufficient to effect a cure, and might therein comprise a "magic shot".


While autohemotherapy as a distinct entity enjoyed a well documented period of popularity during the first half of the 20th century, it also represents the culmination of a fundamental thread weaving through the healing arts for at least a few millennia.  Such diverse traditional practices as bloodletting, acupuncture, coining and moxibustion, and modern-day plasmapheresis, innovations in bone marrow transplantation (use of autologous marrow; and use of stem cells from blood in place of marrow), and to some extent even autotransfusions - all involve the manipulation of one's own blood or blood-components and the possibility that benefits may at least in part be due to a forced defensive response within the body's tissues against harmful substances in the circulating blood.  In this light, autohemotherapy may be viewed as simply the direct application of such a process, made possible by that grand technological advance

- the hypodermic needle.

Bibliography: "OVERVIEW, ACTION, SCOPE, FREQUENCY"

1.  Ravaut, M. Paul, "Essai sur L'Autohématothérapie dans Quelques Dermatoses", Ann. De Derm. et Syph. 4:292-6, May 1913.

2.  Chiyoda S and T Morikawa, Japanese Journal of Clinical Hematology, 1993 Jan, 34(1):39-43; Donskov SI, et al., Human Immunology, 1982 Jul, 4(4):325-333; Khodanova, RN, et al., Journal of Hygiene, Epidemiology, Microbiology and Immunology, 1989, 33(4):463-9;  Kwak, L.W., et al.., New England J. of Medicine, 1992 Oct 22, 327(17):1209-15; Manucharov NK, et al., Biulleten Eksperimentalnoi Biologii i Meditsiny, 1992 Oct, 114(10):395-8; Mascarin M, et al., Pediatria Medica E Chirurgica, 1993 Jul-Aug, 15(4):349-52. (ITA); Sokov EL, Zh Nevropatol Psikhiatr, 1988, 88(4):57-61; van Laar, JM, et al. Journal of Autoimmunity, 1993 Apr., 6(2):159-67; Vizcaino G, Diez-Ewald M; Arteaga-Vizcaino M, Torres E, Invenstigacion Clinica, 1992, 33 (4):165-74.(SP)

3.  JAMA 111 (1938), Editorial, p. 343 38-1.HTM

4.  Jones, J.W., & M.S. Alden, South.M.J. 30: 735-737, July '37

5.  Colella, R & G Pizzillo, Ztschr.f.d.ges.Neurol.u. Psychiat. 152: 337-344, '35: also, Med.argent. 14:1-5, Jan. 35; also, Riv.di pat.nerv. 45:116-127, Jan.-Feb. 35, also, Forze san. 4:212-219, Feb. 10, 36; also, Wien.med.Wchnschr. 85: 341-344, March 23 '35; also, Presse med. 43: 574-576, April 10, '35

6.  Burgess, N., Brit.J.Dermat.  44: 124-131, March '32

7.   Rosenow, E.C., JAMA 44:871-873, (March 18) 1905, 871-3; Jour. Infect. Dis. 17:403-408, 1915; Jour. Infect. Dis. 16:240-268, 1915; Jour. Infect. Dis. 19:333-384, 1916; Jour. Dental Res. 1:205-267, 1919, p. 243; Proc. Staff Meetings of Mayo Clinic 8:500-502 (Aug. 16) 1933 (with Charles Sheard and C. B. Pratt); Proc. Staff Meet., Mayo Clin. 12: 252-256, April 21, 1937 (with Heilman, F.R.); Am. J. Clin. Path. 15: 135-151, April 1945; Postgrad. Med. 2: 346-357, Nov. 1947; Postgrad. Med. 124-136, Feb. 1948; Postgrad. Med. 3: 367-376, May 1948; Ann. Allergy 6: 485-496, Sept.-Oct. 1948; South Dakota J. Med. and Pharm. 5: 243-248; 262; 272, Sept. 1952; South Dakota J. Med. and Pharm. 5: 304-310; 328, Nov. 1952, p. 309; Ohio M.J., 53(7), July 1957, p. 783-5.

8.  Nicolas, Gate and Dupasquier, COMPT. REND SOC. DE BIOL.,
PAR., 1923, lxxxviii, 211; Saxon, L. & J. E. Stoll, Illinois MJ
75:352-355, April '39; Kondo, K. and H.,

Okayama-Igkkai-Zasshi 53:886-887, April '41; Ross, B., and P.J.
Richeson, U.S. Nav. M. Bull. 47:154-155, Jan.-Feb., 1947; Poth,
D.O., Arch. Dermat. & Syph. 69:636-638, Oct. 1949.


9.  Shakman, S.H., "Cuyugan's Malaria Treatment; Aid vs. AIDS?"
AAAS Pacific Division Proceedings Vol. 7:42 (1988).


10. Bocci V., Medical Hypotheses, 1992 Sep, 39(1):30-4.


ORIGINS OF AUTOHEMOTHERAPY


   As in the case of the ancient practice of bloodletting, no
definite date can be assigned to the origination of
autohemotherapy.  If to some extent the reported beneficial
action of bloodletting may be attributed to resorption of some of
the blood being let, then autohemotherapy is as old as
bloodletting; or alternatively, bloodletting may be viewed as the
earliest form of controlled, intentional autohemotherapy.

   Even the origin of the "modern" (early 20th century) field of
"autohemotherapy" is somewhat muddled, emerging within the
subject area of "serum therapy", along with two types of
"autoserotherapy" as well as "autotherapy".

   Within the INDEX MEDICUS's "serum therapy" subject area, "autoserotherapy" first appears as an item as early as 1905, and as a
separate sub-category in 1911 with 6 entries. Through this early
period the term exclusively referred to "Gilbert of Geneva",
1894, and his subcutaneous reinjection of autogenous serous fluid
in pleural effusions.  According to Austin [11E2], Gilbert's
method had evolved from research in 1890-1 which was based on
Debove and Remond's demonstration of tuberculin in exudates of
tuberculosis victims.  Reference to "Gilbert's method" of
serotherapy continued, by name, at least into the 1930s, and, in
substance, into modern times as discussed in Chiyoda and Morikawa
1993.

   In 1993 Chiyoda S and T Morikawa discussed the reinfusion of
concentrated autogenous ascitic fluid in the case of a patient
with: leg edema and ascites, common cold-like symptoms, and
diagnostic findings suggesting systemic lupus erythematosus.
"His ascitic fluid disappeared and complements and albumin in his
serum normalized. ..."


AUTOTHERAPY PRECEDES, AND EVEN ENCOMPASSES AUTOHEMOTHERAPY
   Within the "autoserotherapy" sub-category or listed separately,

between 1911 and 1919, is found the term "autotherapy"; this term primarily referred to the works of Charles Duncan or derivatives thereof, and is treated in detail, separately, in Chapter 6. AUTOTHERAPY.  In summary Duncan regarded "autotherapy" as encompassing all self-generated therapeutic methods; he advocated injection of filtered toxic products from alimentary or pulmonary ailments, and oral ingestion of products of other infections. Duncan acknowledged the influence of Gilbert.

Prior to but apparently not a precedent for Gilbert, Kitasato Shibasaburo and Emil von Behring's work in 1890-1 on tetanus and diphtheria had given rise to the field of "serum therapy" and the concept of "passive immunization".


## AUTOSEROTHERAPY WITH BLOOD-SERUM - NOTES ON SERUM THERAPY

The popularization of the practice of reinjection of autogenous blood-serum was given particular impetus by the 1913 works of Spiethoff (autoserum) [13E6, 13E7].  Spiethoff cited precedents involving the reinjection of others' presumed "immune serum", and the injection of a mother's serum to treat a child, which practices in turn had evolved within the Kitasato/Von Behring tradition.


Long before Spiethoff but not cited by him, Jez in 1901 [01H1] reported the subcutaneous reinjection of autogenous blood-serum drawn from a vein in the treatment of erysipelas, Browning [05E1] discussed theoretical considerations based on Jez's experiments, and Bier also reportedly reinjected venous blood-serum [05H1 per Tillman 35B14].  Even earlier, in 1898, Elfstrom and Grafstrom had successfully treated croupous pneumonia with reinjected autoblood from leeches as early as 1898; they had also attempted the use of venous blood-serum in one (failed) instance, and then reverted to exclusive use of leech-drawn autoblood.


## RAVAUT AND THE RISE OF "CLASSICAL" AUTOHEMOTHERAPY
## ORIGINAL METHOD - SIMPLE INTRAMUSCULAR REINJECTION

Autohemotherapy as a distinct field is generally considered to have originated with Ravaut in 1913 [13H2], despite the existence of prior work by Elfstrom and Grafstrom in 1898 and Landsmann in 1912.  Ravaut's work described the utility of autohemotherapy in treating some dermatoses, and came immediately on the heels of Spiethoff's report on the similar use of autogenous serum [13E6 (11 March 1913)].  Ravaut's method [13H2] involved taking from 10cc to 25cc of blood from a vein in the arm and immediately injecting it into the buttock muscle.

Reacting a bit like he had been upstaged, Spiethoff fired back with an article [13E6] discussing both autoserum and autoblood, claiming to have used autoblood earlier than Ravaut, and giving recognition for prior work not to Ravaut but to Praetorious.

THE HISTORICAL LITERATURE

Posturing aside, the sum result of these various influences was a fair measure of popularity for the therapeutic use of autogenous blood or serum during the first half of the current century. This is evidenced in the nearly 700 listings under "serotherapy" or "serum therapy", in the "Quarterly Cumulative Index Medicus", published by the AMA from 1916 through -1956. These include intravascular as well as extravascular (intramuscular and subcutaneous) methods, although it is the extravascular methodology that originally and generally has been categorized as autohemotherapy.

Through the years, autohemotherapy has been reported effective in a wide range of diseases, most commonly skin diseases and allergies, but also diseases as diverse as schizophrenia. (See the APPENDIX A: AUTOHEMOTHERAPY CHRONOLOGY for various selected discussions; see APPENDIX C: AUTOHEMOTHERAPY BIBLIOGRAPHY for a comprehensive listing.)


AUTOHEMOTHERAPY:   DEFINITION, DESCRIPTION, RECOMMENDATIONS

Within the various series of medical indices published during the 20th century, the term "autohemotherapy" is not listed independently (under the "A"s, but instead appears (except in a single isolated instance) as a sub-category within "serum therapy". This "autohemotherapy" sub-category often comprised the majority of "serum therapy" items. Most of these autohemotherapy items involved subcutaneous or intramuscular reinjection of 3-10cc of freshly drawn autologous blood, and appear to have descended from Ravaut [13H1: ANN. DE DERM. ET SYPH. 4 (May 1913), p. 292].


Despite a uniformly favorable history and lack of negatives, the simple intramuscular reinjection method of autohemotherapy was not covered in the modern American medical curriculum of the late Twentieth century. Nonetheless some older dermatologists and allergists are familiar with it, and its use continues to be common in some European countries, notably Germany and Russia.


The term "autohemotherapy" has also been used to refer to both (a) local application and (b) intravenous reinjection of autologous blood that has been defibrinated or treated with an anticoagulant. In recent years, while overall use of the term "autohemotherapy" has diminished in any case, these secondary meanings appear to be in vogue; to avoid any possible confusion, the "classical" method involving intramuscular or subcutaneous reinjection may herein be so qualified or referred to as "extravascular", "classical" or, as per one recent author, "minor" (Bocci, 1993). In no case in this work will an unqualified "autohemotherapy" be intended to refer to intravenous injection.

INTRAVASCULAR VS. EXTRAVASCULAR

As mentioned above, <u>intravenous</u> reinjection of one's own blood
is referred to by some contemporary and some historical writers
as autohemotherapy; occasionally the two methods have been used
somewhat interchangedly by some writers:  Robertson [16H6]
attempted both intravenous and subcutaneous reinjection, noting a
preference for the former.  Fox [14H2] used subcutaneous and IV
injections interchangeably, without stating a preference for one
or the other; Kaiser [17H1] used IM reinjections, and intraspinal
in chorea; Thomas [41A6] and Marks [42B1] used subcutaneous
autoserum; Woo [37A1] subcutaneously reinjected autogenous
blister-serum.   [see THEORY for further discussios].

It should be reemphasized, however, that

(1) the term "autohemotherapy" has historically been used
primarily in conjunction with extravascular methods of
reinjection (intramuscular or subcutaneous); and

(2) the safety of such extravascular methods (intramuscular or
subcutaneous) has been repeatedly asserted, whereas an element of
far greater risk is known to accompany intravascular injection.
[see discussions of SAFETY below]

DETAILS:  DOSAGE, EXTERIORIZATION, FREQUENCY, LENGTH OF COURSE

DOSAGE

In the 1920s and 1930s 10 cc was a commonly used dosage [e.g.,
Nicolas et al. [23A3]; J.W.Jones and H.S.Alden [37B3, p. 735]; L.
Saxon [38B2, 191]; and L.Clendening, METHODS OF TREATMENT, 1943,
p. 65.].  Smaller doses of 3-5 cc were also used, subcutaneously
or intramuscularly, and continue to be so used at least in Russia
(personal communications, Dr. S. Tasker, Los Angeles) and Germany
(personal communications, Marcus Krump, San Francisco) up to the
present time.

EXTERIORIZATION - TIME OUTSIDE BODY

In 1941 E. Cuyugan reportedly obtained particularly good
results with a single treatment in a series of 40 cases of
malaria, all of which were presumably in the acute stage.

Clendening 1943 has noted that benefits of autohemotherapy may
be temporary.  This observation and the need for repeated
treatments in many diseases could be explained by the continued
existence of a focal infection in accord with the work of
Rosenow, etc. [see *REFERENCE MANUAL ROSENOW ET AL*]

## EXPLANATION OF BENEFICIAL ACTION OF AUTOHEMOTHERAPY

Regarding actions which may be operative with autohemotherapy, we may consider the common-sensical view that the invader is swamped by oxygen when exposed to the air, encased within the coagulating blood, and then deprived of oxygen when reinjected into the tissues; i.e., drowned in oxygen, immobilized by coagulating blood, and finally suffocated in an uninhabitable environment such as bodily tissues.  The body as a whole may then acknowledge the demise and identity of the invader, and a system-wide defense may be mounted.

As discussed by Dr. Cuyugan's son Roberto and others, the blood may contain some appropriate antigenic form of a harmful organism; hence autohemotherapy acts as a very specific "vaccine" against that organism.  This agrees with N. Burgess [33B10, p. 340] who suggested that "it is possible that the blood in these patients contains antigens, and that the injection of blood or serum therefore leads to desensitization".  Such an explanation is in agreement with the pioneering work on the use of autogenous vaccine-therapy by Sir Almroth Wright early in the 20th century; and also with his assertions that in the case of serum therapy, the disease-causing agent is carried through the circulation to tissues where antibodies are formed. [see Chapter 7. THEORETICAL CONSIDERATIONS].

In particular, Dr. E.C. Rosenow's work was initially reviewed by the writer in the context of autohemotherapy, although Rosenow himself is not known to have employed it, insofar as Rosenow showed how a causative organism is indeed to be found in the blood in a wide range of otherwise mysterious disease conditions, particularly in active stages of disease.  Rosenow's authoritative bacteriological findings in turn may be viewed as exhaustive evidence that the action of autohemotherapy may at least in part be attributed to the presence of antigen in the blood; i.e., that autohemotherapy may act as a therapeutic vaccine.  (Some Rosenow excerpts indicating presence of antigen in blood are provided below).

Autoserotherapy, autopyotherapy, etc. (i.e. the reinjection of autogenous serum, pus, etc.) are assumed to act on the same principle.


That autohemotherapy has not customarily been considered a form of vaccine therapy seems largely attributable to separate origins, the former having evolved in part from so-called "serum therapy" as discussed above, and herein lies the dilemna.  Serum therapy, generically the intravenous injection of "immune" serum from an immune person or animal, supposedly conveys "passive immunization"; whereas vaccine therapy attempts to directly elicit immunity in an individual, and hence is referred to as "active immunization".  They're supposed to be different!  So if autohemotherapy is actually a form of vaccine therapy, what does this say of autohemotherapy's supposed serum-therapy/passive-immunization roots?  This is not a new question; very early in the 20th century when serum therapy was a relatively new concept, Wright said of it:  "The whole body of beliefs rests, I am convinced, upon a foundation of sand. ... many of the successful results which have been achieved by serum therapy would find their simplest explanation in the assumption that the sera which were exploited operated as bacterial vaccines."  [see VACCINES - THE WRIGHT STUFF and THEORY]


SOME ROSENOW EXERPTS INDICATING PRESENCE OF ANTIGEN IN BLOOD

PNEUMONIA-SECONDARY TO BLOOD INFECTION; NOT LOCAL  [05R1]

Dr. Rosenow demonstrated "That the pneumococcus [of lobar pneumonia] is not only present, but present in large numbers in the blood ..... In no instance could I demonstrate pneumococci in leucocytes. ... Invasion of the blood in this present series  ... supports ... the view that pneumonia may be the secondary localization of a primary blood invasion and not a local disease." [JAMA 44:871-873, (March 18) 1905, 871-3]


STOMACH ULCER CAUSED BY STREPTOCOCCI IN BLOOD  - 16R8-334

ULCER, INFECTIOUS ORIGIN OF  - HISTORICAL PRECEDENTS

"The infectious origin of ulcer, while not generally accepted, has had adherents for many years."  Dr. Rosenow recounts various studies from 1857 involving the experimental production of stomach ulcer following intravenous injections of various organisms, and demonstrations from 1874 of bacteria in edges and floors of ulcers, which bacteria generally had been considered secondary invaders.  Dr. Rosenow asserts "It is a well known fact that ulcer in the stomach in man occurs not infrequently during severe or fatal infections of various kinds, particularly streptococcal infections. ... Bolton [Ulcer of the Stomach, 1913, p. 59] states that probably the commonest cause of necrosis of the mucous membrane and resulting acute ulcer of the stomach is bacterial infection, that the infection occurs through the blood stream, and that the necrosis is due to the direct effect upon the tissues of the bacterial poison, alone or together with the gastric juice."

"The supposed relation between infected tonsils or gums and gastric ulcer may be due not to the swallowing of bacteria, as is usually supposed, but to the entrance into the blood of streptococci of the proper kind of virulence to produce a local infection in the wall of the stomach.  Many other observations may be cited, such as associated infections of the gall bladder and appendix, which suggest that gastric ulcer may be due to streptococci."  [J. Infect. Dis. 19:333-384, 1916]

ORAL INFECTIONS - DAMAGE THRU BLOOD/LYMPH, NOT SWALLOWING

"It should be emphasized ... that the chief harm from these conditions [infections of the gums and enveloping membranes about the roots of teeth] comes from the absorption of the bacteria and their products into the lymph stream or blood, especially if drainage is inadequate, not from swallowing the infectious material... " [Jour. Dental Res. 1:205-267, 1919]

ANTIGEN IN BLOOD IN ACTIVE STREPOCOCCAL INFECTIONS - PRECIPITIN REACTION

"Patients with active streptococcal infections often appear to have free bacterial antigen in the blood which gives a precipitin reaction with the specific or related antiserum." [Heilman, F.R., and Rosenow, Proc. Staff Meet., Mayo Clin. 12: 252-256, April 21, 1937]


STREPTOCOCCUS IN NASOPHARYNX, PULPLESS TEETH, SOMETIMES BLOOD IN SCHIZOPHRENIA AND EPILEPSY

Conclusions:  "the consistent isolation of alpha streptococci in studies of idiopathic epilepsy and schizophrenia, the reproduction in important respects of the disease pictures in animals, the proof of their serologic specificity by the special methods employed, and the data obtained in these studies indicate: (1) that persons suffering from epilepsy and from schizophrenia harbor in nasopharynx, in pulpless teeth, and sometimes in their blood, specific types of alpha streptococci of low general but high and specific 'neurotropic' virulence; (2) that the streptococci produce neurotoxins which have predilection for certain structures in the brain and thus may play a role in pathogenesis and (3) that attempts to combat such inapparent infections specifically by passive and active immunization with the respective antigens and antibodies are indicated in addition to present-day methods of prevention and cure."

[So. Dakota J. Med. and Pharm. 5: 243-248; 262; 272, Sept. 1952]


ANTIBODY ADMINISTRATION, EFFECT ON ANTIGEN IN BLOOD

Polio, multiple sclerosis, epilepsy, schizophrenia:

"It has been found in previous studies that subcutaneous or intramuscular injection of respective thermal streptococcal antibody in therapeutic amounts is followed by a prompt improvement in symptoms and a diminution in specific streptococcal antigen and an abrupt increase in antibody titer in skin or blood of persons having influenza or other respiratory infections, poliomyelitis, multiple sclerosis, and epilepsy and schizophrenia. ...

"The antibody solution injected subcutaneously was prepared by autoclaving at 17 lbs pressure, a suspension of NaCl solution containing 0.4% phenol.  Two or three ml of the solution of antibody and of NaCl solution in controls depending on the age of patients were injected subcutaneously immediately after the primary intradermal tests had been made ...   South Dakota J. Med. and Pharm. 5: 304-310; 328, Nov. 1952, p. 309]

## CUTANEOUS TEST RESULTS - MS

Dr. Rosenow conducted extensive series of skin tests, wherein reactions to injections of antibody (which indicated the presence of antigen in the blood) and antigen (which indicated presence of antibody) were measured and compared, as listed in Table 2-1 below (Table 2-1 corrects Rosenow's 1957 Table 1 to conform with his narrative discussion, as also provided below:

Table 2-1 (Rosenow's 1957 Table 1). Erythematous cutaneous reactions (sq. cm.) in persons having MS to the intradermal injection of thermal antibody-indicating antigen and of antigen-indicating antibody prepared respectively from streptococci isolated from the nasopharynxes of persons who had MS, neuroses, and arthritis:

| Persons who had M.S. | Cases | Reactions in sq.cm. to injection of: | | | | |
| --- | --- | --- | --- | --- | --- | --- |
| | | Antibody-indicating antigen | Antigen-indicating antibody | | | |
| Type of strain: | | Multiple-sclerosis | | | Neurosis | Arthritis |
| Stain or case #: | | 8125 | 8125 | 7700 | 8126 | 8134 |
| Not receiving vaccine or | 23 | 5.75 | 7.31 | 9.63 | 3.14 | 1.43 |
| thermal antibody | 20 | 6.25 | 8.07 | | 5.04 | 2.15 |
| Receiving antibody and vaccine | 13 | 7.86 | 3.15 | | 3.85 | 1.86 |

"Cutaneous erythematous reactions indicating antibody (5.75 and 6.25 sq. cm.) were significantly less in persons not receiving such therapeutic injections than in persons receiving such treatment (7.86 sq.cm.). ...

"It will be seen that the immediate erythematous reactions to the intradermal injection of streptococcic antibody (taken to indicate specific circulating streptococcic antigen in patients not receiving antibody or vaccine therapeutically) were far greater (7.31, 8.07, and 9.63 sq. cm.), respectively, than in persons receiving therapeutic injections of antibody and vaccine (3.15 sq. cm.). ...

"Erythematous reactions following intradermal injection of
control antibody solutions were uniformly minimal, but in each of
the three groups having multiple sclerosis reactions were greater
to injections of 'neurotropic' (8126) streptococcic thermal
antibody than to corresponding injections of "arthrotropic"
(8134) antibody prepared respectively from streptococci isolated
in studies of diseases of the nervous system and arthritis."

Numerous other Rosenow articles discussed an organism in blood
in various diseases, including Postgrad. Med. Feb. 1948, 124-136
(blood culture method), Nov. 1947, 346-357, and May 1948,
367-376; Jour. Infect. Dis.: 16:240-268, 1915, and 17:403-408,
1915; Proc. Staff Meetings of Mayo Clinic 8:500-502 (Aug. 16)
1933. (With Charles Sheard and C. B. Pratt.); Am. J. Clin. Path.
15: 135-151, April 1945;  Ann. Allergy 6: 485-496, Sept.-Oct.
1948.

THE SAFETY OF AUTOLOGOUS BLOOD - HISTORICAL/MODERN ASSESSMENTS

Historical assessments - safety of autoblood-IM injection:
    The historical literature on "autohemotherapy" contains
numerous references to the safety of IM autoblood injections,
e.g., according to L. Clendening in Methods of Treatment, 1943,
p. 65, "The greatest advantages of autohemotherapy are its
simplicity and safety."  And Poth [49B1] states:  "No reactions
or contraindication to treatment were encountered" in
successfully treating 154 cases of herpes zoster with
[intra-muscular] autohemotherapy."

Historical assessments - risk confined to I.V. reinjection:
    On the specific question of hazards from reinjection of
autologous blood encountered in the historical literature, these
have been associated with intravenous reinjection exclusively.
We are reminded of Sir Almroth Wright's warning of disadvantages
of "autoinoculation" (which would seem relevant not only to
intravenous autohemotherapy) as compared with the use of
(extravascular) "bacterial vaccines" (which might be held as
relevant to intramuscular autohemotherapy); including a greater
risk of intoxication from the former and greater prospects for
the manufacture of beneficial substances from the latter.
    On the other hand, just as Wright had acknowledged some
potential benefits from serum therapy which he attributed to its
acting like a vaccine, so might some corresponding beneficial
side effects be derived from autologous transfusion, beyond
questions of safety and reduced risk of contamination.  In this
regard, one might expect to find similarities, in terms of
potentially beneficial action and underlying causes, in the
procedures known separately as serum therapy (particularly

"autologous"), autologous transfusion, and auto-inoculation
(particularly "induced", as discussed by Wright.  Specifically in
the case of autologous transfusion, Baliazin et al., 1990, have
documented the "immunocorrective properties" of autologous
transfusion as compared with donor blood.


Contemporary assessments - safety of autologous transfusion:

In recent years the use of autologous blood in transfusions has
gained in popularity, partly due to the possibility of
contamination in the blood supply.  As a result the question of
safety of autologous blood from the perspective of blood
reactions, irrespective of the problem of contamination, has also
received renewed attention - and universal affirmative praise.
Typical is this assessment by the American Association of Blood
Banks:

--"Autologous blood and components are the safest transfusions a
patient can receive.  The absence of risk of alloimmunization to
erythrocyte, leukocyte, platelet or plasma protein antigens
significantly reduces the risk of adverse reactions." [Sandler,
S. G., & A. J. Silvergleid, Eds., AUTOLOGOUS TRANSFUSION, 1983,
Arlington, VA: American Association of Blood Banks, page 12.]

Such universally favorable findings as concerns the relative
safety of IV injection of autologous blood may be viewed as
supportive of and consistent with the notable lack of unfavorable
comment in the historical literature as concerns the safety of IM
injection of autoblood; and even moreso in view of generally
acknowledged dangers of IV injection, as with "serum therapy".


ANTICOAGULENT,RECOMMEND AGAINST


Historical assessments - safety of citrated blood:

Although several operators through the years have used a small
amount of sodium citrate as an anticoagulant, in order to keep
the blood from coagulating prior to reinjection, there appears
sufficient reason to avoid their use for reasons discussed in
some articles specifically addressing the topic.

While Kaiser had advocated the use of citrated convalescent
serum as early as 1917 (17H1), the previous year Unger had warned
against the use of such anticoagulants in blood to be used in
transfusion, citing two disadvantages:  "1. the alteration of the
coagulation time of the recipient's blood, and 2., the danger of
causing high temperatures and chills."

Specifically as concerns the use of anticoagulants in
autohemotherapy, in 1938 Dean noted that Descarpenties had
"emphatically" denounced the use of anticoagulants (e.g., 23E6,
in subcutaneous autohemotherapy), arguing that the inhibition of
coagulation must also inhibit the blood's ability to defend

against infection.  Nonetheless Dean himself used citrated blood in intravenous autohemotherapy.  And 1955 Reddick (55C2) used citrated blood in intramuscular autohemotherapy for mental illness.

In 1965 Bacskulin and Bacskulin [65F1] sternly warned against the use of citrated blood for subconjunctival autohemotherapy in corrosions of the eye, citing good results with uncitrated blood.
 [see APPENDIX A: AUTOHEMOTHERAPY CHRONOLOGY]


Arguments against the use of anticoagulants are also further arguments against intravascular reinjection of autoblood, which procedure commonly requires either the use of anticoagulants or defibrination of blood as a practical matter; for example, in modern times, intravascular autohemotherapy in conjunction with ozonization of blood is normally carried out with citrated blood or with the use of other anticoagulants [Bocci 1993; see APPENDIX A: AUTOHEMOTHERAPY CHRONOLOGY].  (A possible exception was the work of Vorschutz in the 20s and 30s, wherein the patient was prepped for immediate reinjection; however, in any case this procedure was far more complex and potentially hazardous than extravascular autohemotherapy.)


AUTOHEMOTHERAPY USED AS LAST RESORT

Autohemotherapy has traditionally occupied the position of "treatment of last resort; if nothing else works, try autohemotherapy; it won't hurt and might help.

For example, as per Jones and Alden [37B3, p. 736], "this method of treatment has served us extremely well as an aid in the intractable cases of psoriasis. We have been somewhat unfair to autohemotherapy in that we have reserved its use for the most difficult cases. ... The average number of injections required for relief is approximately 10. ... it cannot be said that it is curative, although the intervals between attacks have seemed to be lengthened."

That autohemotherapy has occupied the position of treatment of last resort may be partly due to a lack of a generally-accepted explanation of why the procedure might be beneficial.  To the extent that there is a consensus, the beneficial effects of autohemotherapy would appear due to the existence of some antigenic form in the blood which when injected intramuscularly invokes a specific response.  This would support the argument that autohemotherapy is actually a form of autogenous vaccine therapy.

Autohemotherapy repeatedly has been noted to fulfill the most basic Hippocratic doctrine of "do no harm", and was never discredited, but rather seems to have been squeezed out of modern medical curricula by the overwhelming mass of information on new technologies that have become available in the second half of the 20th century.

Nonetheless, it would appear that autogenous therapy methods continue to comprise treatments of last resort, as evidenced in the preponderance of such methods in cancer therapy.  [see Chapter 10: AUTOLOGOUS THERAPY FOR CANCER]

Moreover, immigrants from Europe, notably Germany and Russia, have related that autohemotherapy continues to be routinely used for a variety of ailments.  For example, San Francisco resident Marcus Kremp grew up in Germany, and recalls his family doctor withdrawing blood from the arm, shaking it up for a few seconds, and reinjecting it in the buttock muscle.  Mr. Kremp had received the treatment for headaches following a head fracture, his brother annually for hay fever allergy, and he is aware that his 80-year-old aunt had also received this therapy.  He said he personally believes the treatment works, but hasn't said much about it because he feared people would think he was a bit crazy.


DISAPPEARANCE OF AUTOHEMOTHERAPY - CNIDIAN SYNDROME?


Perhaps in part due to the lack of a universally accepted explanation for reported beneficial effects of autohemotherapy, and certainly in part as a consequence of the advent of antibiotics, references in the medical literature to "classical" autohemotherapy have declined and virtually disappeared.

Other factors contributing to the decline of autohemotherapy's popularity would appear to be:

 (1) an overwhelmed medical education system which, in seeking to encompass the latest information, has inadvertently allowed some valuable lessons of history to be dropped; autohemotherapy is no longer taught in medical schools, hence modern doctors have simply not been educated on the subject.  The demands of the game of drug roulette don't leave much time for consideration of the root causes of diseases and consequent rational therapeutic approaches.  Crushed on the one hand by an ever-expanding Physicians' Desk Reference of pharmaceuticals (soon to outweigh the grossest of telephone directories), and on the other by explosively-growing mountains of genetic detail and genetics's virtual monopoly on future-thought as regards prospects for ultimate mechanical control of metabolic processes, the poor physician-in-training-or-practice's mind simply does not have the time or mandate to consider broader perspectives including unfamiliar historical approaches, or so it would appear.

 (2) the modern medical tendency toward specialization and away from generalized practice; autohemotherapy is clearly a general therapeutic approach.  While unquestionably there is a valid role for specialists in many fields, a tendency toward possible over-specialization might be seen as aligning our moderns with the Cnidians of Hippocrates' time.  As Durant 1939 has noted, "The Cnidians, disliking Hippocrates' penchant for basing 'prognosis' upon general pathology, insisted upon a careful classification of

each ailment ... ."  We may thus view the Cnidians as an early trade union for medical practitioners - their position may not have resulted in better treatment for their patients, but it certainly resulted in more jobs for more Cnidians.

(3) the advent of "wonder" drugs in the 1940s and 1950s, which somewhat diminished the need for the autohemotherapeutic "treatment of last resort", and also diminished the perception of its continued value.  As Lederberg noted in 1988, "Some of the great successes of medical science, including the 'miracle drugs', the antibiotics of the 1940s, have inculcated premature complacency on the part of the broader culture."

(4) the advent of improved culture conditions, which in fortunate instances allowed for formulation of potent specific vaccines; however for the most part progress in development of vaccines, both prophylactic (preventive) and therapeutic, also fell victim to the drug-craze era of most of the latter half of the 20th century.

(5) the gross commercialization of the modern business of medicine, involving major business interests of pharmaceutical companies (e.g., note the importance of advertising to medical journals), health providers (e.g. note a recent trend of HMOs to contract out services to pharmaceutical companies), and the insurance industry.


With all due respect to advocates of various reigning contemporary medical fads, and with prayers that one might somehow stumble on a path to quantum progress in eradicating human disease, it may be nonetheless be incontrovertibly asserted that autohemotherapy can continue to usefully augment even the most significant of more recent medical advances.  Indeed, autohemotherapy merits recognition on its own as a landmark achievement of 20th century medicine - one that can serve humanity well into the twenty-first century and perhaps even beyond to a day when all disease is "history".  This may have particular bearing on diseases whose causative agents are known to be (1) carried in the blood, and (2) whose variability may frustrate vaccine development, e.g., malaria.


RECOMMENDATIONS/INDICATIONS

1.  That autohemotherapy be adopted as a treatment of first resort, so that the patient might begin immediately to fight whatever the ailment may be, while the doctor tries to figure out what it is.  This is not an original recommendation; for example, in 1934 Tillman [35B14] asserted that autoblood deserves the very first place of treatment methods for treating uncomplicated lung congestion, this based on 10 years' experience.

2.  That whenever blood is drawn for blood tests, a small amount be reinjected subcutaneously or IM for therapeutic purposes.  The very need for blood tests speaks to the propriety

of such therapy.  Such practice finds precedent in Colella and Pizzillo, 1935 [35A14], p. 344, who noted "Autohemotherapy helps with cerebral hemorrhage, during and after the attack.  It is absolutely indicated as preventive treatment in cases of established hereditary disposition to high blood pressure."

3.  That currently-existing needle-exchange programs be expanded and promoted for self-administered autohemotherapy, for therapy and/or prophylaxis as required.

AUTOHEMOTHERAPY PROPOSED TREATMENT OF FIRST RESORT: MALARIA, EBOLA, AIDS

It is noted that autohemotherapy has been used successfully to treat malaria, a disease that has otherwise been particularly problematic due to the variability of the malaria parasite.  See particularly APPENDIX C: 88H1, "Cuyugan's Malaria Treatment"; and APPENDIX A: 30B13, Padoan and Frizziero.  For additional literature citations mentioning malaria, see APPENDIX C: 29B8, 32A13, 34A4, 38B12, 43B1, 53B2.  Thus autohemotherapy would appear appropriate for use on a large and continuing scale in Third-World countries where malaria continues to be prevalent, until universally applicable vaccines or other measures are successfully developed.

Similarly, other diseases in which the causative organism disseminates through the blood, including the newly-emergent ebola, seem appropriately likely targets for wide-spread use of autohemotherapy as a safe, low-tech, and immediately available therapy of first resort.  Beyond this, the inclusion of autohemotherapeutic instruction in first-aid and survival training would also appear to merit consideration.  This would allow for prompt administration of autohemotherapy under emergency conditions for the wide range of ailments against which it has reportedly been effective, as well as for newly emergent mysterious conditions.

Chapter 3: BLOODLETTING, VENESECTION, ETC.


ORIGINS: VENESECTION VS. AUTOHEMOTHERAPY - CHICKEN OR EGG?


Bloodletting, bleeding, venesection, phlebotomy:  A truly "barbaric" practice - seemingly absurd in the context of what it was supposed to do, i.e. cure a sickness.  Yet how could it be that so great a medical authority as Hippocrates (460-377 BC) afforded it "first place in conducting the treatment" of many diseases that "do not admit of resolution, if treated at first by medicine."?

And then there's Galen [2nd Century A.D.], whose "influence on medical theory and practice was dominant throughout the Middle Ages and during the Renaissance".  [Encyclopedia Brit. 1987] Certainly to some extent Galen's successes helped to establish even more firmly the widespread use of bloodletting, and its continuing advocacy even into the 20th Century.  But can Galen's successes be attributed simply to his having slandered his competition, as argued by a contemporary historian, Brain 1986? [Brain, Peter, Galen, on Bloodletting, Cambridge U. Press, 1986]

Notwithstanding recurring arguments over moderate- versus liberal- versus abstinence from- bloodletting, for all those hundreds of years, was humanity essentially one succession of lemmings to the sea, as far as venesection goes?  Or is it possible that venesection often actually has worked - it has cured or somehow benefited patients who otherwise would not have survived?

Within this context, it might even be speculated that the substance of autohemotherapy may be older than, and the inspiration for, venesection, with ancestry of both practices logically traceable to the commonly seen phenomenon of a cure of a disease following an unrelated accident or injury.  Hippocrates was heir to the already-existing tradition of venesection.  Galen was an aggressive bleeder, and his instincts were apparently good enough to establish him as the unrivaled ruler of medicine for almost forever, at least for most of the current era (AD).

Then came the modern era, with the pendulum swinging away from bleeding and toward the germ theory, antisepticism, antibiotics, etc. - and the primitive practice of bloodletting has finally been abandoned. Or has it?

Ironically part of the success of one of the components of modern medicine, invasive surgery, may be creditable to autohemotherapy; insofar as exploratory surgery has often resulted in cures, a phenomenon best explained by inadvertent autohemotherapy, is it not possible that in at least some surgeries it is the act of cutting and bleeding, moreso than the surgical intent, that results in an autohemotherapeutic cure? And then there's plasmapheresis - son of venesection. [see BLOODLETTING'S PROGENY - PLASMAPHERESIS, below].

A BRIEF HISTORY OF BLOODLETTING, THROUGH THE 19TH CENTURY

Abel 1915 reviews the long and pervasive history of bloodletting, which "seems to antedate all systems of medicine and to have been one of the earliest therapeutic procedures applied by primitive races."  Its influence was strong long before Hippocrates.  [Separate sections on Hippocrates' and Galen's' bloodletting practices follow.]

Abel notes that leeches have been used for bloodletting since "earliest times", particularly in India.

In the 12th century the "Regimen Sanitatus Salerni" or "code of health" was widely circulated and translated; bloodletting was prescribed for acute diseases for patients in their middle ages, but children and elderly were to be treated cautiously.

During the latter part of the Middle Ages astrology strongly influenced the practice, which "was carried out to great excess."

In the 16th and 17th centuries considerable controversy was encountered between advocates and opponents of bloodletting, and between followers of "Hippocratic" vs. "Arabian" theories.  The Hippocratic tradition advocated bleeding for a vein as near as possible to the diseased part in order to directly remove "foul and stagnant" blood; whereas the Arabian tradition argued that removal from a distant vein "prevented good blood from accumulating in the diseased part."  In the early 16th Century, Pierre Brissot (1478-1522) revived the Hippocratic method based on his own Parisian clinical experience with an acute lung epidemic in 1514.  Opponents of Brissot were able to have his method outlawed by the French Parliament, forcing him from Paris and his professorship.

Toward the end of the 16th century, Leonardo Botallo advised venesection to the limit, probably due to his experience as an army surgeon with generally robust patients; whereas in the early 17th century J.V. Van Helmont condemned venesection altogether. Later in the 17th century Guy Patin was an ardent bleeder and purger, in contrast to Franciscus de le Böe (Sylvius) who preached moderation and caution.  The 18th century "Satire of Gil Blas" presents this picture of 17th century excesses - a notary, brought in to make out a patient's will, rushes to complete his work when he learns the identity of the doctor, a notorious venesectionist.

Nonetheless, as noted by McManus [1963, p. 72] "A leading and most popular textbook of medicine about 1840 said 'Of all the treatments in medicine, the most efficacious is the letting of blood; stand the patient upright and bleed from the ante-cubital vein until syncope occurs.'"

In the late 18th and early 19th centuries, the French and Italians were especially staunch advocates; however, by the mid-

19th century, the rise of new concepts of disease and medicine led to the near-abolition of bloodletting. These included the rise of the cell theory, discovery of bacteria, hydrotherapy, and analgesics and anesthetics. Yet, as per Abel 1915: "the common man, especially in Germany and France, still held firmly that benefits did follow the use of the wetcup, the lancet, and the leech. Tenaciously the old practices were upheld. If physicians refused to bleed, there was always the barber surgeon, fully competent, as in teeth pulling, to give relief. ... Was it not true and known to all stock breeders that the domestic animals could be fattened by judicious bleeding at certain fixed intervals? And it appears now that the common man was right, after all. An empirical method of treatment which has been practised by nearly all races since before the day of Hippocrates almost certainly contains a basis of truth. This is now admitted and physicians are again saving lives by the judicious and timely use of bloodletting."

BLOODLETTING THRU THE 20TH CENTURY

In 1910 Schrup advocated bloodletting "where its indications and limitations are clearly recognized. The incentive for this paper came from the good results which I have observed in the last year in 5 cases, and, in at least 3 of these, life was saved, temporarily, if not permanently, by its use." These 5 cases included: a 55 year-old man, unconscious, with increasing edema of lower extremities and scrotum; a hemiplegic 64-year old man; an 82-year-old woman with a severe attack of la grippe followed by sudden heart collapse; a 57-year-old woman with exopthalmic goiter and increasing cardiac insufficiency; and a stout plethoric 30-year-old woman whose blood was intentionally allowed to flow during breast amputation. Schrup noted that other authors had advised venesection for uremia, eclampsia of pregnancy, nephritis, and pneumonia, which last condition some authorities claimed had greatly increased in mortality due to the neglect of venesection. Also noted were uses in some neuroses, gynecology, rheumatism, pulmonary emphysema, pellagra and liver congestion.

TECHNIC FOR VENESECTION: "... the surest, quickest and easiest way to incise the vein wall, after going through the skin, is to grasp it in a rattooth forceps, feel that he has the vein in its grasp and then cut away the bite, preferably with a sharp scissors. ... The amount of blood that can be drawn at any one time varies from 10 to 30 ounces. The danger of shock is very slight, the flow being regulated automatically by the lowered pressure in the vein and the coagulability of the blood." [Schrup, p. 532]

Also in 1910, Stern summarized the history of bloodletting in children, particularly the 19th century experience, and concluded "that bloodletting in proper cases is probably the most potent single remedial measure which we possess ..."

In 1916-7 Spiethoff, a key figure in the history of autosero- and autohemotherapy as Ravaut's immediate precedent, continued to advocate venesection, alone or in combination with autoserotherapy [17A1]. In 1917 he presented evidence that venesection could be repeated rapidly in robust persons without permanent contraindicatory consequences.  From a robust young woman with eczema but otherwise healthy, he withdrew 100 cc of blood 7 times within 13 days; for less robust persons he suggested that not more than 30-50 cc be removed.


## BLOODLETTING IN THE 90S - THE 1990S

Bloodletting has by no means disappeared from the modern literature.  As a "subject" in MEDLINE, "bloodletting" aka "phlebotomy" or "venesection" sports 462 entries between the years 1990-1994 inclusive.  For this same period, searching for "keywords", numbers of citations in MEDLINE are 484 "bloodletting", 287 "phlebotomy" and 67 "venesection".


### USE OF LEECHES STILL HANGING ON

Lohr, 1988, p. A11, noted the growing use of leeches in Europe and the U.S. after microsurgery to reattach body parts, in order to prevent unwanted blood congestion in tiny blood vessels. Hirudo medicinalis, a small European leech, sucks a small amount of blood from the clogged vessels, and the anticoagulant in its saliva causes the wound to continue draining small amounts of blood for hours afterwards.

In addition, modern researchers are investigating the possibility of using anti-coagulant enzymes in leech saliva might be used for therapy of heart attacks and strokes.  Hirudin, from the European leech, keeps blood from clotting, while hemetin, from an Amazon leech, dissolves blood clots.  Another substance, orgelase, might prove useful in treating glaucoma, as well as in helping with circulation of blood around clots in the heart.

This anticoagulant quality of the "remarkable substance" hirudin was recognized early in the current century as providing a "new use" for leeches, augmenting their traditional use in bloodletting. [Abel 1915]


## BLOODLETTING PROGENY - PLASMAPHERESIS

It is noted that as of 1994 the practice known as plasmapheresis continued to comprise a component of contemporary medical therapy for such disease conditions as myasthenia gravis (see "AUTOIMMUNE DISEASE - MUCH ADO ABOUT NOTHING").  It may be useful for modern critics of past medical practices, such as bloodletting, to bear in mind that plasmapheresis is clearly descended from, and an intended refinement to, the practice of venesection aka bloodletting.

In 1915 Abel confidently predicted :  "Venesection, then, will probably never again be entirely excluded from medicine, as it was during the last quarter of the past century, nor need we fear that the practice will again be misused." [p. 140]

But Abel cautioned about one particular drawback of venesection, the ill effects of overbleeding, which he suggests must be attributed primarily to the loss of red corpuscles.  To counteract this, Able proposed "the speedy return into the body of the red and the white corpuscles instead of throwing them away as hitherto has been our custom.  The only thing that would be removed from the blood of a person bled in this way would be its fluid part - the plasma. ... We have named the procedure plasmapheresis." [141]

Thanks at least in part to Abel's own invention, plasmapheresis, his prediction that "venesection ...  will probably never again be entirely excluded from medicine" continued to hold true through the last quarter of the 20th century.


## TRANSFUSIONS NO PROBLEM FOR INCAS

Arrhenius 1907 has noted "Since the earliest times the injection of the blood of animals into the veins of the human sick has been practised for therapeutical purposes." [p. 218]

According to the ENCYCLOPEDIA BRITANNICA, in Europe attempts at transfusions were made as early as 1628 by the Italian physician Giovanni Colle.  This was the same year in which William Harvey's monograph on circulation of the blood was published, although his findings had announced in 1616.  By 1665 Richard Lower was performing transfusions on dogs, and by 1667 both he and Jean Baptiste Denis in France had transfused lambs' blood into human subjects.  In 1667,  a Denis cross-transfusion resulted in a human death, causing Denis to be imprisoned for a year.  England outlawed transfusions in 1668.  Overall so many patients died from transfusion incompatibility reactions that the process was banned in France, England and Italy after the late 17th Century.

Nonetheless, and notwithstanding some notable historical failures, we find the use of lamb's blood in humans discussed in the medical literature early in the 20th century by Bier (1901), with intravenous injections of small amounts 1-1/2 to 20cc.  "Of the various animal blood types, lamb's blood is one of the least poisonous to man." [Bier 1901]

We are also reminded that the conventional field of serum therapy traditionally involved the use of horse-serum, and as such a degree of cross transfusion has carried into modern times.

Regarding human to human transfusion, the Incas had apparently practiced blood transfusion successfully long ago; incompatibility reactions were apparently not a problem as nearly all South American Indians are of blood type O-Rh-positive.

James Blundell in 19th century England advocated the use of human blood for transfusion, sparking a mini-revival in interest. This interest diminished during the last quarter of the century, however, concurrent with the introduction of injections of saline solution to treat shock, and following Landois's 1875 demonstration that mixing of different types of blood usually resulted in clumping and sometimes hemolysis. It was not until 1900 that Landsteiner discovered the ABO blood-type groups, enabling modern-day transfusions. [Wien p. 1629; Encyclopedia Britannica, 1986; Bier 1901]

BLOODY (INJECTION) HORROR STORIES:

Two 19th Century instances of whole-blood-injection that were not part of the historical evolution of autohemotherapy were clearly not intended to inspire replication, but rather to demonstrate that the materials injected did not convey disease-causing agents for the diseases in question. That neither of these instances resulted in a fatality could, nonetheless, be explained by the principles of prophylactic or therapeutic vaccine (which explanation also might be invoked to explain autohemotherapy):

- In 1804 an American undergraduate medical student, Stubbins Firth, "injected himself with blood, urine, sweat, black vomit, and other material from yellow fever victims. He then swallowed this material along with all manner of other repulsive substances taken from patients dying of yellow fever. ... he did not become ill." [Lehrer, EXPLORERS OF THE BODY, Doubleday, 1979, p. 360-1]

(Yellow fever is caused by a virus transmitted by a mosquito). Here it may be suggested that the act of swallowing the same materials that had been injected (presumably extravascularly, although Lehrer did not specify) might, in concert with Duncan's discussions of autotherapy, cancel out the potential ill effects which might have been conveyed through injection, or vice-versa. Kind of a mechanical ying-yang sort of thing.

- In 1894 a British medical officer, David Bruce, identified the protozoa and tse tse fly carrier responsible for an African animal infection, "nagana"; later he sought to prove that they also caused African sleeping sickness and Gambian fever in humans. "To refute Bruce, a German named Taute working in Portuguese East Africa injected himself with five cc of blood from animals dying of nagana and allowed himself to be bitten with nagana-carrying tse-tse flys -- and lived." [Lehrer, 250] Here even if nagana and the human diseases had turned out to have the same cause (Lehrer did not address this), the (presumably extravascular) injection of 5 cc of blood from dying animals could have acted like a prophylactic vaccine comprised of an attenuated organism, aborting the possibly-harmful effects of the tse-tse bites.

## GALEN ON BLOODLETTING, ETC.

The place in history of Galen of Pergamum, Greece (131-201 AD), is nothing short of astounding, with his medical theory and practice dominating European medicine though the middle ages and Renaissance - the better part of two millennia!  As McManus 1963 noted, p. 95, "Galen's views on medicine and physiology prevailed until the time of Harvey [1578-1657] and after."  Son of an architect, Galen studied in Smyrna in Asia Minor, Corinth in Greece, and Alexandria in Egypt, before returning home to Pergamum in the year 157 at age 28 to serve as chief physician for the gladiators.  In 161 he moved to Rome and built a considerable reputation owing to his success as a physician, his willingness to take on patients others thought incurable, and through public lectures and dissections.

[We may briefly note an interesting parallel between Galen and the 16th century Leonardo Botallo, both of whom were ardent venesectionists and both of whom gained their experience with generally robust patients; Galen with gladiators, Botallo with soldiers.]

GALEN ON:

PLEURISY

[per Brain, p. 90]  "In pleuritic patients, phlebotomy on the same side as the affected rib has often shown the clearest benefit, while if it is on the opposite side, the benefits are either quite indefinite or are seen only after some time has elapsed.  Phlebotomy on the affected side has often checked, within an hour, the severest pains in the eye, when the vein known as the humoral is cut.  It is better, and might be tried in all diseases, after moderate amounts of blood have been let, to perform the procedure called epaphairesis, sometimes on the same day when this is practicable, and sometimes on the following one..."

EPIPHAIRESIS

[per Brain, p. 134] "The full amount [of blood] to be taken is not necessarily removed at one operation; it is sometimes desirable to divide it among several, especially when there is an accumulation of crude humours.  this is known as epiphairesis (repeated removal), and the venesections may be performed on the same day or on successive ones.  If blood is let twice on the same day, the first evacuation should be smaller.

[Sensitization?  As in vaccine-therapy, initial dose is small, then larger; same also often practiced with autohemotherapy]

INFLAMMATION; Prophylactic venesection

[per Brain, p. 125-7] "One of the dangers of plethors is inflammation. ... The plethors, and subsequent inflammation, were to be dispersed by emptying the veins. ... Erasistratus proposed to empty the veins by starving the patient; Galen, in his first work on bloodletting at least, believed that the quickest and most effective way to empty them was by venesection. ... [Galen] says that the evacuation of the residues of nutriment is of crucial importance.  If the residues accumulate they become hotter and more acrid, and so give rise to inflammations, erysipelas, herpes, carbuncles, fevers, and numerous other conditions. ... The ill effects of inflammation are so great that the physician is justified, not only in letting blood when it is established, but in using venesection prophylactically before the plethos exists, for instance immediately after an injury.  [as in prophylactic autotherapy?]

### SUPPRESSING/BRINGING ON MENSES

[per Brain, p. 130]  "according to Galen, venesection in the arm checks the menstrual flow by revulsion, and the Hippocratic writers, he assays, recommended scarifying the ankles to bring on the menses."

### CONDITIONS APPROPRIATE FOR BLEEDING

Brain [p. 129] lists a number of specific conditions in which Galen had used and recommended venesection, including: angina and peripneumonia with suffocation, synache, suppression of the menses and of the haemorrhoidal flux, ophthalmic, anorexia nervosa, dementia from vitiated humors, hypermotility from heat, torpor from cold, gout, arthritis, epilepsy, melancholia, haemoptysis, scotomatic diseases, pleurisy, and hepatitis.  Here, Brain notes "It is essential to apply the treatment on the side of the body on which the condition being treated is situated ... ."  Yet elsewhere, p. 130, Brain notes, "As a general rule, a vein should be opened as far as possible from the spot where the blood collects in plethors. ... however when [inflammations] have become established a part as near as possible to the affected one should be used."

### GALEN'S SUCCESS

Brain [p. 173] asks "Why did Galen succeed in his practice?" and then suggests it may have been because  "he had no hesitation in violently attacking his medical opponents", "proclaimed himself to be above all sects", and "some of his more unlikely opinions ... had not failed him".

While Prof. Brain may have correctly characterized Galen's attacks and proclamations, nonetheless much of Galen's success in his practice must be credited to successful results; without such success his practice and legacy could not possibly have survived.

### GALEN'S COMPETITION

Brain [p. 16, Note 6] likens the method of Chrysippi, teacher of Erasistratus who was the object of Galen's criticism, to the modern practice of autotransfusion.  Chrysippi used bandaging to reduce the amount of blood in the region of the chest.  Says Brain, "His method is an interesting anticipation of the modern practice of auto-transfusion, and the even more modern medical antishock trousers, which squeeze blood out of the legs so that the vital centers get more of it."

## HIPPOCRATES - ON BLOODLETTING

### PRESCRIPTION FOR BLEEDING [Adams 1886, 261]

"Bleed in acute affections, if the disease appear strong, and the patients be in the vigor of life, and if they have strength. If it be quinsy or any other of the pleuritic affections, purge with electuaries; but if the patient be weaker, or if you abstract more blood, you may administer a clyster every third day, until he be out of danger, and enjoin total abstinence if necessary"

### CONDITIONS CALLING FOR VENESECTION [262]

"Hypochondria inflamed not from retention of flatus, tension of the diaphragm, checked respiration with dry orthopnoea, when no pus is formed, but when these complaints are connected with obstructed respiration; but more especially strong pains of the liver, heaviness of the spleen, and other phlegmasiae and intense pains above the diaphragm, diseases connected with collections of humors, -- all these diseases do not admit of resolution, if treated at first by medicine, but venesection holds the first place in conducting the treatment; then we may have recourse to a clyster, unless the disease be great and strong; but if so, purging may also be necessary; but bleeding and purging together require caution and moderation. ...

"When a person suddenly loses his speech, in connexion with obstruction of the veins, - if this happens without warning or any other strong cause, one ought to open the internal vein of the right arm, and abstract blood more or less according to the habit and age of the patient.  Such cases are mostly attended with the following symptoms: redness of the face, eyes fixed, hands distended, grinding of the teeth, palpitations, jaws fixed, coldness of the extremities, retention of airs in the veins."

[Adams points out that "these symptoms are descriptive of congestion in the brain, threatening an attack either of apoplexy or epilepsy."  It is noted that numerous reports are listed in the INDEX on the use of autohemotherapy for apoplexy (and cerebral hemorrhage) and for epilepsy; and further that Rosenow's work identifies a blood-borne microbial cause for epilepsy emanating from oral foci.]

# HIPPOCRATES - SOME HISTORICAL NOTES

## PLATO'S "ASCLEPIAD OF COS" (460-377 BC)

Hippocrates was born into a family which had produced well-known physicians for generations, the Asclepiads, and was called "the asclepiad of Cos" by his younger contemporary Plato.  During his career Hippocrates traveled throughout Greece and Asia Minor, and often taught at the medical school at Cos.  He is traditionally regarded as the "father" of medicine. [Encyclopedia Britannica 1987]

## "UNMERRY WAR":  HIPPOCRATES AND THE CNIDIANS

Durant 1939:  "Secular medicine in 5th Century Greece took forms in four great schools: at Cos and Cnidus in Asia Minor, at Crotona in Italy, and in Sicily. ... At Cnidus the dominating figure was Euryphron, who composed a medical summary known as the Cnidian Sentences, explained pleurisy as a disease of the lungs, ascribed many illnesses to constipation, and became famous for his success as an obstetrician.  An unmerry war raged between the schools of Cos and Cnidus; for the Cnidians, disliking Hippocrates' penchant for basing 'prognosis' upon general pathology, insisted upon a careful classification of each ailment, and a treatment of it on specific lines.  In the end, by a kind of philosophical justice, many of the Cnidian writings found their way into the Hippocratic collection."

## HIPPOCRATES - MORE ON BLOOD

## LEG ULCERS, ETC.

The most recent innovation in the treatment of leg ulcers, as of the mid 1990s, involves the external application of a salve made from autogenous blood.

Although Wien [25E7d] has dated the first use of blood in therapy as occurring in 47AD, Hippocrates (and predecessors) had clearly advocated the use of blood in therapy long before.  This included not only the practice of bloodletting, or venesection, but also the therapeutic value of blood on skin ulcers:

"In every recent ulcer, except in the belly, it is expedient to cause blood to flow from it abundantly, and as may seem seasonable; for thus will the wound and the adjacent parts be less attacked with inflammation.  And in like manner, from old ulcers, especially if situated in the leg, in a toe or finger, more than in any other part of the body. For when the blood flows they become drier and less in size, as being thus dried up.  It is this especially which prevents such ulcers from healing: by getting into a state of putrefaction and corruption." [THE

TEACHINGS OF HIPPOCRATES, Adams edition, p. 326].

### BENEFITS OF HEMOSORPTION

As is noted in some of the autohemotherapy literature, some spontaneous cures following exploratory surgery or an unrelated injury are thought to have resulted from the action of autohemotherapy, whereby some errant blood may have found its way to tissues in sufficient quantities so as to comprise autohemotherapy.  Some contemporary articles utilize the term "hemosorption".  [See Chapter 9: MEDLINE UPDATES ...].

In the same vein (no pun intended), Hippocrates correlated the absence of some diseases with hemorrhoids and varicosity, which circulatory conditions might be seen as fostering increased absorption of blood by one's tissues; notably these include diseases for which autoserotherapy or autohemotherapy (IM) has been reported beneficial, including pleurisy, mental illness and skin diseases; as well as conditions of baldness and hump-back.

### PLEURISY, PNEUMONIA, ULCER, BOILS, SWELLINGS, SKIN DISEASES

"Sufferers from hemorrhoids are attacked neither by pleurisy nor by pneumonia, nor by spreading ulcer, nor by boils, nor by swellings, nor perhaps by skin-eruptions and skin diseases. However, unseasonably cured, many have been quickly caught by such diseases, and, moreover, in a fatal manner.  All other abscessions, too, such as fistula, are cures of other diseases. So symptoms that relieve complaints if they come after their development, prevent the development if they come before." [Humours XX]

It is noted in asserting that varicosity relates inversely to baldness, hump backs, and madness, the Hippocratic writings seemingly place these conditions with more conventional diseases like pleurisy, etc.  Hippocrates also stressed the relation between blood and intelligence. [See BALDNESS, HUMPBACKS, MADNESS, BLOOD AND INTELLIGENCE below.]


### HIPPOCRATES -  FROM AIR-BORNE DISEASES TO VARICOSE VEINS


### AIR-BORNE DISEASES

" ... diseases are all the offspring of air"  [Jones 1922, Vol. 2, Ch. V., p. 233]


### ALL DISEASES "ONE ESSENCE AND CAUSE"

"Now of all diseases the fashion is the same, but the seat varies.  So while diseases are thought to be entirely unlike one another, owing to the difference in their seat, in reality all have one essence and cause.  [Jones 1923, Vol. 2, p. 229, "Breaths", Ch. II, (p. 229)]

AUTOTHERAPY

Durant 1939, p. 345, attributes to Hippocrates:  "In any cure nature, i.e. the powers and constitution of the body - is the principal healer. ..."  [Will Durant, The Life of Greece, Simon and Schuster, N.Y., 1939, p. 343]

BALDNESS AND VARICOSE VEINS

"Bald people are not subject to large varicose veins; bald people who get varicose veins grow hair again.  [Jones 1923, Vol. IV, Aphorisms, Sixth Section (VI), #XXXIV]

BLOOD AND INTELLIGENCE, IRREGULARITIES

"...no constituent of the body in anyone contributes more to intelligence than does blood.  So long as the blood remains in its normal condition, intelligence too remains normal; but when the blood alters, the intelligence also changes. ... The progress of the blood through the body proving irregular, all kinds of irregularities occur.  [Jones 1923, II, 249]

BLOODLETTING - Jones 1923, I, 126:  Hippocrates's views on bloodletting are discussed above in ON BLOODLETTING.

DRUGS: "JUST SAY NO"

Of Hippocrates, Durant notes: "His teacher, Herodicus of Selynbria, formed his art by accustoming him to rely upon diet and exercise rather than upon drugs." [Will Durant, The Life of Greece, Simon and Schuster, N.Y., 1939, p. 343; Hippocrates, Jones 1923, II, 59]

FEES:

"This piece of advice also will need our consideration, as it contributes somewhat to the whole.  For should you begin by discussing fees, you will suggest to the patient either that you will go away and leave him if no agreement can be reached, or that you will neglect him and not prescribe any immediate treatment.  So one must not be anxious about fixing a fee.  For I consider such a worry to be harmful to a troubled patient, particularly if the disease be acute.  For the quickness of the disease, offering no opportunity for turning back, spurs on the good physician not to seek his profit but rather to lay hold on reputation.  Therefore it is better to reproach a patient you have saved than to extort money from those who are at death's door."  [Jones 1923, Vol. 1, p. 317, "Precepts, Ch. IV]

FEVER AND ABSCESSED JOINT - Jones 1923, II, p. 49
 " ... If a fever be protracted, although the patient is in a

state indicating recovery, and pain do not persist through
inflammation or any other obvious cause, you may expect an
abscession, with swelling and pain, to one of the joints,
especially to the lower ones.  Such abscessions come more often,
and earlier, when patients are under thirty.  You must suspect at
once the occurrence of an abscession if the fever last longer
than twenty days; but in older patients it is less likely, even
if the fever be more protracted."

## FOCAL INFECTION & SYSTEMIC DISEASE

"One may observe in medicine many ... examples of violent
lesions which are without harm, and contain in themselves the
whole crisis of the malady, while slighter injuries are
malignant, producing a chronic progeny of diseases and spreading
widely into the rest of the body."  [Jones 1922, Vol. 3, transl.
by ET Wittington, Wm. Heinemann 1927, Vol. 3, p. 307, "On
joints", Ch. XLIX]

## FOCUS OF INFECTION:  ERYSIPELAS FROM TRIVIAL ACCIDENT OR INJURY

"Many were attacked by erysipelas all over the body, when the
exciting cause was a trivial accident or injury." [Adams, 127]

## HEADACHE WITH FEVER - Jones 1923, II, 241

"Headache with fever arises in the following manner.  The blood
passages in the head become narrowed.  The veins in fact are
filled with air, and when full and inflated cause the headache;
for the hot blood, forcibly forced through the narrow passages,
cannot traverse them quickly because of the many hindrances and
barriers in the way.  This too is the reason why pulsations occur
about the temples."

The correlation of blood constriction with headache, in
conjunction with the known anticoagulant effect of aspirin, is
compatible with the view that headache is caused by miniclots in
the brain. [see also HEADACHE]

## HOMOSEXUALITY AS DISEASE

Homosexuality arises from horseback riding and cutting of an
ear vein.  It is no more or less divine than other disease.
[Jones 1923, Vol. 1, p. 127, XXII; Adams edition, 38]

## HUMP-BACK AND VARICOSE VEINS

"Some of those [hump-back conditions] lower down are resolved
when varicosities form in the legs, and still more when these are
in the vein at the back of the knee."  ["On Joints, XLI
(Hippocrates/Jones, Vol. 3, 1928, 1968, p. 279)]

LIFE
"Life is short, and the art long; the occasion fleeting; experience fallacious; and judgment difficult." [Adams edition, p. 292]

MADNESS
"Varicose veins or hemorrhoids supervening on madness remove it" [Aphorisms VI,XXI (Hippocrates, Jones 1931, 1967, Harvard U. Press, Vol. 4, p. 785)]

"Madness, dread and fear, sleeplessness, mistakes, aimless anxieties, absent-mindedness ... These things that we suffer all come from the brain, when it is not healthy, but becomes abnormally hot, cold, moist, or dry, or suffers any other unnatural affection to which it was not accustomed. Madness comes from its [the brain's] moistness. When the brain is abnormally moist, of necessity it moves, and when it moves neither sight nor hearing are still, but we see or hear now one thing and now another, and the tongue speaks in accordance with the things seen and heard on any occasion. But all the time the brain is still a man is intelligent." [Jones 1923, Vol. 2, Ch. XVII, p. 175; Adams, 347, 358]

PHYSICIAN
"The intimacy also between physician and patient is close. Patients in fact put themselves into the hands of their physician, and at every moment he meets women, maidens and possessions very precious indeed. So towards all these self-control must be used." [Jones 1922, Vol. 2, p. 313]

QUACKERY - Jones 1923, I, xii,8,310,320-2,328

RACES - THE "LONGHEADS"
"There is no other race at all with heads like theirs. Originally custom was chiefly responsible ... . Those that have the longest heads they consider the noblest, and their custom is as follows. As soon as a child is born they remodel its head with their hands, while it is still soft and the body tender, and force it to increase in length by applying bandages and suitable appliances, which spoil the roundness of the head and increase its length. ... as time went on the process became natural ... .
If bald parents have for the most part bald children ..., squinting parents squinting children, and so on .., what prevents a long-headed parent from having a long-headed child? [Hippocrates, Translated by WHS Jones, Wm Heinemann Ltd., London, 1923, Vol. 1:

p. 111, "Airs Waters Places", Chapter XIV - the "longheads".]

SACRED DISEASE (epilepsy)
Re "the disease called sacred", Hippocrates attributes this to the same cause as apoplexy and dropsy [Jones 1923, II, 249]

"... it has the same nature as other diseases, and the cause that gives rise to individual diseases.  It is also curable, no less than other illnesses... .  Its origin, like that of other diseases, lies in heredity."  [WHS Jones, 1923, Vol. 2, p. 139, "The Sacred Disease", Chapter V, p. 151]

"the disease called the sacred arises from causes as the others, namely those things that enter and quit the body ... [Adams, 360]

SEASONALITY OF DISEASE - Adams ed., 300
Spring:  maniacal, epilepsy, bloody flux, quinsy, coryza, hoarseness, cough, leprosy, lichen alphos, exanthemata ulcerative, tubercles, arthritis
Autumn:  sciatica, asthma, epilepsy

TEETH - See Adams edition, 128

THROAT ULCERATION
"An ulcerated throat with fever is serious... [Jones 1923, II, 46-47, 242; Adams, 55]

TONSILS, ULCER ON - Jones 1923, II, 326-8

UVULA, RED/ENLARGED - Jones 1923, II, 49:
"It is dangerous to cut away or lance the uvula while it is red and enlarged, for inflammation and hemorrhage supervene after such treatment; but at this time try to reduce such swellings by the other means.  When, however, the gathering is now complete, forming what is called "the grape," that is, when the point of the uvula is enlarged and livid, while the upper part is thinner, it is then safe to operate. ..."

VARICOSE VEINS - Jones 1923, I, 86; see BALDNESS, HUMP-BACK, MADNESS, above.

Chapter 4: BONE-MARROW TRANSPLANTATION

AUTOLOGOUS BONE MARROW TRANSPLANT  = I.V. AUTOHEMOTHERAPY

In recent years the use of bone marrow transplantation in the treatment of blood and other diseases has grown steadily.  Two major trends within the bone marrow transplantation field are particularly notable in that they expose the underlying beneficial action as perhaps intimately related (or identical) with that underlying autohemotherapy, and at the same time signal possible evolution of the field as a whole into a form of (intravenous) autohemotherapy.  These two trends are (1) increased popularity of autologous transplantation, and (2) the use of blood stem cells from the circulating blood (or even whole circulating blood) vs. stem cells from the marrow.

The first of these trends is clearly apparent from a view of overall statistics concerning bone marrow transplantation from 1966 through 1993, as summarized in Table 4-1, "MEDLINE - BMT TRENDS & PROJECTIONS".  It is noted that the percentage of citations involving the keyword "autologous" increased from 11.6% during the period 1966-1975 to 27.3% for the period 1990-1993. The obvious impetus for a move towards autologous methods derives from difficulties in matching marrow and dangers from mis-matched marrow.

Some recent writers have expressed a preference for peripheral blood stem cells over bone marrow, not only in terms of ease of collection, but most importantly in terms of effectiveness.  Chao and Blume 1990 note, among other advantages, that the time to engraftment is shorter with peripheral cells than with marrow; and Ossenkoppele GJ et al. 1994 assert that the use of peripheral stem cells "has the advantage of dramatically accelerating haematopoietic recovery."  Ossenkoppele et al. went a step further (or further backwards, if you will) and "in place of the more complicated, expensive and time-consuming procedure" of withdrawal and processing 7 liters of blood, collected 1 liter of blood and reinfused it unprocessed after 24 hours.

These are not isolated instances.  Indeed, J. Goldman, editor of Bone Marrow Transplantation, has indicated [July, 1994, 14:1] "A change of name to 'Blood and Marrow Transplantation' is probable"; and forecasts "It seems more than ever likely that blood-derived stem cells will replace marrow for many indications".  Two additional studies in this same journal issue refer to the use of such peripheral cells (Brice P et al and Sheridan WP et al.).

Goldman refers to changes in bone marrow transplantation, its use in lymphomas and solid tumors, notably breast cancer, and "perhaps the most unexpected success story of the last decade ... the introduction to clinical practice of haemopoietic growth factors."

As projected in Table 4-1, by the year 2010 most bone-marrow transplantation will be autologous:

Table 4-1:  MEDLINE - BMT TRENDS & PROJECTIONS

MEDLINE subject: BONE MARROW TRANSPLANTATION;
MEDLINE keyword: AUTOLOGOUS

|  | PROJECTED AUTOLOOUS | | | | | | |
|---|---|---|---|---|---|---|---|
|  | 66-75 | 75-79 | 80-84 | 85-89 | 90-94 | 95-99 | 00-04 | 04-09 |
| Total BMT | 1760 | 1524 | 2527 | 4988 | 7251 | | | |
| #-autologous | 205 | 199 | 366 | 975 | 1989 | | | |
| %-autologous | 11.6% | 13.1% | 14.5% | 19.6% | 27.3% | 35.0% | 42.7% | 50.4% |
|  | \ / | \ / | \ / | \ / | \ / | \ / | \ / | |
| autologous-%  increase: | | 1.5 | 1.4 | 5.1 | 7.7 | 7.7 | 7.7 | 7.7 |

---

It is noted that if %-autologous were to continue to increase at a sustained rate of 7.7% from a 1990-94 level of 27.3%, by the year 2010 the majority of blood-marrow transplants will be autologous; at an increasing rate (as has in fact been occurring, i.e., from 1.4% increase to 5.1% to 7.7%, between reporting periods), this will occur even sooner.  Coupling this with Bone Marrow Transplantation editor Goldman's suggestion that blood-derived stem cells "replace marrow for many indications"; and working in the suggestion of Raina et al. 1996 and Ossenkoppele et al. 1994, that unprocessed whole blood be used in the place of peripheral blood progenitor cells (PBPC) [see WHOLE BLOOD... below]; the simple fact is that a sizeable portion of bone-marrow-transplantation is soon to become (IV) autohemotherapy.

Thus, it may be useful to take a summary view of reported uses bone-marrow-transplantation; to note that many related conditions have already been reported treated by autohemotherapy [e.g. leukemia, anemia, sclerosis, lymphoma; see INDEX]; and to suggest that insofar as many of these conditions seem destined to be treated by a (more expensive and complicated) form of autohemotherapy in future years, that the "classical" and simplest form of autohemotherapy (extravascular, i.e. intramuscular or subcutaneous) might be undertaken expeditiously, in controlled clinical trials as well as by individual practitioners, at a minimum of cost and without risk of harm.

DISORDERS IN WHICH BONE MARROW TRANSPLANTATION HAS BEEN USED:

- Leukemia: acute; chronic granulocytic; hairy-cell
- Anemia, aplastic; Fanconi's
- Myelosclerosis - acute "malignant"
- Non-Hodgkin's lymphoma [primarily autologous]
- Hodgkin's disease [primarily autologous]
- Multiple myeloma
- Osteoporosis
- Tumors (breast and testicular cancers)
- Thalassemia major

[sources: Chou NJ, et al., West. J. Med. 151 (Dec. 1989) 638-43; Gorin NC, Comptes Rendus des Seances de la Societe de Biologie et de Sesfilialie, 1993, 187 (4), 452-86; Buchsel PC and Kelleher J [Nursing Clinics of N. America 24, Dec. 1989, 907-938]


AUTOLOGOUS BONE MARROW TRANSPLANT V PERIPHERAL STEM CELLS

Chao NJ and Blume KG, West. J. Med 152 (Jan. 1990), summarize the unique aspects of autologous bone marrow transplantation:

1. The harvested bone marrow usually needs to be stored, to allow time for myeloablative therapy to be administered and for any drug to be metabolized and excreted. The time period may vary from several hours to months or even years. Prior to cryopreservation red blood cells and granulocytes should be removed.

2. An attempt is made to remove ("purge") obvious or possible contaminating tumor cells from the marrow.

3. The use of peripheral stem cells. "Peripheral stem cells, especially when collected at the time a patient is recovering from standard chemotherapy, are able to fully reconstitute the marrow of patients who have had myeloablative therapy. In fact, the time to engraftment from these peripheral cells is shorter than when using marrow. ... [This idea] has several attractive features. Cells can be collected by repeated apheresis, and there is no need for marrow harvesting and possible general anesthesia. This is especially useful for some patients who have no harvestable marrow ... [or] with possible marrow disease ..."

The authors discuss the use of autologous bone marrow transplantation in conjunction with therapy of a number of diseases: diffuse large cell lymphoma, Hodgkin's disease, high-grade (Burkitt's, lymphoblastic) and other lymphomas, solid tumors and leukemias.

"... Clearly, the primary concern of autologous bone marrow transplantation for leukemia is reinfusion of clonogenic cells. The assumption is that when marrow is harvested from a patient in complete remission, it is contaminated with a small number of leukemic cells. The mechanical handling and the freezing and thawing may eliminate a good fraction of these cells, and small numbers reinfused may not necessarily lead to leukemia relapse. Several pilot studies have been done with encouraging results."

The authors mention several types of tumors which have "shown some response to transplantation", including sarcomas, melanomas, small-cell lung cancer, colon cancer, multiple myeloma, neuroblastoma and breast cancer ("in unfavorable groups of patients, the results are encouraging, but it is still quite early.")


WHOLE BLOOD - BETTER, SIMPLER, CHEAPER, FASTER THAN MARROW


At least two recent articles have

- indicated that the use of reinjected whole blood is comparable to the use of stem cells from the blood, thus preferable in view of its far greater simplicity and ease of rapid administration; and

- asserted that the use of either whole blood or stem cells is preferable to bone marrow:


Raina, V., et al., Cancer, 77 (6), 1073-8, March 15, 1996, per MEDLINE ABSTRACT, discuss the contemporary practice whereby "chemotherapy can be supplemented with autologous haemopoeitic blood cells; cryopreserved bone marrow has conventionally been used for this, but blood stem cells are now in common use. ... Results with whole blood are similar to conventional blood stem cell transplants, but much better than autologous BMT [bone-marrow transplantation]. ... It has the potential of becoming an alternative to autologous marrow and peripheral blood stem cell transplantation in patients with MM [multiple myeloma]."


Ossenkoppele GJ et al., Bone Marrow Transplantation 13 (Jan) 1994, discussed the use of unprocessed whole blood in the place of peripheral blood progenitor cells (PBPC).

The authors noted that "infusion of mobilised PBPC after high-dose chemotherapy is associated with markedly accelerated platelet and neutrophil recovery compared with autologous BMT [bone marrow transplant], as has been shown recently in a number of studies."

However, in this study, in place of the more complicated, expensive and time-consuming procedure of collecting PBPC involving the withdrawal and processing of 7 liters of blood, "we mobilised peripheral blood stem cells by G-CSF [growth factor granulocyte colony-stimulating factor] only, collected 1 liter of blood by phlebotomy and reinfused the blood unprocessed after 24 hours. ... two phlebotomies of 500 ml each were ... [each] collected in a ... polyvinylchloride bag with 70 ml CPD as anticoagulant. ... Immediately after blood collection, high-dose melphalan was infused in 10 min.   After 24 hours the two bags of blood were reinfused over 4 hours."

".... In addition to avoiding the sequelae associated with BM [bone marrow] harvesting, infusion of mobilised PBPC has the advantage of dramatically accelerating haematopoietic recovery."

The authors concluded that their "encouraging results are most probably due to the reinfusion of G-CSF-stimulated whole blood."


PRESS REPORTS ON COST, EFFECT. OF ABMT FOR BREAST CANCER

Bazell R, in The New Republic, 203, 9-10+ (Dec. 31, 1990), "Topic of Cancer", discusses the controversy over whether autologous bone marrow transplant is helpful for breast cancer, citing high costs of $100,000 to $200,000, and data showing 5-20 percent of patients die from the procedure itself. It is noted that Blue Cross and Blue Shield had offered to finance clinical trials and negotiated a price drop to $80,000. (v. cost of autohemotherapy - syringe).

Zamichow N, Los Angeles Times Dec. 19, 1991, A40, discusses the nationwide clinical trials of autologous bone marrow transplantation for breast cancer. Bone marrow is removed with a needle, treated with an anti-cancer drug and frozen. The patient is then given 3-6 times the standard amount of chemotherapy in an attempt to eradicate the cancer cells, and the frozen marrow is thawed and infused into the patient. Reportedly in a Harvard Medical School study at 13 medical centers, 58 percent of patients receiving this treatment had no cancer after one year, compared to 30 percent of patients receiving only conventional therapy.


Postscript 2004: It is noted that the field of stem cell therapy has become prominent as the cutting edge of medical science in the early years of the new millennium, with the practice of autologous stem cell therapy at the forefront. For more information, check the Medline Index under keywords: autologous stem cell.

Chapter 5: VACCINE-THERAPY


OVERVIEW: VACCINE THERAPY - THE WRIGHT STUFF


The term "vaccine" originated in Jenner's reference to cowpox
as "variolae vaccinnia", and the transference of this disease to
humans as a prophylactic against smallpox.  Jenner had noted that
milkmaids did not contract smallpox, apparently gaining immunity
by having become infected on their hands with a milder form of
disease from cows with cowpox.  Jenner obtained material from the
lesion of such a milkmaid, and transferred it to a scratch on the
arm of a young boy, thereby inducing cowpox as a prophylactic
against smallpox.  The term "vaccine" first came to be used to
describe this prophylactic procedure, and subsequently came to be
commonly used in reference to similarly-employed measures aimed
at preventing a wide range of infectious diseases.


IMMUNIZATION AGAINST ANY FOREIGN AGENT IS POSSIBLE

-- p. 23-4  "...From studies thus far, it is reasonable to
assume that fowls and mammals can be immunized against any
foreign antigenic agent, whether it is a simple protein material
..., or complex cellular material and infectious agents such as
red blood cells, viruses, bacteria, and animal parasites."
[Cushing, JE and DH Campbell, Principles of Immunology, McGraw-
Hill, New York, 1957.]


The concept of therapeutic vaccines originated with Sir Almroth
Wright early in the 20th Century:  "Sir Almroth Wright extended
the principles of active immunization to include not only the
prevention but also the treatment of infectious diseases."
[Encyclopedia Britannica 1972, "Vaccine Therapy"]  The concept of
vaccine-therapy is once again gaining adherents as the limits of
drug-therapy have become increasingly evident.  [see VACCINE-
THERAPY UPDATE in MEDLINE UPDATES]

We shall visit in this chapter with Wright and his vaccine-
therapy concept, his stellar staff, some enthusiastic followers,
and details of his programme.

Additionally, it is noted that the works of C. H. Duncan and
E.C. Rosenow were in good part inspired by Wright.  In turn
Duncan's works comprise the major portion of Chapter 6:
AUTOTHERAPY; and Rosenow's works comprised the inspiration for
research into, and motivation behind, the separate volume:
*REFERENCE MANUAL ROSENOW ET AL.*


SIR ALMROTH WRIGHT

"best known for advancing vaccination through the use of
autogenous vaccines .. and through antityphoid immunization

with typhoid bacilli killed by heat." [Encycl. Brit. 1990]

As noted in the INTRODUCTION, although Sir Almroth Wright is not known to have used autohemotherapy, his "STUDIES OF IMMUNIZATION" nonetheless provides precedents for virtually all aspects of Cuyugan's method of treatment and for autohemotherapy in general. [see INTRODUCTION, ABSTRACT for summary overview, and THE WRIGHT STUFF below for details.]

Wright was one of the top immunologists around the turn of the century (19th to 20th), and served as inspiration for Bernard Shaw's play The Doctor's Dilemna: "It will be evident to all experts that my play could not have been written but for the work done by Sir Almroth Wright in the theory and practice of securing immunization from bacterial diseases by inoculation of vaccines made of their own bacteria. etc." In 1897 Wright had introduced a vaccine prepared from killed typhoid bacilli as a means of preventing typhoid. During WWI, nearly all persons in the British Expeditionary Force were vaccinated. For vaccinated persons, rates of infection and death were 2.35 and 0.139 per 1000, resp., compared to 104 and 14.6 for the unvaccinated.

Wright's work is not without controversy, even in his own time inspiring the somewhat playful use of the mocking moniker "Sir 'Almost' Wright". And as recently as 1979, pop-med-writer Steven Lehrer in his Explorers of the Body seems to have been seduced by his own prosaic propensities when he offered that "Perhaps Wright managed to miss the immunologic boat with the opsonin theory because his real abilities lay in the realm of literature rather than science."

In fact Wright's work continues to serve an integral role in the foundation of modern immunology theory. For example Ivan Roitt, somewhat revered in contemporary immunology as the spiritual godfather of "Autoimmunity" (unfortunately exposed herein as pure myth), places Wright's work in his "top-ten" list of immunology-history highlights. And according to William Clark, *Experimental Foundations of Modern Immunology* [(1986), 416.], "it seems that the major role of IgG and IgM antibody in the elimination of bacteria is opsonization for phagocytosis." [The relations between "opsonins", antibody, and coagulation are discussed further in Chapter 7: THEORETICAL CONSIDERATIONS.]

THERAPEUTIC VACCINES

- AUTOGENOUS OR STOCK?

Theoretically, a strictly prophylactic vaccine could not be autogenous, insofar as the candidate to be protected is presumably not infected - thus the causative organism presumably does not reside therein. In contrast, the fact that the causative organism by definition does reside in an infected individual makes the autogenous vaccine not merely possible, but clearly preferable under most circumstances.


## PREFERABILITY OF AUTOGENOUS 1916; 1972

The preferability of autogenous (self-generated) vaccines over stock vaccines was integral to the vaccine-therapy work of Sir Almroth Wright, particularly emphasized by him, and universally recognized up to modern times.  For example:

Dumke in 1916 wrote:  "...it would look as though it would be a difficult matter to make stock serum where a coccus is the offender and so many families and changes are possible. Consequently, where there are so many strains of practically the same germ, it would be better to obtain a vaccine from a strain direct from the patient."

The Encyclopedia Britannica 1972, in its section on "Vaccine Therapy", noted:  "Autogenous vaccines are prepared from the actual microorganism isolated from the particular patient being treated.  Such preparations are superior to even polyvalent stock vaccines in the treatment of chronic infections, such as sinusitis and some skin eruptions, since all the antibodies that develop are specific for the particular agent causing the disease."


## DANGERS OF STOCK VACCINES; ASTHMA CAUSED BY BACTERIAL VACCINES

Hektoen 1929 referred to several cases of untoward, harmful and fatal effects from subcutaneous application of polyvalent stock vaccines.  Hektoen also noted:  "If asthma is due, in certain cases, to sensitization to bacterial protein, it would seem that asthmatic attacks might follow prolonged courses of bacterial vaccines in persons who have been free from asthmatic symptoms. ...  Seventeen cases of asthma are reported by 14 physicians as having followed courses of bacterial stock vaccines, injected subcutaneously ... [into] patients who previously were not known to have suffered from asthma."  [p. 868]


## POSSIBLE EXCEPTION TO PREFERABILITY-OF-AUTOGENOUS

In the case of some acute epidemic-disease conditions, the proper advance preparation of highly specific stock therapeutic-vaccines may allow for the requisite, more-timely-than-autogenous-vaccine response, as Drs. Rosenow and Rappaport have demonstrated in the case of poliomyelitis. (See POLIO in *REFERENCE MANUAL ROSENOW ET AL*)


## AUTOHEMOTHERAPY INCORPORATES BOTH IMMEDIACY AND SPECIFICITY

Autohemotherapy, while clearly possessing a lesser potency potential than vaccines (either autogenous or stock), offers the attributes of unquestionable specificity and unrivalled immediacy.

As Roitt 1977, p. 1, has noted, "Memory, specificity and the recognition of 'non-self' - these lie at the heart of immunology."


## EXCUSES FOR SLOW DEVELOPMENT OF VACCINES; THERAPY IMPLICATIONS
## WHY IMMUNIZATION AGAINST ALL IMPORTANT DISEASES NOT PRACTICED

As noted above, Cushing and Campbell 1957 have offered: "...The failure to practice immunization [against all important infectious diseases] may be due to one or more of the following reasons:  (1) the causative agent is not known; (2) the causative agent is not available in sufficient quantities to be of practical use; (3) the antigen available is too toxic to be administered in practical amounts; (4) important antigens are lost on artificial cultivation; (5) the antigen does not produce protective antibodies; (6) the number of strains of the infective organism is too variable; and (7) the control of the disease by sanitation methods is more practical than immunization."

Without specifically discussing vaccine-therapy, the authors refer to the use of autogenous vaccines within discussions of bacterial vaccines; of course, autogenous vaccines are by definition therapeutic. [Cushing and Campbell 1957]


## ANTIBIOTICS CAUSED LOSS OF INTEREST IN BACTERIAL VACCINES

In recent years, Encyclopedia Britannica, 1991, 12 p. 228 has noted, "Interest in bacterial vaccines slackened with the introduction of antibiotics in the mid-20th century, but vaccines remain a mainstay in the fight against many infectious diseases."


## VACCINE BOTTOM LINE: VACCINES "NOT MONEY-MAKERS"

In a survey of leading researchers around the world, Science magazine [Cohen, J., Science 265 (2 Sept. 1994), "Bumps on the Vaccine Road"] has sought to identify major obstacles to the development of new vaccines.  "Predictably money -- or rather, lack of it - was one of the most frequently mentioned obstacles. Even though vaccines are among the most cost-effective medical interventions ever devised, they are not big money-makers.  A recent study for UNICEF estimates that the entire global vaccine market is only $3 billion.  By comparison, the anti-ulcer drug Zantac, the best-selling pharmaceutical, last year took in $3.5 billion by itself.  'The major stumbling block [in vaccine R&D] is there's not enough money to bring basic science up through development of a vaccine,' says Scott Halstead, the Rockefeller Foundation's deputy director of the Health Sciences Division.

"Companies can make money on a vaccine - if it's used in developed countries.  ... for diseases that don't afflict developed countries, there is scant commercial interest in vaccines.  Malaria ... is a telling example."

This example of malaria seems particularly appropriate for autohemotherapy, in view of the "scant commercial interest" in a prophylactic vaccine, and moreover the fact that no one has figured out how to devise a prophylactic vaccine in any case.]

While the prime focus in Cohen's discussion is on preventive rather than therapeutic vaccines, one might understand how suppression of interest in the former might extend to the latter. In the case of vaccine-therapy, big investor profits would not be expected, insofar as each vaccine is personalized and thus mass production of a single cure is problematic. [One possible approach to making strides in this direction might involve a sort of "Fotomat" for personalized vaccines; once the organism is obtained, e.g. from a nasopharyngeal swab or a properly preserved pin-prick, the remainder of the process might be automated.]

## ANTI-VIRAL VACCINES REQUIRED CULTURE ADVANCES OF THE 50S

Lederberg 1988: "The basic principles of vaccination were established long ago, but practical means of production of vaccines for viral infection like polio had to await the cell and tissue culture advances of the 1950s." [Lederberg, J, JAMA 260 (Aug. 5, 1988), p. 684-5]

Beyond the obvious case example of polio, one might suggest that such advances in general, among other factors, served to divert attention from Dr. Rosenow's work and the role of focal infection, and from autohemotherapy.

## HEKTOEN 1929 - VACCINE SURVEY, CRITICISMS

Although some meticulous practitioners such as Rosenow and followers consistently attained good results; mixed results of vaccine-therapy, as reflected in Hektoen's 1929 survey, Table 5-1 below, have left a legacy not void of skepticism, as expressed by Wahrer, Sandström and Wigzell, 1993, "Differences in opinion may exist as to whether the principles of therapeutic vaccines have been solidly established."

Hektoen 1929, 867, noted "From 1906, the date of Wright's introduction of vaccine treatment, the number of papers on vaccines in medical journals constantly increased until it reached a formidable volume around 1912. From this time on the interest in the treatment evidently declines, for the number of papers on vaccine-therapy recorded by the Index Medicus steadily shrinks until today they form a small part of the articles listed." [Autovaccines peaked in the late 1920s see Table i-1.]

## REASONS FOR FAILURES OF VACCINE-THERAPY

Wright suggested that in cases where vaccine-therapy failed, this may have been due to (a) the selection of an inappropriate microbe, and/or (b) alteration-beyond-usefulness of an otherwise appropriate microbe in preparing the vaccine (which occurrences seemingly recommend the use of autohemotherapy).

HEKTOEN SURVEY RESULTS

Table 5-1. Autovaccine results
          (Hektoen 1929 survey)
          1261 physicians reporting.

| Disease | Good | Negative | Variable |
|---|---|---|---|
| Mastoiditis | – | 6 | 7 |
| Osteomyelitis | – | 6 | 8 |
| Otitis media | 5 | 16 | 10 |
| Nephritis | 1 | 2 | 0 |
| Acne | 25 | 28 | 25 |
| Asthma | 11 | 9 | 25 |
| Bronchiectasis | 1 | 2 | 2 |
| Bronchitis | 18 | 10 | 15 |
| Carbuncle | 12 | 3 | 2 |
| Colds | 7 | 4 | 15 |
| Cystitis | 8 | 4 | 8 |
| Erysipelas | 2 | 2 | 0 |
| Furunculosis | 91 | 30 | 79 |
| Genito-urinary | 2 | 3 | 2 |
| Gonorrhea | 2 | 5 | 2 |
| Pyelitis | 9 | 6 | 15 |
| Rheumatism | 8 | 10 | 16 |
| Sinusitis | 9 | 5 | 10 |
| Sycosis | 2 | 2 | 1 |
| Throat Infect. | 4 | 1 | 1 |
| T.B. | 3 | 3 | 1 |
| Pneumonia | 5 | 3 | 0 |
| Septicemia | 3 | 4 | 1 |
| | | | |
| TOTALS | 229 | 164 | 245 |

## THE WRIGHT STAFF

### FLEMING - PENICILLIN; FLEMING NEVER ABLE TO REPRODUCE ORIGINAL RESULT

Unquestionably the best known of Sir Almroth Wright's junior associates was Alexander Fleming of penicillin fame. While it has been suggested that the association with Wright may have limited Fleming [H. Hughes in D. Wilson, 1976], the contrary suggestion seems as defensible, i.e., that Fleming could have been long-forgotten except as a footnote to penicillin and Wright, were it not for the efforts of Sir Almroth. The two men worked together for forty years, from 1906 to 1946. [H. F. Dowling, 1977.]

Without Wright's aggressive promotion, Fleming might have been remembered as a man who stumbled over penicillin and couldn't make it work. Reportedly "Fleming himself was never able to reproduce his original result", "had classified penicillin with lysozome" and "regarded it as hopeless." [T.I. Williams, Howard Florey, Oxford U. Press, 1984, p. 65, 209] As late as 1939 Fleming was inclined to write off penicillin as an antibiotic. [Dowling, 1977, 135.]

It was Florey who figured out how to produce useable penicillin and proved its effectiveness, and Chain who led the way to chemical extraction; and in 1940 the two published the findings of their Oxford group regarding the chemotherapeutic attributes of penicillin (British J. of Experimental Pathology).

The London Times (Aug. 30, 1942) subsequently reported on the miracle of penicillin, without crediting Fleming. Sir Almroth Wright immediately submitted a letter which the Times published, which claimed primary credit for Fleming and St. Mary's. Although authorities at Oxford objected to Wright's characterization, the "myth" of Fleming and penicillin was established. [Dowling/Williams]


### FLEMING - VACCINE-THERAPY

Whatever his role in the penicillin affair, Fleming continued to be associated with vaccine-therapy. In 1934, he and G. F. Petrie of the Lister Institute wrote Recent Advances in Vaccine and Serum Therapy for "The Recent Advances Series" [P. Blakiston's Son & Co., Inc., Philadelphia 1934]. Therein is found these observations:

VACCINE THERAPY FOR VIRAL INFECTION: "... there is no essential difference between the immunity mechanism which is set in motion by viruses and by bacteria when they are introduced into the body of an animal; ... in conformity with experience in bacterial immunity, the most efficient vaccine against a virus disease is the living attenuated organism, although the killed virus may in some instances have a prophylactic value."[201 - Petrie]

VACCINE PREPARATION - KEEP IT SIMPLE:  "... it must be remembered that any complication of the method of [vaccine] preparation increases the possibility of contamination."

THE BEST VACCINE:  "... if it were possible to obtain all the useful antigenic components of the bacteria in solution and at the same time accurately standardize the antigenic content, this would form the best type of vaccine."[252]

ADVANTAGE OF AUTOGENOUS VACCINE:  "... when it is certain that the microbe recovered from the patient is really the infecting agent, there is little doubt that in most cases an autogenous vaccine has theoretically an advantage over a stock vaccine."[253]

HOWEVER: "in the case of infections of the alimentary or respiratory tracts ... an autogenous vaccine may easily be made from the wrong microbe."

"AUTOLYSATES:  These have been recommended as vaccines, and with some bacteria, such as staphylococcus, they are probably effective, but sometimes the breaking down process proceeds too far and the immunizing power is lost."

Fleming's continuing interest in vaccine-therapy is noted in his 1939 publication, "Serum and vaccine therapy in combination with sulfanilamide ...", Proc. Roy. Soc. Med. 32:911-920, June 1939.


FREEMAN, JOHN - ALLERGIES;
SIR ALMROTH'S "SON IN SCIENCE"

   In Wright's discussion of the genesis of his interest in autogenous vaccine therapy, John Freeman's observations of autoinoculations are credited with having provided the initial impetus.  (see WRIGHT, AUTO-INOCULATION below)

Wright had reportedly once referred to Freeman as his "son in science", although by 1928 their relations were reportedly strained as a result of Wright's alleged "insistence on putting his name on Freeman's most important scientific publication", this concerning the study of allergies. [Wilson, D., 1978]


FREEMAN ON ALLERGIES

Freeman's key work was a continuation of Leonard Noon's 1910 studies of hay fever and other allergic diseases.  Freeman grouped together hay and other pollen fevers, animal and human asthmas, and "food idiosyncrasies", terming them first "toxic idiopathies", and later "protein idiopathies":

Freeman, J.,"Toxic Idiopathies", The Lancet, July 31, 1920, 229-35.

Freeman, John, "Skin reactions in asthma", protein idiopathies. The Practitioner 116:73-8, January 1926.

Freeman is credited with having established the modern view

that hayfever is an allergy to windblown pollen [Wilson, D., 1978]


## WILLIAM BOAG LEISHMAN - LEISHMAN'S STAIN, LEISHMANIASIS, ETC.

Leishman (1865-1926) worked under Sir Almroth Wright at the Army Medical School, Netley, succeeding Wright as professor when Wright transferred to London in 1902.  Leishman remained at Netley until 1919.  With Wright he worked on prophylactic inoculations in India, which work paid off during the First World War.  Leishman's work is well-remembered: Leishman's stain, Leishmaniasis and Leishman-Donovan body are named after him. [Parish 1965]


## LEONARD COLEBROOK - SULFONAMIDES

In retrospect we may consider Leonard Colebrook to have been Sir Almroth Wright's most dedicated protege.  In 1952 Colebrook produced a bibliography of Wright's published writings; and in 1954, some four decades or so following Wright's reign, Colebrook authored Almroth Wright, Provocative Doctor and Thinker.  In this work Colebrook projected the possibility that "in the future, with more knowledge at our disposal, medicine will turn again to Wright's conception of 'calling up the latent forces of the organism.' The physician of the future may yet become an immunizator".

It is interesting that Colebrook himself, as well as Fleming via penicillin, played a significant role in overcoming a limitation that had frustrated Wright and his contemporaries - the inability to chemically treat an internal infection.

Wright had asserted that antiseptics in the interior of the body would cause more damage to the body than to infecting bacteria.  [see WRIGHT, MISCELLANY, ANTIBIOTICS below]  Similarly von Behring, with whom Wright would otherwise vehemently differ with respect to the operative mechanism underlying so-called "serum therapy", had said "inner disinfection is a vain dream", which viewpoint prevailed through the mid 1930s [Dowling p.106]

(Much later, regarding the use of iodine and mercurochrome for infection, and antiseptics in general, Roseburg 1969 asserted "they do no good, and they may do harm." [p. 199, Theodor Roseburg, Life on Man, Viking Press 1969)

Then in 1935 the German Gerhardt Domagk reported the discovery of "Prontisil", which had cured mice of lethal doses of hemolytic streptococci.  This was initially greeted with skepticism by the likes of Ronald Hare, a leading British bacteriologist.  However, Hare's chief at Queen Charlotte's Hospital, London, happened to be Colebrook, who decided to investigate the new drug himself. Colebrook obtained samples in late 1935, and used the drug to treat 64 cases of puerperal sepsis in 1936.  The fatality rate was 4.7%, much lower than the 29% experienced during the previous 4 years.  The significance of this result was immediately recognized by the editor of <u>The Lancet</u>, which then led to the publication of more than 5000 articles on sulfonamides in the next decade and a half. [Dowling, Harry F., <u>Fighting Infection</u>, Harvard U. Press, 1977, 106-122].

Nonetheless, in an October 25, 1955 lecture, Colebrook cautioned that puerperal sepsis "is still with us.  There is still, indeed, more infection than there should be ... and further, that even though puerperal fever was then largely curable", that a mother who has recovered from streptococcal infection is very often sterile; and such sterility may be a cause of lifelong unhappiness." [Marks 1976, p. 221-2]

In view of Colebrook's prominent role in demonstrating the utility of sulfonamides, his continuing belief in vaccine-therapy notwithstanding seems worthy of particular note.


THE WRIGHT STUFF - OVERVIEW
[Excerpts, Wright, A.E.,  <u>Vaccine therapy</u>, 1919]


THEORY:
"... it is within our power to immunise against every variety of microbe, provided that we have at our disposal a vaccine which is affiliated to that microbe and have at disposal the means for arriving at the proper dosage." [p. 329]


PRINCIPLES OF THERAPEUTIC IMMUNIZATION
"On the two broad principles which ought to guide us when we set ourselves to combat bacterial infection by the agency of the protective elements which are furnished by the organism" ...

"Principle 1.  Therapeutic immunization should be resorted to in every case where the antibacterial power of a patient's blood falls below the standard which is attained when the organism is making an effective response to infection.

"Principle 2.  Where the blood is rich in antibacterial elements a fuller lymph stream should be determined to the affected part..."  [p. 347]


VACCINE-THERAPY


TO TREAT BACTERIAL DISEASE
Regarding "the treatment of bacterial disease by vaccine-therapy":  "The essential feature of this method is the scientific exploitation for therapeutic uses of the protective machinery with which the organism is equipped." [p. 324]


STOCK VACCINES

Regarding the preparation of vaccines, "while it would seem probable that in all cases the best results would be obtainable by the use of vaccines prepared from the original patient, and while such vaccines ought, wherever possible, to be resorted to in dangerous or obstinate infections, in the ordinary case, stock vaccines give very satisfactory results." [p. 375]

## AUTOGENOUS STAPHYLOCOCCUS VACCINE

Regarding treatment of chronic staphylococcus by inoculations of a staphylococcus vaccine, "... it is advisable in obstinate cases to resort to a vaccine made with the particular strain of a micro-organism which has acclimatized itself to grow in the patient's organism. [(1906) p. 254]

## SEPTICAEMIC INFECTIONS AND BACTERIAL VACCINES

Regarding " ... the possibility of bacterial vaccines rending a useful service in connection with the treatment of septicaemic infections, I have to confess that the idea that bacterial vaccines could here play a useful role was only a short time ago very uncongenial to my preconceived notions.  I conceived that when bacteria found access to the blood and generalized themselves in the system the machinery for immunization which is at the disposal of an organism was fully called into action.  In accordance with this I assumed that to inoculate bacterial vaccines in such circumstances would be to add fuel to the fire without contributing anything to the elaboration of those bacterial elements which serve to extinguish the conflagration. [p. 310]

... in the reasoning which I above rehearsed, the possibility of a different effect being produced by bacterial elements introduced into the blood stream and the same bacterial elements introduced directly into the tissues was overlooked.  Yet consideration will show that there maybe quite important differences, first in the matter of the toxic effects exerted, and secondly with respect to the immunizing response elicited by one and the same quantum of bacterial elements.

... The general toxication effect ... may be expected to be greatest where, as occurs in these infections, bacterial derivatives find direct access to the circulating blood, and least where, as would be the case in the inoculation of a vaccine, the bacterial elements are introduced into the tissues." [311]

... In the case where bacteria are, as in septicaemic conditions, found in the bloodstream ..., the bacterial derivatives are of necessity diluted by the whole volume of the blood and lymph before they can come into application upon the tissues in which, we may take it, the machinery for the derivation of protective substances is located. ... [p. 311]

"Can inoculations with bacterial vaccines be undertaken in ...
the case where the infecting microbes are cultivating themselves
in the circulating blood, or in direct anatomical relation to
this, producing 'spontaneous auto-inoculations' whenever the
bacteriotropic pressure of the blood falls"? ("case of
generalized infection with spontaneous auto-inoculations")  [p.
352]

"In the case of a septicaemia which fails to evoke any, or
which evokes only very unsatisfactory immunizing responses, I
would suggest that an attempt should be made to call forth
immunizing responses by inoculation of bacterial vaccines. ...
the employment of vaccines in these cases is not the unreasonable
proceeding that it might at first sight appear... . [p. 353]

INTRAVENOUS v. SUBCUTANEOUS/ INTRAMUSCULAR INJECTION

FOR SEPTICEMIA

"If ... the bacteriotropic substances are manufactured in the
tissues at the seat of inoculation, ...conditions for successful
immunisation must be less favorable when the vaccinating elements
are thrown into the circulating blood than when they are
inoculated directly into the tissues. ...

COMPARATIVE INTOXICATION FROM VACCINE INTO TISSUES v. BLOOD

"There still remains the objection that the inoculation of
bacterial vaccines might aggravate his intoxication. ... the
incorporation of an aliquot quantum of vaccine into the tissues
must produce less intoxication than the inoculation of that same
quantum of vaccine directly into the blood stream. ...

"I would put to you that in view of these considerations that
the question as to whether vaccine-therapy can, or cannot, be
successfully employed in connexion with septicaemic disease is a
question which ought not to be prejudged.  It is a question which
can be decided only by actual trial."[p. 350]

COMPARATIVE PRODUCTION OF PROTECTIVE SUBSTANCES

" Where a bacterial vaccine is inoculated directly into the
tissues, the bacterial products will come into application with
these in a very concentrated form, calling forth a
correspondingly larger production of protective substances. ...
Such larger production of protective substances is, in point of
fact, regularly achieved in the horse in connexion with the
production of diphtheria antitoxin, when, in lieu of intravenous
inoculations, subcutaneous and intra-muscular inoculations are
resorted to ... . " [p. 311]

## AUTO-INOCULATION

### SPONTANEOUS, SPONTANEOUS CURE

"...intoxication phenomena and immunizing responses exactly similar to those which supervene upon the inoculation of a bacterial vaccine, must in the ordinary course occur whenever bacterial products, or as the case may be bacteria, escape from localized foci of bacterial infection and pass into the circulation. ... it must be by the agency of immunizing responses to such auto-inoculations that spontaneous cures are achieved." [p. 342-3]

### ARTIFICIALLY INDUCED

Beyond spontaneous autoinoculations, Wright discussed "artificially 'induced auto-inoculations'". Based on "an illuminating observation by my collaborator, Dr. J. Freeman, in connexion with the effects produced on the blood by massage of a gonococcal joint, we have at St. Mary's Hospital during the last twelve months devoted ourselves to a systematic study of the conditions under which auto-inoculations can be produced in persons affected with localized bacterial infections."

### EXERCISE, MASSAGE, SURGERY, ETC. AS AGENTS OF AUTOINOCULATION

" ... auto-inoculations follow upon all active and passive movements which affect a focus of infection, and upon all vascular changes which activate the lymph stream in such a focus ...," and may be produced "by massage and extirpation operations affecting tuberculosis glands; by passive extension, massage, and divers surgical operations affecting tuberculosis and gonococcal joints; and by scraping operations undertaken in connexion with tuberculosis caries and staphylococcal osteomyelitis." under varying circumstances, auto-inoculations have been brought about by the following activities: breathing deeply, reading aloud (laryngeal affection), walking, hot fomentations, by agency of massage, active muscular movements, Biers bandaging ... . [p. 345]

"Where we have to choose between lowering the bacteriotropic pressure of the circulating blood by an excessive auto-inoculation, and leaving the bacteria in a localized focus of infection for the nonce unmolested, we ought unhesitatingly to elect for the latter alternative [to assure] the safeguarding of the citadel of the circulating blood..." [p. 350]

### AUTO-INOCULATION v. BACTERIAL VACCINES

### ADVANTAGES OF AUTO-INOCULATION

"In the following respects auto-inoculation would appear to

have an advantage over inoculations of bacterial vaccines:

"(a) Where we are employing auto-inoculations we must invariably be employing the correct vaccine, or in the case of a mixed infection the correct mixture of vaccines.

"(b) Our therapeutic operations are not - when we proceed by the method of auto-inoculation - as they are when we proceed by the method of vaccine-therapy - limited by our power of cultivating the infecting micro-organisms on artificial media.

"(c) Treatment by auto-inoculation may in every case be begun without any preliminary diagnostic work, and without the delay which is inevitable where a special vaccine has to be prepared."

"(d) The draining off from the focus of infection of the lymph that is impregnated with bacterial products and its replacement by lymph freshly derived from the blood stream, may be expected to exert a beneficial effect upon that focus." [350-1]


## DISADVANTAGES OF AUTO-INOCULATION

"These advantages are, however, more than outweighed by the following disadvantages:

"(a) In the case of auto-inoculations we operate with living cultures. The activated lymph stream may accordingly carry into the bloodstream not only bacterial products but also living bacteria.

"(b) In the case of auto-inoculations we are operating with unmeasured, and therefore often ill-adjusted, doses of bacteria and their products. ...

"(c) Auto-inoculations are not everywhere practicable. ..."

"(d) As compared with immunisation by bacterial vaccines hypodermically inoculated, immunisation by auto-inoculations is, it would seem, always more expensive to the patient - expensive in the sense that the patient obtains for one and the same equivalent of intoxication a smaller yield of bacteriotropic substances.

"(e) Finally: The demands which are made upon the patient's time, and the work which is thrown upon the physician are, in the case where auto-inoculation methods are employed under the control of blood examinations, much more serious than in the case where the patient is inoculated with bacterial vaccines." [p.351]


## SERUM THERAPY


## FOUNDATIONS

"The whole system of serum-therapy, except where it is a question of the neutralization of a poison like diphtheria toxin by the aid of an anti-toxic serum, appears to me to rest upon very insecure foundations."  [(1906) p. 301]

"...The whole body of beliefs rests, I am convinced, upon a foundation of sand."  [p. 302]

## SERUM THERAPY AS VACCINE THERAPY

"I suggest to you that many of the successful results which have been achieved by serum therapy would find their simplest explanation in the assumption that the sera which were exploited operated as bacterial vaccines." [p.311]

Wright illustrates some of the major inconsistencies of the concept of serum therapy with a discussion of the reportedly successful experience of M. Chantemesse in the case of typhoid fever, and Wright's own personal experience with an anti-Malta fever serum from the Army Medical School, Netley.  In both instances there was immediate exacerbation of symptoms, lasting from 3-5 days, followed by improvement, a pattern which is logically explained by the continued presence in the serum of toxic elements which on reinjection cause the serum to act as a bacterial vaccine.

Moreover, Chantemesse had advocated very small doses, reduced proportionally with the severity of symptoms, and if necessary reinoculation is undertaken only after passage of several days (e.g. 16-21).  Of this, Wright says "it becomes clear as noonday that the scheme of dosage employed is the exact reverse of that which would be apposite if we were dealing with a true 'antiserum' ... . Rather does one, where a true antiserum is to hand, give in each case ... large doses of serum.  Again, in the more serious cases one ... gives larger and larger doses [and] one does not allow a long interval to elapse before reinoculation." [312-314]


## PROBLEMS WITH SERUM THERAPY

(1) omits investigation of blood and

(2) assumes: (a) animal (horse) that supplies serum had responded with immunizating reaction, (b) that this would work in man, and (c) that "very high dilution in which the serum comes into application" will exert a therapeutic effect.

"Let it be noted that where vaccine-therapy is the form of therapeutic immunisation which is employed, the antibacterial substances which are obtained are native to the patient's organism; further, that the total yield of these substances can be brought to bear on the infection in the concentration in which they are available in the blood." (Of course, the easiest way to assure this is to use the blood itself as vaccine, ergo autohemotherapy, but Wright didn't use it). [348]


## MISCELLANEOUS

## ANTIBIOTICS

"it is now all but universally recognized that it is futile to attempt to check bacterial growth in the interior of the organism by antiseptics which have - as our present antibiotics have - a greater affinity for the constituent elements of the body than they have for any bacteria [20N4, 319].

## COAGULATION AND IMMUNITY

"alterations in the anti-bacterial power of the blood" are associated with a "diminution in the coagulability of the blood".

## OPSONINS

"We have here conclusive proof that the blood fluids modify the bacteria in a manner which renders them a ready prey to the phagocytes.

"We may speak of this as an 'opsonic' effect (opsono - I cater for; I prepare victuals for), and we may employ the term 'opsonins' to designate the elements in the blood fluids which produce this effect." [(1903) p. 83]

Wright's method involved the mixing and incubation of bacteria along with washed corpuscles, adding blood serum, and comparing individual rates of uptake of bacteria with rates for "normal" serum. The resultant relative rate comprises the opsonic index for an individual at a given point in time, and is used as a definitive guide for the administering or withholding of vaccine.

For details the reader is kindly referred to the original [20N4].

## PROGNOSIS, WHEN SEAT OF INFECTION BECOMES HOT/RED:

Regarding "prognosis and therapeutics of local bacterial infections", ..."The prognosis will ... be 'pro tonto' good whenever the seat of infection becomes hot. For this local rise of temperature and the bright red colouration will be indicative of an increased afflux of arterial blood and of a correspondingly increased lymph flow." [(1899) p. 41]

## PHAGOCYTIC POWER OF BLOOD, OVER TIME/IN AIR

"Even after a lapse of 3 days .... the phagocytic power has not declined to less than one-half or one-third of that of the blood freshly drawn. We have found no indication of a variation within the space of a few hours." [p. 79]

Wright also demonstrated that the phagocytic power of the blood was not diminished by exposure to the air.

## TREATMENT BY THE EXTIRPATION OF THE OBTRUSIVE FOCUS OF

INFECTION

Wright discusses advantages of extirpation in cases of extreme live-endangering infection, where all infecting bacteria can be removed without danger, or where extirpation removes a useless organ which is specifically subject to infection, but emphasizes "assuredly these are not the conditions under which the majority of scraping and extirpating operations are undertaken." [321-2]

Wright here does not specifically refer to oral foci; however it is noted that his reference to removal of "a useless organ which is specifically subject to infection" invites consideration of infected tonsils and teeth.


ON WRIGHT: OHLMACHER; ALLEN; ROBERTSON; AND BEYOND


OHLMACHER (1907)

WRIGHT'S MODESTY: In 1907 Ohlmacher praised recent (4-5 years') vaccine-therapy work of Wright, as "an accomplishment of far-reaching humanitarian importance" which had not received deserved "immediate and extensive proclamation throughout civilized world." largely due to "the principal investigator's natural modesty. ...


WRIGHT'S METHOD: SMALL DOSE, LONG INTERVAL BETWEEN INOCULATIONS

"Compared with all similar essays in the direction of artificial bacterial inoculations two features of Wright's methods are prominent - the comparatively small dose and the long interval between inoculations. ...

AFTER VACCINE: NEGATIVE PHASE, THEN POSITIVE PHASE OF 5-7 DAYS

"... following the events subsequent to the introduction of a bacterial vaccine ... [is a] negative phase [-] the constitutional depression and aggravation of the local lesion [and then a] positive phase [-] the improved general tone and healing in the local lesion" which generally lasts 5-7 days.

OPSONIC THERAPY RULE: RE-INOCULATE AS POSITIVE PHASE FADES

"An imperative rule in opsonic therapy is not to reinoculate during the negative phase, and the time of election for a new treatment is just after the positive phase begins to fade. ...

"The vaccines are 'corresponding' or, better still, they are autogenous, that is, prepared from the patient's own lesion."

Ohlmacher cites successful applications in a range of diseases, from acne to gonorrheal rheumatism, staphylococcus infections to pneumococcus emphysema.


ALLEN (1908) [RW, <u>Vaccine Therapy and Opsonic Method of Treatment</u>]:

"To Wright ... is due the entire credit of originating the idea

of estimating the changes in the opsonic content of the blood as
guidance in the therapeutic use of bacterial vaccines.  ... to
the genesis of a new scientific system of medicine the impulse
has now been given ...   "The surgeon will triumph where now he
fails, and, armed with additional power, he will not fear the
inroads of bacterial invasion."


   ROBERTSON (1916)  Robertson notes that while immunity to
disease by previous sufferers had been known for nearly 3000
years, it was Salmon and Smith in 1886 who first demonstrated
that immunity could be produced with heat-killed microorganisms,
or bacterial filtrates, and not only with living organisms.

   "To Wright we owe the present use of bacterins.  He originally
suggested the use of killed microorganisms as a therapeutic
measure, especially in chronic affections.  This was in 1904.  He
further suggested the advisability of employing autogenous
strains. ... The basic fact ... is that the same organism which
begets the infection, brings about the cure when recovery
occurs." [16H6]


   AUTOSENSITIZED VACCINES: AUTOBLOOD & AUTOVACCINE COMBINED
(incorporating "autoserobacterins", "autoserovaccine")
   Auto-sensitized vaccines, vaccines comprised of a combination
of autoblood and autogenous vaccine, seemingly offer the
advantage of "covering all bases" so to speak, and also defy a
simple "active" vs. "passive" characterization.  On one hand, if
a vaccine happens to be inadvertently comprised of the wrong
organism or phase, serum or blood with which it is merged may
contain the proper antigen anyway.  And where the correct
pathogen is incorporated into a therapeutic vaccine, allowing for
increased control over dosage, merger with autologous serum or
blood might help inactivate the pathogen in a natural manner.


   C.H. Pierce [15N3, 416], in a 1916 article on "the practical
value of autogenous vaccine-therapy referred to the then-recent
work of "Kreuscher, of the Murphy staff" on auto-sensitized
vaccines:

   "By using blood serum of the patients in culturing the
organisms, and later more inactivated serum for the menstruum of
the vaccine, the dose in units may be increased from millions to
billions without reaction and with much greater efficiency than
the straight vaccine. ... It is the perfection of the
vaccinetherapy, such as we hardly hoped for, and yet is hardly
practicable in the office of the general practitioner.  The
technic is somewhat laborious, and the waiting hours, 158 in all,
make the use of the autosensitized product out of the question in
the severe acute conditions ... ."
   While Pierce omits reference to Sir A.E. Wright, the originator

of the field of autogenous vaccine therapy, he acknowledges two
of his "students", who shall receive particular attention in this
writer's work - Charles H. Duncan and Edward C. Rosenow.

Duncan is acknowledged for having usefully augmented the
original work of Gilbert on serotherapy, in the case of purulent
serous fluid.  Duncan's work is discussed in detail below in
Chapter 6: AUTOTHERAPY.

Rosenow is lavishly praised for having "reversed the opinions
of the highest medical authority of the world and thrown to earth
the false theories of older medicine".  Indeed he has, and no one
seems to be paying attention [see *REFERENCE MANUAL ROSENOW ET AL*]


Bibliography - Autosensitized vaccines:


-- Bazy, L. and L. Cuvillier, Sensitized autovaccine, PRESSE
MÉD. 26:219, April 25 '18; ab. JAMA 70: 1898, June 15, '18
-- Cecil, R.L., Sensitized vaccine in prophylaxis and
treatment of infections, Am. J. M. Sc. 155: 781, June 1918
-- Dumke, E.R., "Vaccine and serum therapy", N. W. Medicine
XV(5):168-171, May 1916.
-- Golovine, S., autobacteriotherapy; attempt at replacing
vaccine therapy by method better suited to use in colonial
medicine, Presse med. 43:579-581, April 10, '35
-- Kreucher, P.H., Auto-sensitized autogenous vaccines.
(Preliminary report.)  SURG. CLIN., CHICAGO, 1914, iii,
1119-1122.
-- Lopes Ferreira, Autogenous vaccine in association with serum
and sulfonamide, GAC. MED. MEXICO, 1943, 73:41-3 [1076 cd]
-- Mulford, H. K.. Company, report from, Serobacterins
(sensitized bacterial vaccines), CHINA M. J. 35: 131, March 1921
Fairbanks Barbarosa, J., Vaccinotherapy and serotherapy in
otorhinolaryngology, REV. BRASIL. OTORINOLAR., 1943, 11: 215-243.
-- Vallet, G., "Vaccinothérapie par les autovaccins
auto-sensibilisés." COMPT. REND. SOC. DE BIOL., Par., lxxxiv
(1921), 5-7.
-- Wohl, M.G., Autosensitized vaccines.  MED. REC., N.Y., 1916,
lxxxix, 770-772.
-- Wohl, autoserobacterins in, AM. J. M. SC. 152: 262, Aug. '16

Chapter 6: AUTOTHERAPY

## ORIGIN OF AUTOVAMPIRISM

Considering that the classical tradition of autohemotherapy, as based on and derived from Ravaut, predominantly involves either intramuscular or subcutaneous injections, one might be tempted to define classical autohemotherapy as "extravascular" (in contrast to "intravascular" or "intravenous"); except that classical autohemotherapy does not appear to have utilized, let alone embraced, the concept of "oral" administration of autologous blood.

However, if at least some of autohemotherapy's reported beneficial action is attributable to its function as an autologous vaccine, it may be noted that in the case of "vaccine", "oral" administration is by definition included. (Moseby's Medical Dict.)  [Furthermore, it is noted that Dr. Rosenow, who specifically came to refer to "intramuscular" and "subcutaneous" somewhat interchangeably - as either/or, was also associated with oral vaccine-development in the case of influenza and colds.  See *REFERENCE MANUAL ROSENOW ET AL*]

So if autohemotherapy is really a form of vaccine, the question might logically be raised as to why not include "oral" application within autohemotherapy's scope?  Call it "AUTOVAMPIRISM".  And employ it for any disease where it is known that the causative organism disseminates through the bloodstream.  Now be a good, that is, well, person and DRINK YOUR BLOOD.

Perhaps a novel concept, but not a new one.  In the early 20th century Charles H. Duncan seems to have prescribed a form of at-least-occasional autovampirism when he discussed the proven-beneficial practice of dog-catchers sucking on their wounds.  Similarly, Duncan's prescribing oral autotherapy in cases involving a bleeding wound also must be viewed as having comprised to some extent oral autohemotherapy - or AUTOVAMPIRISM:  Duncan had his patients sucking on the soiled bandages of their festering wounds. [15E7, p. 1001]  As with classical autohemotherapy, a mixture of blood and causative organism are introduced to a tissue-medium in which the organism cannot survive; although of course in the case of a wound the organism is being taken at its point of entry, whereas with classical autohemotherapy it is taken downstream from "unknown" sources (very often oral foci). [see *REFERENCE MANUAL ROSENOW ET AL*]

Of course, as Duncan points out, the dogs themselves knew this long before he did; any animal that licks his bleeding wound is to some extent performing autovampirism.

Prophylaxis (disease prevention) through the use of oral vaccine is particularly well known in modern times from our experience with poliomyelitis.  Therapeutical oral vaccines are also employed in modern times, as is seen in the case of oral "antigen" currently being utilized in the case of arthritis, encephalomyelitis and uveitis [Marx J, in Science 252, 27-8 (Apr. 5, 1991)].  This current work is based on the finding that such therapy can suppress disease conditions in laboratory animals.

So once again, if autohemotherapy is really a form of autogenous vaccine-therapy, the process of reinjecting freshly-drawn autoblood might be simplified:  DRINK YOUR BLOOD.

## YING-YANG DILEMNA OF ORAL AUTOTHERAPY

Lick a wound and it gets better.  Oral autotherapy.  As discussed by Duncan and others, it seems to work, but why?  Is it due to a vaccine principle, i.e., organisms introduced to tissues where antibodies are formed?  Of can we credit the antibacterial properties of saliva?  Articles written long after Duncan's time suggest elements of both may be involved.  For example:

### Oral autotherapy as active immunization:

ORAL AUTOTHERAPY MS ARTHRITIS ENCEPHALOMYELITIS UVEITIS-Marx 91

Marx J, in Science 252, 27-8 (Apr. 5, 1991) discussed the testing of "oral antigen therapy" for so-called "autoimmune" diseases, based on the finding that such therapy can suppress disease conditions in laboratory animals with experimental allergic encephalomyelitis, arthritis, and uveitis.  The very existence of "protein antigens that trigger the abnormal immune reactions" might be viewed as a contemporary confirmation of Rosenow's demonstration of a bacterial cause for these diseases (see *REFERENCE MANUAL ROSENOW ET AL*), while the oral feeding of these antigens to sufferers clearly resembles Duncan's oral autotherapy methods of 70-80 years ago, as discussed below.

### ORAL AUTOTHERAPY FOR DOGBITES, IN THE TALMUD - Boetcher 1964

Boetcher, 1964, p. 67, notes a "remarkable therapeutic measure from the Talmud consisted of the remedies that were prescribed against rabies.  People who were bitten by mad dogs were advised to eat the dog's own liver.  This advice merely repeats what was well known to the doctors of antiquity, which is still practiced today among primitive people."

Boetcher proposed that "The success of this form of treatment obviously is connected with the liver's function as an organ producing immune bodies.  The antibodies that have been developed within the sick animal are employed to help the human patient."

It seems at least as logical to propose that the causative organism, as captured and somewhat attenuated in the liver of the dog, comprises an oral therapeutic vaccine for the dog-bite-victim, stimulating that person's production of antibodies to counteract the rabies infection.  Presumably this same mechanism would be operative in the case of Duncan's discussions of how New

York City dogcatchers avoid rabies (by licking their dogbites) and Duncan's and French's recommendations that poison ivy infections be treated by eating leaves from the offending plant (below).


LAB ANIMALS INTUITIVELY PRACTICE AUTOTHERAPY - ROSENOW 1953

Dr. Rosenow's half-century of working with laboratory animals afforded these fascinating observations: "The mice that become ill are not allowed in the huddle or they voluntarily remain apart and are not molested while life lasts. But after death, the well mice if cannibalistic almost invariably eat the diseased organ, such as pneumonic lungs produced by cerebral and/or nasal inoculation of 'pneumotropic' streptococcus or virus of influenza. In sharp contrast if death was due to encephalitis following inoculation of the streptococcus or virus of encephalitis, they remove the skull and eat the diseased brain."

Rosenow, E.C., Streptococci in etiology of diverse diseases, including diseases of nervous system, J. Nerv. and Ment. Dis. 117: 415-428, May 1953 [53R1]. (See also *REFERENCE MANUAL ROSENOW ET AL*).


Oral autotherapy and antimicrobial substances:

"LINGUAL ANTIMICROBIAL PEPTIDE": AUTOTHERAPY? Schonwetter 1995

Schonwetter et. al. (1995) note that "Antimicrobial peptides have ... been detected in barrier epithelial cells of several mammalian species, including mice, cows, and humans. ... Although abrasions to the surface of the tongue occur often, invasive infections in a normal host are rare, remain localized, and heal rapidly." The authors assert that naturally occurring antimicrobial and antifungal substances markedly increase around tongue lesions, and conclude that "elucidation of the regulatory mechanisms responsible for stimulation of [these substances] ... may have therapeutic applications in enhancing mucosal immunity."

The authors suggest that a "lingual antimicrobial peptide ... is a key component of the mucosal [tongue] response to injury".

If such a substance is activated against invading microbes at the site of an injury to the tongue, is it not also possible or even necessary that this might also occur to some extent in the case of invading microbes at the site of an injury elsewhere on the body? For example, in the case of licking a wound. The very existence of antimicrobial, "naturally-occurring" epithelial excretions supports the notion that the therapeutical action of licking one's own wounds, etc., may be attributed at least in part to such excretions, over and above that attributable to oral "vaccination".

[Schonwetter, BS, ED Stolzenberg, and MA Zasloff, "Epithelial Antibiotics Induced at Sites of Inflammation", Science 267, 1645-8]

AUTOTHERAPY FOUNDER
- CHARLES DUNCAN


AMERICAN MEDICAL DIRECTORY, 8TH ED. 1923, AMA, Chicago: Duncan, Chas. H. (H) N.Y.9,'05; l'07; F7 - 2612 Broadway; 11-12, 6-7

POLKS MEDICAL REGISTER AND DIRECTORY, Polk, Detroit, 1917:

Duncan, Charles H, M D, New York Homo Med Coll, NY City, 1905; Formerly Attending Surgeon Volunteer Hosp; Mem Co, State and Natl Homo Med Socs; Discoverer and Founder of Autotherapy; Specialty Rheumatism and Lung Infections; Hours 11 a m - 12 m and 6-7 p m; Tel 6432 Riverside; 2612 Broadway


AUTOTHERAPY: CONCEPTUAL, PHILOSOPHICAL, POLITICAL - DUNCAN

AUTOTHERAPY AS UNIFYING PRINCIPLE OF MEDICINE - DUNCAN 12E1

In 1911 Duncan endorsed a comprehensive autogenous approach, acknowledging the precedents of both Gilbert of Geneva and Wright.  Duncan declared the field of "autotherapy" to encompass "any method or system of medication that employs all of the autogenous toxic substance developed during the course of the disease to cure disease". [12E1, p. 481]

"Autotherapy is the keystone in the arch of the great medical superstructure that has been raised by both dominant schools of medicine.  As the keystone fills out the arch, joining the two leaning sides, so auto-therapy joins the two great schools of medicine by strengthening and beautifying each. ...

"Auto-therapy is natural therapy, or as the name implies, self-therapy.  Autotherapy employs nature's weapons in combatting disease; we cannot go behind it."

"... restoring normal equilibrium is the all-important factor in the treatment of disease." [17E2, p. 325]

"The fresh unmodified toxic substances developed during the course of an infection are the substances nature utilizes in autoimmunizing the patient; these are also the substances the physician employs in treating the patient autotherapeutically." [17E2, p. 328]


STATE OF THE MEDICAL PROFESSION - DUNCAN 14H5

In 1914, Duncan offered this commentary on the medical profession:

"In its innumerable adjustments, our therapeutics of the past resemble in many respects the fashion supplement of some modern trade journals.  What is new today is often old tomorrow. Commercialism runs rampant throughout the various ramifications of medicine."

"... Demonstrated results should not be despised nor ignored because they do not seem to coincide with the doctrines or theories of men who may be temporarily in exalted positions, and who assume the rôle of virtuous infallibility. [A prime example of THE an individual is discussed below in "THE VENERABLE MEDICAL TRADITION OF ARROGANCE"]

"... Until we know all possible changes that can transpire in complex organic chemistry and biology, it is becoming that we be more humble and broadminded. Indifference to demonstrated results is an intolerable attitude." [14H5, p. 411]


NATURE OFTEN CURES WHERE SCIENCE UTTERLY FAILS - DUNCAN 17E2

In 1916 Duncan suggested to critics of his methods: "The criticism of the autotherapeutic remedy as unscientific is unjustifiable unless we desire to be scientific in preference to being effective in the treatment of our patients. Nature often cures where science utterly fails." 17E2, 332


AUTOTHERAPY THEORY


AUTOTHERAPEUTIC INJECTIONS & LEUCOCYTES - DUNCAN 14E5

"... When the patient is injected into comparatively healthy tissues with the unmodified filtered toxins from the focus of his infections, leucocytes are attracted to the point of injection in large numbers, and they are stimulated by the development of specific antibodies to perform a very specific function - to destroy that microorganism only to whose toxins they responded, the microorganism from which the patient suffers. There being none of these microorganisms at the point of injection, the specific leukocytes pass on into the circulation to the focus of infection, where they combat or route out that microorganism from the soil of its recent adoption." [14H5, p. 409]


BLOOD AS CONTAINING DISEASE AGENT - DUNCAN 13E1, 1218

MORE ANTIBODIES DEVELOP IN SUBCUTANEOUS - DUNCAN 13E1, 1218

AUTOTHERAPY: PHYSICIAN HELPS NATURE PERFORMS CURE - DUNCAN 13E1

"Again, in serious infectious disease, when autoinoculation takes place by the natural processes within the body, we believe it is because the toxines of the disease escape into the blood stream. (Duncan's italics) Now experience in the laboratory in the preparation of antitoxines shows conclusively that more antibodies are developed when the toxines are placed in the subcutaneous tissues rather than in the blood stream; for these reasons, autotherapy, or the physician's method of assisting Nature to perform a cure, has distinct advantage over the natural processes of cure."

## BACTERIAL ORIGIN OF DISEASE   DUNCAN 12E1

Duncan offered that "The opinion is fast gaining ground that practically all diseases will eventually be proved to be of a bacterial origin..." [12E1, 475]  Such an origin establishes the propriety of vaccine-therapy.

## STOCK VACCINE IS UNSCIENTIFIC, SHOTGUN THERAPY - DUNCAN 14E4

Duncan asserted that "Administration of stock, conglomerate vaccine is shot-gun therapy, pure and simple, and is wholly unscientific." [14E4,552]

## HAZARDS OF MANIPULATION OF VACCINE - DUNCAN 12E1

"When any of the toxic substances developed during the course of the disease, as the bacterial toxic substances, for example, have been changed (as by heat or when grown in culture media outside of the body tissues, or by time) their therapeutic value is lessened in proportion to the change that takes place in them by the various processes which they undergo. ..."

"The fresh nascent toxic substance of the bacteria grown in the patient's own tissues is one of the substances nature employs in auto-inoculation or when a natural cure is made." [12E1, p. 473-8]

## WRIGHT'S VACCINES CRITICIZED AS NOT AUTOGENOUS - DUNCAN 17E2

"... the autogenous vaccine prepared according to Wright contains only one [of several possibly-involved] toxins, and it is of altered or lowered therapeutic value; furthermore, it may not be the right one or we may not be able to grow it outside the body tissues." [14H4, 146]

Duncan points out that such vaccines "do not include tissue toxines that correspond to each bacterial toxine ... nor do they include the toxines of the other microorganisms that frequently complicate severe infections." [13E4, 1221]

Duncan asserts that Wright's autogenous vaccine "strictly speaking is not autogenous, for Wright's vaccines are not the parent organism developed within the patient's body, but they are their grandchildren which have been developed on agar-agar, Bouillon, animal's blood, etc.  The autotherapeutic remedy is the only strictly autogenous therapeutic preparation we have at our command in fighting disease and death.

"Wright's partial toxin complex is distinctly modified by every step in the laboratory through which it passes.  If his vaccines cure, such cure is not because of the laboratory manipulation, but in spite of it."

"The superiority of the autotherapeutic remedy over Wright's old and faulty vaccine is at once apparent and not open to controversy." [17E2, p. 331-2]

DUNCAN - TECHNIQUE: GENERAL RULE; COROLLARY; VARIATIONS

GENERAL RULE: HYPODERMIC INJECTION, TOXIC PRODUCT DUNCAN 12E1

"In intra-alimentary and intra-pulmonary diseases if the toxic product of the disease be placed in healthy tissues outside of these systems, it will tend to develop specific antibodies." In these cases, Duncan recommended filtering the discharge of the disease through a Berkefield filter and injecting it hypodermically. Thus he claimed to have successfully treated several advanced cases of phthisis pulmonalis "by hypodermically injecting their filtered sputa." [12E1, 473; see "DISEASES, ACUTE BRONCHITIS below, for specific details.]


"COROLLARY": ORAL ADMINISTRATION, TOXIC PRODUCT - DUNCAN 12E1

Duncan asserted that "In extra-alimentary and extra-pulmonary diseases, if the toxic product is placed in the mouth it will tend to develop specific antibodies" (even including such conditions as snakebite and rabies). ... "There can be no doubt that Lux, a homeopathic horse doctor, a pioneer of this method of treating disease, made a big reputation about 1822 by curing many flocks of sheep and many shepherds by giving autogenous virus by the mouth [diluted product of a sheep that had come down with the disease]. But Lux failed to recognize the great importance of the autogenous product, and drifted to using stock solution of the heterologous product. For this reason he failed, and his system of medication passed into history ..." [12E1, p. 473]


ARTIFICIAL BLISTER/BURN DUNCAN 12E1

LOCUS MINORIS RESISTENTIAE

In 1911, Duncan built on a method Wright had used to obtain sufficient quantities of a causative organism in order to produce a therapeutic vaccine. Duncan quotes Wright (<u>Proc. Royal Soc. Med.</u>), discussing his action in 3 desperate cases of Pruritus Ani:

"In each case I have found that a platinum loop applied to the seat of irritation brought away quite astonishing numbers of microbes, invariably staphylococcus, pseudo-diphtheria and occasionally tetragenus, and in each of these cases life has been rendered comfortable, or, at any rate, quite tolerable, by the use of proper vaccines."

Duncan advocated that "an artificial point of least resistance may be made by means of a burn or blister" to which will be attracted the causative microorganism which might then be used for autoinoculation purposes. (Duncan claimed this had never previously been attempted, arguing for doing so on logical grounds; he was apparently unaware that Jez had done this as early as 1901, in order to obtain fluid for autoinoculation.)

"Healthy tissues are usually able to resist an invasion of pathological microorganisms, but a lowered vitality coupled with exhaustion or fatigue, lack of proper nourishment, etc., are etiological factors that are recognized as predisposing to a successful invasion of pathological bacteria.  Especially are pathological microorganisms likely to find lodgment in the tissues under these conditions, if there is a point of least resistance in the body.  Weak lungs are predisposed to pulmonary infections, etc.  The locus minoris resistentiae, or point of least resistance, about which so much has been recently written, is pretty well understood.  The experiments of Baumgarten are well known.  He crushed the testicle of healthy rabbits and then injected tubercular bacilli in the jugular vein.  The tubercular bacilli were invariably demonstrated in the testicles.  It was the point of least resistance and the bacteria were attracted to it." [12E1,475-6]

### AUTOBLOOD AS CULTURE MEDIUM, MENSTRUUM - DUNCAN 12E1

Duncan [1911 (12E1] discussed the use of autoblood or autoserum as "the ideal culture medium for autogenous vaccination"; he also suggested that after obtaining an offending organism by "filtering the discharge of the disease ... if a menstruum is needed to dilute it, use the patient's own blood."

### SUBCUTANEOUS AUTOHEMOTHERAPY, AFTER GILBERT - DUNCAN 17E2

In 1916 [17E2, p. 331], without reference to Ravaut or the by-now blossoming field of autohemotherapy, described a method of autohemotherapy which employed a technique similar to the autoserotherapy method that Gilbert had employed with serous fluid in pleural effusion:  "... the writer has cured infections by simply puncturing a vein with a hypodermic needle, drawing the blood into the syringe that already contains sterile physiological salt solution, and then withdrawing the needle till it is just beneath the skin and inject the contents there."

Duncan noted the probable connection between this procedure and some accidental cures:  "... the probable efficacy of a trauma that results in extravasation of blood into the subdermal tissues in a patient suffering with some chronic infection is apparent."

In a succeeding article [NYMJ, Sept. 9, 1916], Duncan noted that in systemic infections "or those in which the pus pocket is not accessible, cure will result from the subcutaneous injection of small doses of the patient's own blood diluted with physiological salt solution."

### AUTOTHERAPY UNDERLIES MANY PRACTICES - DUNCAN, VARIOUS SOURCES
### BIER'S HYPEREMIA TREATMENT - DUNCAN 13E4
### HOT FOMENTATIONS AS AUTOTHERAPY - DUNCAN 13E4, 1218

"We are all autotherapists, humiliating as it may be to acknowledge it; it is this natural autotherapy that is exploited by the time honored custom of applying hot fomentations, Bier's hyperemia treatment, etc.

ELECTRO-STIMULATION AS AUTOTHERAPY - DUNCAN 17E2

IRRADIATION THERAPY AS AUTOTHERAPY - DUNCAN 17E2

Duncan [17E2, p. 329] was first led to suspect that electrostimulation by high-frequency current might actually comprise autoinoculation, by the similarity in reported cures of chronic catarrhal conditions to those cures he had obtained with autotherapy. Subsequently he found that benefits attributed to Roentgen irradiation in cases of psoriasis, lupus and eczema were also similar to those of autotherapy. "What more natural than to suppose that the patient himself furnishes the necessary unmodified toxin complex under the stimulus of Roentgen irradiation!"

Additionally, Duncan discussed cures in 3 cases of acne and one of psoriasis, treated by high-frequency waves, x-rays and/or ultraviolet light, that appeared to constitute evidence of autoinoculative action.

"One of the greatest arguments in favor of the autoinoculation hypothesis is the latent period which follows Roentgen or radium irradiation and which precedes the amelioration. The ominous pause, to my mind, is eloquent; and indicates that the resources of the patient are gathered to react to the toxins; it appeals to everyone familiar with reactive medication as the negative phase preceding the positive phase. The reaction is not merely a physical or chemical one, but a biological action in which the energy of the reaction may exceed the energy of the attack."[17E2, p. 330]

INJECTION OF SEA PLASMA, ETC. AS AUTOTHERAPY - DUNCAN 17E2

Duncan argues that the subdermal injection of large quantities of fluid, such as isotonic quantities of fluid, such as isotonic solutions of sea plasma, sterile water, etc., "must necessarily rupture some minute blood vessels, and therefore produce some extravasation into the tissues. The toxins would now be diluted with a physiological salt solution within the loose cellular subdermal tissues where we know the greatest amount of antibodies are developed. With this explanation it is apparent that this [sea plasma] process is nothing more or less than an autotherapeutic procedure." [17E2, p. 330-1]

SCARIFICATION AS AUTOTHERAPY - DUNCAN 12E1

"Then there remains vaccination with the toxic product of the disease by scarification, or placing the crude discharge on a healthy raw surface. ... This practically is auto-inoculation. ... It is the way nature cures the tissues." [12E1, 479-80]

Duncan adds this cautionary note: "No one would think of putting the crude chancroidal virus on a raw surface or give it by the mouth. A skilled appreciation of the nature of the infection should always be the guide in administering autogenous products."


URINE, THERAPEUTIC USE   DUNCAN 14E3

Occasionally when discussing autogenous therapy methods, the subject of therapeutic use of urine has come up. As early as 1913 [14E3] Charles Duncan discussed the use of urine as a form of "autotherapy". While this writer has not specifically sought out reference to such experiences, we note two references in the autohemotherapy literature regarding the effects of autohemotherapy on the urine and on the blood: 35B3 (chlorides in urine), 35B4 (diastases in).

The therapeutical use of autogenous urine, whether administered orally (which the writer has heard of) or inoculated (as Duncan did), could be logically explained something like this:  Although a patient may not mount a sufficiently adequate response to gain the upper hand against a given disease, in any case some of the invaders may be expelled from the patient via the urine in some form, either intact, attenuated or destroyed. When returned to the patient in a manner which does not allow for the survival or rejuvenation of the invaders, the patient's physiology is given an augmented opportunity to identify the invader and then mount a system-wide defensive response against it, hopefully rooting out its cousins which otherwise would continue unchecked to wreak havoc or worse. In other words, drinking one's own urine may be tantamount to an oral therapeutical vaccine.

For the record, perhaps when this writer reads more of the benefits and successes of drinking one's own urine, he may do so. But as of now, it's not on the menu. Nonetheless, it does make sense, and certainly involves a far-less complicated procedure than even the relatively low-tech procedure of drawing one's blood and reinjecting it intramuscularly.


SOME SPECIFIC DISEASE DISCUSSIONS - DUNCAN, VARIOUS SOURCES

ACNE, BOILS, INFECTIONS, OZENA, RHEUMATISM, TONSILLITIS - 14H5

Dr. Rierson, Dixon, CA:  "I have treated more than 110 cases with autotherapy; boils, rheumatism, infections, etc. [including ozena, tonsillitis, acne] with results that have been a revelation to me and to my patients. ... The writer has had no failures when this infection [tonsillitis] is treated early, and he has treated many."


BRONCHITIS, FURNACLES, GONORRHEA, IRITIS, RHINITIS, TB - Rose in

Duncan 14H5

Henry W. Rose, M.D.:  "During the past year I have cured many infections with autotherapy that have apparently resisted all other methods known to me.  This includes many cases of chronic rhinitis with sinus involvement, acute and chronic bronchitis, acute and chronic conditions in the female pelvis, acute gonorrhea in the male, furnacles and pulmonary tuberculosis.

"One case that I diagnosed as acute iritis responded quickly with this treatment. ... We have a weapon in autotherapy the power of which we have little dreamed."  [17E2, p. 333]


BRONCHITIS; TREATED WITH FILTERED SPUTUM - DUNCAN 13E4

Duncan claimed that acute bronchitis could be cured in 24 hours, and chronic bronchitis often in 2 weeks, with hypodermic injections of filtered sputum:  "The following technique was closely followed:  Sputum, 1 dram; distilled water, 1 ounce.  Mix in a 2-ounce bottle, shake well, and allow to stand for 24 hours.  Filter through as Berkefield filter.  Inject 20 minims of the bacteria-free filtrate into the loose cellular tissues over the biceps muscle.  Give no further dose until the patient ceases to improve under the preceding dose.  In chronic cases this will often be from the 3rd to the 5th day ...."  [14H5; from NYMJ, 1912 (13E4)]


CANCER, PUS-PRODUCING ORGANISMS - DUNCAN 12E1

"It is believed by many that the pain incident to cancer is caused by the action of pus-producing micro-organisms, and we know when these organisms are given by the mouth, in extra-alimentary and extra-pulmonary diseases, specific antibodies are developed in the serum."  12E1,475


CEREBROSPINAL MENINGITIS, I.M. SPINAL FLUID - HOWARD IN DUNCAN 16H2

In an article published in August [NYMJ, Aug. 19, 1916; 16H2], Duncan discussed a method of treatment that had been used successfully since 1910 in cerebrospinal meningitis, involving "tapping the spinal canal and injecting intramuscularly the spinal fluid thus obtained."  He related a description of a case reported in 1911 by a Dr. C. C. Howard of N. Y., at the Metropolitan Hospital, in which the patient "was cyanosed, his pulse was erratic, he was bathed in a cold sweat, rigidity was marked, and there was a loss of all reflexes.  The case approached so near death, that [Dr. Howard] decided to see what results would follow injection of the spinal fluid under the skin.  He made a spinal puncture, drew off quite a large amount of fluid, and injected some of it into the muscles of the back.  In the course of 3 or 4 hours the temperature fell from 105 degrees to 102 F.  Four injections were given in a similar

manner.   the man had absolutely nothing remaining as a result of
the attack and was perfectly well when he left the hospital."


## CHOLECYSTITIS, APPENDICITIS; FILTERED SPUTUM - DUNCAN 13E8

In 1914 Duncan recalled he had "reported a case of colecystitis
cured, and the operation aborted, by injecting the filtrate of
sputum hypodermically."  Encouraged by his success in this and
other similar cases, he employed the filtrate of sputum
successfully in two cases of acute appendicitis, after operation
had been refused, avoiding an operation in each instance.  "In
all of these cases the pain ceased in from 6 to 12 hours, as if
by the action of morphine." [13E8, per 14H5]


## CHRONIC BRONCHITIS - TONEY IN DUNCAN 14H5

Dr. L.C. Toney, in his own personal case of chronic bronchitis:
"I can truly say it has been magical."


## CHRONIC CATARRHAL OTITIS MEDIA - FARMER IN DUNCAN 14H5

Dr. C.E. Farmer, Sacramento, Ca, in chronic catarrhal otitis
media: "I consider this case most remarkable, as nearly
everything known to medical science had been done for the patient
previously without relief."


## DOG BITE, ETC., ORAL AUTOTHERAPY - DUNCAN 12E1, p. 474-8

To further substantiate his position concerning oral
autotherapy, Duncan visited the dog-catching station at East
102nd St. and East River in New York City:  "Seven professional
dog catchers and their drivers were interviewed.  They each told
the writer that they had been bitten by hundreds of dogs and many
times by mad dogs; that they do not fear sepsis or hydrophobia or
tetanus; that they are conscientious in sucking their wounds
immediately upon being bitten by any dog."

"The dog, in licking and curing his wounds .. cleanses the
wound, but by this very act he gives himself a dose of autogenous
vaccine."

Duncan discusses his personal successful experience with
placing autogenous toxic substances, pus or dilutions in the
mouth, in cases of infected wounds; "hundreds of cases of
sepsis"; acne vulgaris (10 cases); styes; furuncles; boils;
abscesses; adenitis, when due to bacteria; puerperal septicemia;
and leucorrhea.

Duncan argues that this manner of treatment might be logically
extended to a number of other conditions, on the assumption that
they may be traced to bacterial infection, including burns, x-ray
dermatitis, urinary calculus, bacteriuria, pruritus ani,
diabetes, rheumatism and even cancer.

"The writer is informed that nearly all undertakers and

embalmers suck a wound when injured in working around the
cadaver.  In the medical school in Philadelphia we were told by
Dr. Weaver to suck any accidental wound we might receive in
dissecting ... " [12E1, 474-8]


### INFLUENZA - BORROWS IN DUNCAN 14H5

Dr. F.B. Borrows, Plainwell, Mich., reporting on a case of
acute influenza: "I have been using autotherapy in my practice
now for over a year with great satisfaction; in all kinds of
localized infections, almost invariably with success."


### INFECTED WOUNDS - DUNCAN 15E7

"The prevention of infection by means of autotherapy is so very
simple and dependable, that it is remarkable that it has
heretofore escaped the attention of the profession.

"The patient should be instructed to lick or suck his wounds as
soon as it is received, and every two to four hours afterwards
for several days.  If this is done there will be no more deaths
from infection, for the wound will apparently heal by first
intention.  If for anatomical reasons the wound is inaccessible
to sucking and licking, infection may be aborted by simply
chewing for five minutes twice daily the blood-stained cloth
covering the wound, swallowing the fluid."[15E7, p. 1001]


### INFLUENZA - RUSH IN DUNCAN 14H5

Dr. Warren Rush, Lake City, Fla., as an influenza patient:
"Autotherapy has done for me what apparently no other medication
could do.  It means that my usefulness in life has been
restored."


### MENTAL ILLNESS - DUNCAN 12E1

"Dementia praecox is very generally supposed to be due to toxic
Substances.  Can it be treated successfully by auto-therapeutic
measures?  Surely the comparative hopelessness of this most
pitiful disease warrants at least a fair trial of this extremely
simple therapeutic measure."  [12E1, 479]


### POISON IVY - DUNCAN 16H2

On Sept. 23, 1916, the NYMJ, 608, prefaced a report by Dr. J.
M. French of Milford Mass., with: "...recipients of this oral
prescription are likely to suspect a practical joke and to
imagine themselves with very sore mouths.  The remedy, however,
seems to be in perfect accord with the theory and practice of Dr.
Charles H. Duncan, who will pounce on this case report as a fine
example of his beloved autotherapy."

The French report discussed "remarkable results in the

prevention and cure of rhus poisoning by chewing the young leaves of the plant and swallowing the juice."

Duncan on November 4 (NYMJ, p. 901 - 16H2) commented that chewing a few leaves of a poison ivy plant being cleared away, as a preventive measure, had been the custom of instruction to park workers in Fairmont Park, Philadelphia, and had been adopted in Bronx Park in the Spring of 1916. Duncan described a case as "the worst spectacle of ivy poisoning the writer had ever seen", when a man living in the country "one evening when defecating in the woods was unfortunate enough to select a spot that was covered with poison ivy." He was instructed to chew a leaf of this particular plant, and within 3 days after doing so, was able to return to work as a butler. Duncan went on to briefly describe similar measures in cases of snake and scorpion bites, and bites from mad dogs.


POLIOMYELITIS - DUNCAN 16H2

SWALLOW TO SUMMER AS STRAW TO THE WIND - DUNCAN 16H2

Based on Howard's reported success with meningitis and a number of similar cases reported by Dr. G. F. Laidlaw of New York, Duncan suggested that poliomyelitis, also being a toxic neuritis, might similarly be amenable to treatment with I.M. spinal fluid.

Duncan reported on the only case he had seen, a 2-1/2 year old boy who had taken sick on July 22: "The case was not seen until the 24th. There was vomiting, stupor, and a temperature of 102 degrees F; slept with his eyes open and rolled up. there was marked twitching of the muscles of the legs and arms. On the 25th there was a partial left-sided facial paralysis and partial paralysis of both legs. On the evening of that day the spinal canal was punctured and about 10cc of fluid withdrawn, and one cc injected hypodermically. Within 12 hours the stupor disappeared and the temperature fell to 99 degrees F. He was sent to the hospital where .5 cc injection of spinal fluid was given. At the present writing, Aug. 7th, temperature and pulse are normal."

Of this result, Duncan noted: "While one swallow does not make a summer, neither does one case ordinarily mean anything, still a straw tells the way the wind blows."


RHEUMATISM/ARTHRITIS; BACTERIA IN BLOOD - DUNCAN 12E1

"When the bacteria are in the blood stream (as it is claimed bacteria have been found there in rheumatism), they develop few antibodies, but when injected hypodermically they develop more antibodies. Injecting animals with vaccines in the laboratory to increase the power of the serum in developing antitoxins clearly proves this." [12E1, 473c]


SCORPION BITE - 16H2

Duncan recommended autotherapeutical measures for scorpion

bite, along with snakebite, dog-bite.

## SNAKEBITE - [12E1, p. 474-8]

Duncan raises the question as to whether the efficacy of sucking snakebite, when possible, is also due to the circumstance that this causes an autoinoculation.

## TETANUS AND OTHER TOXIC NEURITIDES - DUNCAN 16H2

Duncan suggested, based on his and others' experiences with cerebrospinal meningitis and poliomyelitis, "that tests be made in treating tetanus and other toxic neuritides, by the autotherapeutic method."

## WOUNDS - DUNCAN 14E4

In 1914 Duncan prescribed that "wounds of the stomach and lungs must be treated by following the general rule ..." [intradermal injection of toxic filtrate], wounds further down in the alimentary tract might be treated by the 'corollary' [orally]: "It appears that some wounds of the ileum and the large intestine may be successfully treated in this manner. In closed wounds or in some puncture wounds ... a small silver wire inserted for three or four days will tend to lead the exudate to the surface without leaving a large opening."

"In the last analysis it appears, that a patient may abort infection by simply chewing his own bloody dressings twice daily."

Dr. E.F. Mills of NYC reported a case of "one of the most severe purulent infections I have ever seen ... Amputation has been performed for a very much less severe condition." Within five days after oral autotherapy was initiated, the case was discharged cured. [14E4, p. 555-563]

## VENERABLE TRADITION OF ARROGANCE

Two weeks following Duncan's discussions of polio in the NYMJ (16H2), on Sept. 2, 1916, the NYMJ reprinted a N.Y.Times letter by S. J. Meltzer of the Rockefeller Institute which was critical of a method of "autoinoculation" which had been employed by L.C. Ager of the Kingston Ave. Hospital, as reported in the Aug. 12 Weekly Bulletin of the Dept. of Health. Meltzer indicated a far greater concern with this official bulletin than with Duncan's Aug. 19 NYMJ article discussing the "same method of treatment", insofar as Meltzer doubted the Duncan article would have much influence with "discerning medical readers". Having thus vented his arrogance Melzer went on to concede "superficially the method appears to be based on a few indisputable scientific premises. It is based on the assumption that during the active stage of the disease the spinal fluid of the patient contains live virus.

This is indeed a fact, as is shown by the work of Flexner and his associates."

Ager's Sept. 16 response outlined his procedure, which bore a striking resemblance to that of Howard and Duncan: "... the treatment consists of drawing off from 15 to 60, 70, or even a larger number of cc of spinal fluid and reinjecting into the muscular tissues from .5 to 2 or 3 cc of fluid ... ." Ager reported cases "where there appeared to be no hope of recovery, and in which consent was freely given by the parents after the method had been explained. ... In a number of instances the treatment was followed by marked improvement, reduction in temperature, and partial return to consciousness."

On Sept. 23 in the same journal, Meltzer expressed his concern over the safety of withdrawing such large amounts of spinal fluid, but allowed that the intramuscular reinjection probably did no harm. (It may be noted that independent of these discussions, A. Sophian had noted on Aug. 19 (NTMJ) that hydrocephalus was often present in acute stages of polio and was the usual cause of respiratory failure, stating as "imperative" the removal of spinal fluid until the pressure falls to normal.)

In considering the outrageous behavior of Meltzer, seemingly more intent on preserving the phony infallibility of the status quo, we are reminded of the comment of McManus 1963, p. 85, "Someone has said that nothing becomes a scientist less than an aura of certainty ...". Perhaps the critical point here is that the likes of Meltzer are in reality businessmen/politicians, and not scientists. The true scientist: is by definition a seeker of truth and objective presenter of the facts; and very rare.


SOME AUTOTHERAPY TESTIMONIALS


RESULTS NO OTHER MEDICATION HAS GIVEN - VERTES IN DUNCAN 14H5

Dr. Alexander Vertes, Louisville, Ky.: "I am using autotherapy when it is applicable to the exclusion of all other medication, because it gives me results that no other medication has ever given."


THE MOST SCIENTIFIC VACCINE EVER USED - FREEMAN IN DUNCAN 14H5

Prof. William H. Freeman: "Dr. Duncan's autogenous toxin complex is the most scientific vaccine ever used in medicine."


AUTOTHERAPY INEXPENSIVE, LOGICAL, SAFE - NYMJ EDITORIAL 1912

In 1912, the NYMJ [Dec. 21, 1912, p. 1289], "AUTOTHERAPY: We have given considerable space to the results and theories of Dr. Charles H. Duncan in this and the previous issues of the JOURNAL, for the theory involved is of fascinating interest. If the heterogenous vaccines are valuable, as many competent therapeutists maintain, it follows logically that the autogenous are equally if not more so.  The necessary equipment lies ready to every practitioner's hand, there is no expense involved, and the procedure does not contraindicate drafts upon the ordinary materia medica .... Not least among the inducements to try this simple method is the apparent freedom from all danger."


DUNCAN USEFULLY AUGMENTS GILBERT - PIERCE 14H6

In 1914 E.A. Pierce discussed how Duncan's work usefully augments that of Gilbert, noting that in the use of Gilbert' method: "Should the fluid prove to be purulent, do not reinject but treat the case surgically, or according to the method of Duncan by filtration and ingestion."


FORMER NAVY SURGEON PRAISES DUNCAN'S METHODS- PARHAM 16E1

A 1915 Duncan article bore the title: "A positive method of curing purulent infection, an appeal to the army surgeon" [15E8]. Without specific reference to this appeal, former Navy Surgeon J.C. Parham exhaustively praised the effectiveness of Duncan's methods:


DISEASED TISSUE AND "OVERDOSAGE":  "Broadly stated, infectious diseases at least are terminated successfully when the organism reacts and produces a sufficiency of opsonins, agglutinins, precipitins, or whatever we may call them, to neutralize the causative agent of the disease. ... Autotherapy uses the end products of disease processes, toxins, to form antibodies with which to neutralize the organisms responsible for the pathologic condition; it means the production of active immunity.  It is by no means clear why the toxins of disease already subjected to absorption by the body tissues originating them should require removal and readministration hypodermically or per orem to produce antibodies as readily as we require for therapeutic uses unless it is that they can not excite antibody production in tissues whose vitality is lowered as they can in healthy tissues; such appears to be the case, or the question of over-dosage may play a part."

METHOD:  "The wound discharge, pus, sputum or urine containing the responsible organisms to the amount of a few minims or cubic centimeters, depending on the amount available, is added to 50cc of sterile water in a sterile container, which is closed and then set aside for from 12 to 24 hours in an incubator at about 99 degrees F.  A warm room serves the purpose as well ... .

"The container should be vigorously agitated 4 or 5 times during the period of waiting.  Upon the completion of the incubation period the contents of the container are passed through a Berkfeld filter of sufficient fineness to prevent the passage of organisms and the resulting filtrate constitutes the finished product. ... the degree of toxicity [of a filtrate is] in direct ratio to the length of time. ...

"The dose also depends on the amount of discharge or pus used in making the filtrate and the condition of the patient."

In the case of carbuncle, "2 cc of the filtrate was administered per hypodermic."

MAGIC:  "There are some types of infection in which autogenous filtrates act almost magically, among these those of the skin being pre-eminent."  Parham provides a synopsis of cases, including carbuncle, furunculosis, cellulitis, lymphadenitis and like infections.

CELLULITIS:  "When no pus is available, as in the case of cellulitis before resolution or pus formation, my method has been to make free incisions and pack with sterile gauze.  The dressing is kept wet with Wright's solution and at the end of 24 hours removed and the stained portion of the gauze clipped off and sterile water added.  With this the filtrate is made."

CREDIT:

"So far as I have been able to ascertain, the entire credit for this method of treatment must be given to Duncan.  The principles enunciated in this article are his almost without exception."

Chapter 7: THEORETICAL CONSIDERATIONS

COAGULATION & IMMUNE SYSTEM:  DEFENSES

Although we may readily presume Dr. Cuyugan was familiar with the field of autohemotherapy, we do not know the precise motivation behind his having put the blood in a culture dish and allowed it to begin to coagulate, swirling it around in order to keep the action even, and reinjecting it before it coagulated.

Aside from the possible influence of the coagulation process, the act of exposing the blood to the air would also expose the organism in the blood to much more oxygen than is found in the circulating blood; presumably the longer the exposure, the more damage to the offending organism.  Moreover, imply reinjecting blood intramuscularly, even without coagulation or exposure to the air, would seemingly deprive the organism of the environment it requires to survive.


With respect to the coagulation process, in accord with the work of Sir Almroth Wright with which Cuyugan was undoubtedly familiar, the coagulating blood might have been theorized to act as "opsonins", or simply be seen as forcing the adhesion of blood fluids to the malaria parasite.  In any case, it would appear that the initiation of the coagulation process would to some extent immobilize the invader.

At the same time, the process of coagulation involves the formation of defensive substances, injection of which (as in Cuyugan's autohemotherapeutic procedure) might in some fashion "passively" augment the body's own "actively"-generated antibodies.  At least that's what "real" antibody is supposed to do.  (It is noted that Dr. Rosenow used artificially-generated autologous antibody (see ROSENOW RECIPES); however, it is not known how the bio-physico-chemical qualities of coagulating autoblood compare with those of Rosenow's antibody.


The relationship between coagulation and the immune systems is of on-going modern interest, e.g., Ferreira and Barcinski 1986 discussed a "mechanism [that] may represent a link between immunoregulatory phenomena and blood coagulation."

L. Poller addressed the subject in conjunction with "disseminated intravascular coagulation" [L. Poller, <u>Recent Advances in Blood Coagulation</u> 2 (1977)]:

  - p. 26 "The [kinin and complement systems] show similarities to the coagulation system and delineating the interactions between these systems will be an active area of research"

  - p. 52  "Very little is known about the possible interaction of complement components with clotting, although it seems established that the link between the two exists on the platelet level."

- p. 103  "It is now clear they [the kallikrein-kinin, and the complement systems] are all interrelated and that factor XII occupies a key position in the reactions. ... Kinins ... contribute to the inflammatory reaction by ... [among other things] leucocyte migration... . ...it is now fairly well accepted that activation of factor XII is a common trigger mechanism to both [coagulation and kallikrein-kinin systems]".

- p. 300  "Despite the unconvincing evidence of a direct relationship between the coagulation and complement cascade systems, clinical evidence of an association between the two still stands, in particular DIC [disseminated intravascular coagulation] associated with endotoxaemic and immune complex triggers."

Romer (1962) discusses the roles of globulins in both coagulation and immunology:  "One globulin type takes part in the formation of the blood clot from the fibrinogen proteins.  Other globulins of a highly specific nature are sensitive to protein materials of 'foreign' origin... .  Certain globulins are active agents in disease protection as the antibodies effective against invading viruses."  [A.S. Romer, THE VERTEBRATE BODY (1962), 412]


OPSONINS AND SERUM ANTIBODIES


Notwithstanding Steven Lehrer's (1979, Explorer's of the Body) pop-science dismissal of Wright as having missed the boat with his opsonic theory (see VACCINE), the concept of opsonins continues to comprise an integral part of modern immunology theory.  Following are excerpts discussing the opsonic nature of some globulins, and the relationship between antibodies and opsonins.  (see Sabin, Florence, 1938.)


OPSONIC GLOBULINS

--  "Two proteins, one a B-globulin and the other an a1-globulin, are opsonic without the aid of complement.." [Dorland's Illustrated Medical Dictionary (1981)

--  "IgG is the principal immunoglobin of normal human serum ... the major form of antibody produced in the secondary reaction. ... Although some bacteria clearly can be killed directly by antibody and complement 'in vivo', it seems likely that the major role of IgM and IgG antibody in the elimination of bacteria is opsonization for phagocytosis.  ... Although the existence of a variety of nonspecific serum factor opsonins has often been hypothesized, the most important and effective opsonins are various classes of immunoglobulin molecules, and certain components of complement." [William R. Clark (UCLA), THE EXPERIMENTAL FOUNDATIONS OF MODERN IMMUNOLOGY, 3rd Edition

(1986), p. 418]


OPSONIN = SERUM ANTIBODY

Also from Clark, 1986:

- p. 534  "opsonization ... usually involves matching a particular cell with an antibody complement, enabling it to adhere firmly to the surface of a phagocyte".

- p. 6  "...opsonins were soon shown to be identical with serum antibodies."

- p. 147  "The first step in the phagocytic process is the formation of stable contact with the particle to be ingested... . Formation of a stable contact can occur mechanically...".

- p. 416  "... antibody (particularly secretory antibody) plays a key role early in the course of microbial invasions by preventing the establishment of both bacterial and viral infections. ...  IgA antibodies seem to function chiefly by neutralizing bacteria and viruses before they attach to and penetrate epithelial cells. ... IgG antibodies can also be highly effective in neutralizing viruses that circulate in the bloodstream during the course of an infection (e.g., polio virus)."


Blood clotting, opsonins, antibody - all defensive, not the same, but all interrelated.  Thus it would appear that autohemotherapy could involve some degree of "passive" as well as "active" mechanism of action.

CONCEPTUAL DILEMMA:   PASSIVE V.S. ACTIVE IMMUNITY; IV V. XV

The concept of serum therapy, generally considered and treated by MEDLINE as synonymous with so-called passive immunization, assumes that the so-called immune serum of a previously-immunized animal might "passively" convey immunity to another animal.

[BUT:  In the case of autohemotherapy, such an explanation seems inappropriate at first glance; however, if defensive qualities of autologous blood were able to be improved in the process of removal and reinjection (e.g. via initiation of coagulation) and made comparable to an "immune serum", the net effect could be the same.]

As shown in Table 7-1, below, "active immunization" tends to be associated with: intramuscular, subcutaneous, intradermal or oral, rather than intravenous injection; and the opposite is the case for so-called "passive immunization".  From 1966 through 1993, within the MEDLINE subject area "passive immunization", the keyword "intravenous#" is encountered 1516 times, vs. a total of 856 for "intramuscular#", "subcutaneous#", "intradermal#" and "oral"; whereas in the subject area "active immunization", 207 citations are retrieved with the keyword "intravenous#" vs. a total of 2317 for "intramuscular#", "subcutaneous#", "intradermal#" and "oral".

The association of extravascular injection with "active immunity" is similarly reflected in the Moseby's Medical Dictionary (1994) definition of "vaccine" as "a suspension of attenuated or killed microorganisms administered intradermally, intramuscularly, orally, or subcutaneously to induce active immunity to infectious disease."

Thus, injection into the tissues, with autoblood or whatever, would logically (and most ready theoretically) be associated with an attempt to elicit an "active" response from those tissues, rather than "passively" adding to existing stores of protective substances.  [BUT: Rosenow's skin tests with antibody and antigen indicate the latter is also possible; see ROSENOW METHOD/ANTIBODY.]

In the case of autoblood, the situation is further complicated by the fact that IV reinjection (always a hazard) requires the addition of an anticoagulant (always a hazard) or removing coagulants prior to reinjection, either of which might be seen as thereby reducing the defensive qualities of the blood with possible implication of reduced immunity-conveying potential.

Wright's work asserted that any benefit from (intravenous) serum therapy was not the result of a "passive" mechanism, but rather constituted "active" immunization; bacterial derivatives within the "immune serum" may hopefully eventually wend their way through the circulation to tissues in which antibodies are formed.  Wright's position was supported by the observation that, when effective, so-called "serum therapy" involved the application of increasing doses in a similar fashion as with vaccine-therapy. [see VACCINE, WRIGHT]

## SAFEGUARD THE CITADEL OF CIRCULATING BLOOD

Further elaboration on two points might be made - safety and effectiveness - relative to manner of injection.

In considering inoculation into the circulation (IV) vs. into the tissues (IM or SC, etc.), prime considerations would be (1) to not do harm and (2) to do good.  On the first point, dangers of intravenous inoculation have long been recognized, from a number of perspectives.

In 1907 the renowned chemist Svante Arrhenius noted "A mixture which is innocuous to guinea-pigs when injected subcutaneously may kill them when injected intracardially, i.e., directly into the blood"  Arrhenius attributed this to a slower rate of diffusion into the blood in the case of subcutaneous injection, during which "the antitoxin binds the toxin; whereas with IV injection, "the poison is bound by the tissues of the animal before it has time to react with the antitoxin."  [Arrhenius, 1907, p.31].

In the same era, Sir Almroth Wright cautioned as concerns auto-inoculation, specifically referring to the need to "safeguard the citadel of circulating blood".  And in modern times, specifically concerning blood products, Roitt offered that "Isolated *y*-globulin preparations tend to form small aggregates spontaneously and these can lead to severe anaphylactic reactions when administered intravenously ... .  For this reason the material is always injected intramuscularly."

On the question of effectiveness, Wright illustrated the efficacy of intramuscular, etc. injections with knowledge gained from the development of "immune serums" in horses: "a larger production of protective substances is, in point of fact, regularly achieved... when, in lieu of intravenous inoculations, subcutaneous and intra-muscular inoculations are resorted to" [Wright 1909 (09E1)].

This is consistent with and substantiated by Florence Sabin's 1939 landmark "evidence implicating the cells of the reticulo-endothelial system in the formation of antibodies"; Sabin demonstrated that this occurs primarily in the tissues, and that the circulating blood primarily serves a transport function.  And Edward C. Rosenow, a dedicated protege of Sir Almroth Wright in his extensive utilization of autogenous vaccine therapy, came to utilize subcutaneous or intramuscular injections exclusively.

It is clearly beyond the scope of this work to definitively resolve questions raised by Wright concerning the general case of the true nature of the relationship between so-called "passive immunization" and "active immunization".  Against Wright's excellent and seemingly unassailable points, we must urge examination of Rosenow's relevant work.  Rosenow's autologous inoculum was referred to as "antigen" and "antibody", which were injected intramuscularly or subcutaneously (although earlier in his career he had participated in studies employing conventional, IV, "serum therapy").

While his earlier work featured vaccine-therapy, in his later years Dr. Rosenow had come to use "antibody" to a greater extent than "antigen"; however in his last articles he utilized both.


NOT A STICKING POINT - EXTRAVASCULAR INPUT, BUT WHAT ROUTE?

One would have thought the question certainly by now settled - Sir Almroth Wright spoke of injection into the tissues; Florence Sabin established the antibody-producing role of the reticulo-endothelial system; "classical" autohemotherapy primarily has involved intramuscular, but also subcutaneous, injections; vaccines are administered intramuscularly, subcutaneously, intradermally or orally; Rosenow's thermal antibody was administered subcutaneously and also intramuscularly.  So if "classical" autohemotherapy is actually an autoblood-cocktail vaccine, which would be the preferred route -  intramuscular or subcutaneous?

A cursory MEDLINE search for keywords: "compar# intramuscular# subcutaneous# injection" seems to indicate overall that there's not much of a critical difference between intramuscular and subcutaneous injection in terms of bioavailability of either vaccines or drugs - they both in fact do deliver, and consideration of their relative advantages and disadvantages continues to occupy the interest and time of investigators.  In a word, the preferred method would appear to be "extravascular", over "intravascular".

Table 7-2 exhibits the results of this search, grouped by vaccines, hormones, insulin, and other; where both IM and SC are checked, the study indicated that the two methods did not significantly differ; where only one is checked, a preference for that method was indicated.

Table 7-1.   PASSIVE vs. ACTIVE; IV v. IM/SC/ID/Oral

| | | 1966 -'74 | 1975 -'79 | 1980 -'84 | 1985 -'89 | 1990 -'93 | Totals |
|---|---|---|---|---|---|---|---|
| Years: | | | | | | | |
| **Subject: passive immunization** | | | | | | | |
| +keyword: intravenous# | | 71 | 78 | 222 | 711 | 434 | 1516 |
| IM,SC,ID or Oral | | 99 | 146 | 157 | 307 | 147 | 856 |
| (-intramuscular# | (IM) | 26 | 24 | 35 | 65 | 28 | 178) |
| (-subcutaneous# | (SC) | 39 | 61 | 69 | 102 | 37 | 308) |
| (-intradermal# | (ID) | 26 | 33 | 28 | 49 | 20 | 156) |
| (-oral | (Or) | 19 | 42 | 43 | 108 | 71 | 283) |
| **Subject: active immunization** | | | | | | | |
| +keyword: intravenous# | | 56 | 25 | 21 | 42 | 63 | 207 |
| IM,SC,ID or Oral | | 791 | 386 | 350 | 381 | 409 | 2317 |
| (-intramuscular# | (IM) | 109 | 87 | 59 | 75 | 105 | 435) |
| (-subcutaneous# | (SC) | 258 | 131 | 101 | 104 | 81 | 675) |
| (-intradermal# | (ID) | 89 | 50 | 56 | 71 | 53 | 319) |
| (-oral | (Or) | 430 | 186 | 170 | 185 | 228 | 1199) |

## Table 7-2.   INTRAMUSCULAR (IM) vs. SUBCUTANEOUS (SC) INJECTION

                                                               IM SC

   ---VACCINES
Dennehy PH, et al., 1991, varicella vaccine, 166 children  x   x
Suntharasamai P, et al., 1987, rabies vaccine,118 subjects x   x
Wahl M, Hermodsson S, 1987, hepatitis B vaccine

                                         [IM higher serocon]
Lemon M, et al., 1983, hepatitis B vaccine by SC jet       x   x
Jemski JV, 1981, Francisela tularensis vaccine, in rats    x   x


   ---HORMONES
le Cotonnec, JY, et al., 1993, follicle stim. hormone      x   x
Saal W, et al., 1991, human chorionic gonadotropin

                                              [SC slower]
Takano K, et al., 1988, human growth hormone, 20 patients  x   x
Russo L, 1982, human growth hormone

                                           [SC less pain]


   ---INSULIN
Henricksen JE, et al., 1991, insulin, 11 type 1 diabetics
                                          [SC more constant]
Pickup JC, et al., 1981, contin.insulin, brittle diabetes
                                          [SC not effective]
Guerra SM, Kitabchi AE, 1975, insulin, in lean subjects
                                          [IM faster absorp.]


   ---OTHER
Jundt JW, et al., 1993, methotrexate, rheumatoid arthritis x   x
Ronald AL, et al., 1993, morphine absorption, elderly pat. x   x
Sanders P, et al., 1988, chloramphenicol, in cattle        x   x
Pacini A, et al., 1987, tumor necrosis factor, cancer      x   x
Wright FC, Riner JC, 1985, ivermectin, rabbit psoroptes    x   x
Muhlhauser I, et al., 1985, glucagon, 6 nondiabetic men    x   x
Vodos K, 1976, agglutinin formation in exper.infect.poult. x   x

SPECULATION ON:  "EXTRAVASCULAR" AS/AND "PASSIVE IMMUNITY"


   That Dr. Rosenow was indeed injecting "antibody" and "antigen"
is supported by his consistently having separately obtained
properly-indicative respective skin reactions in cutaneous tests
[See:  Rosenow, E.C., South Dakota J. Med. and Pharm. 5: 304-310;
328, Nov. 1952; J. Nerv. and Ment. Dis. 122: 321-331, Oct. 1955].

   Nonetheless, it would appear that the extravascular injection
of antibody would not directly in the short run appreciably add
to stores of existing antibody except at the site of injection.

   As therapeutical measures, Dr. Rosenow injected both antigen
and "thermal" antibody subcutaneously or intramuscularly (into
the tissues, whereas Wright and others have maintained,
antibodies are formed).  In that "thermal" antibody is comprised
of well-oxidized antigen [45R4], might its injection stimulate
antibody development, rather than passing through unaltered to
the circulation?

   But then, how to explain Dr. Rosenow's separate
antigen/antibody reactions?  If Dr. Rosenow's work firmly
establishes that beneficial action of subcutaneously-administered
autologous "antibody" is properly attributed to a "passive
immunization" mechanism, or "serum therapy", it seems to refute
Wright's near-blanket condemnation of serum therapy.  (It is
noted that Wright conceded the "neutralization of a poison like
diphtheria toxin by the aid of an anti-toxic serum", a concession
which might not be necessary if toxins turn out to be markers for
phase transition of microorganisms into smaller forms, as has
been recently demonstrated for an endotoxin [Hurley JC [Lancet,
1993 May 1, 341(8853):1133-5].

   When considering the action of extravascular injection,
analogies of lock-and-key or mirror-image antibody-production
conceivably might be augmented by the concept of "glove-in-
glove", allowing either "antigen" v. "antibody" to evoke a like
response in the form of fostering production of antibody.

   Likewise in the case of autohemotherapy, particularly as
practiced by Dr. Cuyugan (see INTRO) where blood fluids are
purposefully allowed to coagulate about coexisting invaders in
the blood, resultant forms complementary to those of the invaders
also comprise a portion of the intramuscular or subcutaneous
injection.  Do these so-formed globulins then pass unimpeded into
the bloodstream, or do they foster development within the
reticulo-endothelial system of other globulins a.k.a. antibodies
which do so?  That the latter may be the case, as suggested above
for the action of Dr. Rosenow's thermal antibody, might be viewed
as consistent with Pauling's conceptualization of "molecular
complementariness" [Huemer RP ed. 1986], and the above "glove-
into-glove" concept.

   Whatever the motivation or proffered explanations or true
underlying action, methods which involve IM or SC reinjection of

both "antigen" and "antibody" bring to mind a distinct category
of mixed auto-serum-vaccines in the historical literature (see
Chapter 5: VACCINE THERAPY, last item, "Autosensitized
vaccines".)


ARRHENIUS: HEATED BLOOD -  HEMOLYSIN, COAGULATION,
AGGLUTINATION

ON THE INACTIVATION OF HEMOLYSIN  Arrhenius 1907

"If we heat blood-serum containing ... haemolysin to 55 degrees C
for about 30 minutes, we find that it loses its haemolytic power.
 It is said to be 'inactivated'." [p.19]

    ...

   "The normal serum of an animal contains a substance which
haemolyses the erythrocytes of animals of other species, and this
substance was called alexin (protecting substance) by Buchner,
who determined also that the alexin is rapidly decomposed at a
temperature of 55 degrees C or more." [p. 218]


HEAT AND FORMATION OF AGGLUTININ  Arrhenius 1907

AGGLUTINATION AS COAGULATION

   Arrhenius had showed that the velocity of reaction for
agglutinins is proportional to the concentration of the
agglutinin and increases with temperature, and from this
"concluded that the agglutination depends on a chemical reaction
of the agglutinin with some content of the bacterium. In his
excellent work on microbiology DuClaux shows that this chemical
reaction is really a coagulation." [p. 164]


IMMUNOTHERAPY WITH INTERLEUKIN-2 - IV V. SUBCUTANEOUS INJECTION

   Zanbello, R, et. al., Cancer 74 (9) November 1, 1994, 2562-9,
compared IV infusion of recombinant interleukin-2, with
subcutaneous injection, reporting that subcutaneous immunotherapy
"induces a preferential increase in T cells".  With intravenous
infusion, "the absolute number of CD3+ cells was unchanged, and
they showed a low or absent expression of the p55 and negativity
for the p75 IL-2R".  After subcutaneous injection, the absolute
number of CD3+ cells was significantly increased.


BIBLIOGRAPHY - THEORETICAL CONSIDERATIONS


-- Arrhenius, Svante A., Immunology, MacMillan Co. 1907
-- Chase, Allan, MAGIC SHOTS, William Morrow, 1982
-- Clark, William R., THE EXPERIMENTAL FOUNDATIONS OF MODERN
IMMUNOLOGY, 3rd Edition, 1986 (UCLA)
-- Cushing, JE and DH Campbell, Principles of Immunology, McGraw-
Hill, New York, 1957.

-- Ferreira OC and Barcinski MA, <u>Cellular Immunology</u> 101 (1986), 259-265, "Autologous Induction of the Human T-Cell-Dependent Monocyte Procoagulant Activity: A Possible Link between Immunoregulatory Phenomena and Blood Coagulation"

-- Huemer, R.P., ed. <u>The Roots of Molecular Medicine</u>, WH Freeman, New York 1986

-- Poller, L., <u>Recent Advances in Blood Coagulation</u> 2 (1977)

-- Roitt, Ivan M., <u>Essential Immunology, Third Ed.</u>, Blackwell Scientific Publications, Oxford 1977

-- Romer, A.S., THE VERTEBRATE BODY (1962)

-- Sabin, Florence, J. EXPER. MED. 70, 67-82, "Cellular Reactions to a Dye-Protein with a Concept of the Mechanism of Antibody Formation", 1939

## Chapter 8: ALTERNATIVE MEDICINE

### "ALTERNATIVE" MEDICAL APPROACHES

### HOMEOPATHY

#### HOMEOPATHY PERFECTED = AUTOTHERAPY

Smith 1982 notes "Homeopathy is a specialized system of therapeutics, developed by Dr. Samuel Christian Hahnemann, 1755-1843, based on the  scientific and natural law of healing: 'Similia similibus curentur' or 'Likes are cured by likes.'"  Per Smith,  Hahnemann's best known books on medicine are Organon and Materia Medica Pura.  Hahnemann developed his method as a result of noticing, while in the process of translating medical books, that people who took Peruvian bark developed symptoms of malaria, the disease for which it was used as a cure.  "He tried it on himself and then on his family; then he tried other drugs until he was finally convinced that he had discovered a real scientific law of treatment. ... Hahnemann spent six years in proving drugs and verifying his principle before proclaiming it."

In other words, Hahnemann spent 6 years taking drugs that made him sick, and while under their influence, tried to describe what it felt like, so its effect could be matched with disease symptoms.  Of course the ultimate of "similarity" is "being identical", so that the perfect medicine would seem best not the shotgun speculation of homeopathic or allopathic medicine, although the former would most likely do the least harm, from both standpoints of less toxicity and smaller doses.  However, as emphasized by Saxon in 1949 and Duncan in the early nineteen-teens, both M.D.s and also homeopaths, the ultimate homeopathic weapon is autotherapeutic.  Use the actual organism from the patient; nothing could be more similar.

#### HOMEOPATHY - AIDS/ARC AND TYPHOID

Bagley 1987 notes many symptoms are common to both typhoid and ARC/AIDS, suggesting the possible utility of homeopathic remedies historically used for the former in treatment of the latter. Bagley lists the following remedies: Arsenicum, Baptista, Rhus tox, Lachesis, Phosphoric Acid, Mercuris, Nitric Acid, Phosphorus, Muriatic Acid, and Bryonia.

As common symptoms to both illnesses, Bagley lists: insidious onset of symptoms, weight loss, fatigue, loss of appetite, night fevers, diarrhea, leukopenia, red-purple skin lesions, splenomegaly, cough, bronchitis, and delirium.

A major difference is noted in typhoid's evolution over days and weeks, whereas AIDS/ARC progresses over months or years. [see AIDS]

## ALLOPATHY V. HOMEOPATHY

If Hahnemann came back in current times, he wouldn't have to search so hard for substances to make him sick. He could just go to the local pharmacy, or to the Physicians' Desk Reference.

Here he would find that many medicines prescribed by allopaths in modern times are also known to cause side-effects that are exacerbations or mimic symptoms of the diseases they purport to treat.

Thus it is that Prednisone, for example, a drug which has been prescribed to a woman with muscle disease, actually is known to cause muscle weakness and atrophy, and also causes facial erythema and lupus erythematosus.

A particularly horrendous set of examples is found in the array of drugs being used to "treat" mental illness. Several of these, e.g. Haldol, Ativan, and Risperdone, are particularly well-known to cause symptoms that on the other side of the ledger are used to define mental illness.

There is of course some logic in all of this, e.g., that the drugs involved may somehow be related to the causative organisms, and therefore may under the best of circumstances act as a specific vaccine and indeed aid in therapy; or conversely may not elicit a beneficial response but rather worsen the condition. The recent finding [Science 268, June 1995, p. 1850] that common pathogens may infect both plants and animals is consistent with such a suggestion.

The presumed usual (hopefully often and certainly at least occasional) benefits of allopathic and homeopathic medicines cannot be denied; however, a common characteristic of both is that they are generally the result of a "crap-shoot", a grand world-wide treasure hunt. If successful, the hunt will lead to a substance with a specific therapeutic affinity for the organism causing a particular disease. Thus the hunt is well-directed back to where it hopes to lead - to the infected individual wherein is certainly found the causative organism.

## ACUPUNCTURE

### ACUPUNCTURE PROPOSED TO WORK THROUGH NERVOUS SYSTEM

Mann, 1973, p. 5, "In acupuncture, the needle is frequently placed at the opposite end, and possibly opposite side, of the body from that of the diseased organ or site of symptoms. Under certain conditions one of these distant and contralateral pricks can have an effect in one or two seconds. This speed of conduction excludes the blood and lymphatic system (at least in this type of response) and leaves to my way of thinking, the nervous system as the only contender."

## NON-NEURAL THEORIES OF ACUPUNCTURE

Other, "non-neural" theories are also noted, including a special conducting system, a magnetic theory, some involving quantum mechanics, contraction wave theory, electrical discharge al la condenser theory, and release of cortisone or histamine or adrenaline. This last seems most readily correlated with some theoretical attempts to explain the beneficial action of autoblood therapy. [Mann, 1973, Chapter 1, "General Considerations, Neural Theory of the Action of Acupuncture"]

Mann, p. 30, discusses some accidental cures, such as spontaneous cures following exploratory operations where the patient is merely sewed back up, and speculates that these might be due to acupuncture by the surgical knife.

## AUTOHEMOTHERAPY AS ALTERNATE EXPLANATION OF ACUPUNCTURE ACTION

Whatever the value of the acupuncture explanation may be, these instances unquestionably involve autoinoculation of autogenous blood into the tissues, and hence comprise a form of autohemotherapy. This also appears to be the case for two other examples of accidental cures discussed by Mann, one involving a boy who "fell down, hitting his forehead at the root of the nose on the iron bedstead, and was immediately cured of the sinus trouble he had suffered from for 2 or 3 years"; and the other a woman whose nearly daily headache and general malaise of 10 years' duration was relieved when her skin was pricked in the process of getting blood tests.

## ACUPUNCTURE-AUTOHEMOTHERAPY-ROSENOW CORRELATIONS

Mann, p. 207-220, lists purportedly successful results of acupuncture in over 3000 cases, including rheumatic and allied diseases, pulmonary diseases, urology, gynecology, cardiology, digestive tract, neurology, eye diseases, headache, asthma and hayfever, sexual malfunction, psychiatry and trigeminal neuralgia. It is noted that many of these conditions have been treated by autohemotherapeutical means and/or were the subject of Dr. Rosenow's investigations.

## EXPERT CHALLENGES YIN-YANG & ACUPUNCTURE THEORY

Acupuncture-expert Mann, well into his book, challenges conventional acupuncture theory, noting, p. 59: " ... the idea of complementary opposites, the negative and the positive, which the Chinese called the Yin and the Yang ... are at the very root of the Chinese way of life ... ". However, p. 194, it is noted that acupuncture may have a normalizing influence on both the overactive and the underactive, and the circumstance "that the treatment does not differentiate between the two ... jeopardizes the whole idea of polarity, of Yin and Yang [and] in fact much of the theoretical background of acupuncture. ... One might think it difficult to practice acupuncture without a firm theoretical background, but actually this makes little difference for when I treat a patient I know what works and nothing else."

Alas, do not despair professor Mann.  You can have your empirical success and a "firm" theory too - in the characterization of acupuncture as a form of autohemotherapy.

Mann's accounts (p. 3) of primitive and historical examples of acupuncture include methods as or more readily viewed as autohemotherapeutic:  "The Bantu of South Africa sometimes scratch certain parts of the body to cure disease.  In the treatment of sciatica some Arabs cauterize with a hot metal probe a part of the ear. ... Some Eskimos practice simple acupuncture with sharp stones.  An isolated cannibalistic tribe in Brazil shoot tiny arrows with a blowpipe at specific parts of the body.  The only observer ever to return from them thinks that, as the tribe shows distinct Mongoloid features, this might also be related to acupuncture.  [Let us get carried away!!]  Possibly the cautery practiced in medieval Europe is also related to the tradition though this was mainly applied at congested or painful places and would therefore correspond to the simplest form of acupuncture in which only the 'locus dolenti', and not the distant part, is stimulated."

Mann, p. 25, notes: "The Chinese describe the acupuncture points as being quite small - a matter of millimeters.  In my experience this is only true to a limited extent for not infrequently a stimulus anywhere in an area as large as a dermatome (or several dermatomes ... ) is sufficient."  Mann indicates 12 dermatomes running horizontally across the back between the waist and under the armpits.  We may note that such larger target areas argue against attributing the action of acupuncture to hitting the right nerve, and in favor of any beneficial action being due to autohemotherapeutic action (forcing blood into the tissues where antibodies are formed.

Mann, p. 192, "Traditional Chinese works on acupuncture describe about 50 different ways of inserting acupuncture needles [including] inserting the needle 3 or 9 or 81 times", etc.

Mann, p. 193, asserts that the size of the stimulus increases with: a fat needle, deeper insertion, more movement, more acupuncture points, and repetition of treatment.  We may note that insofar as all of these would also likely increase exposure of blood to tissues, these also would involve increased autoinoculations.


COINING; YOGA, MASSAGE, EXERCISE; CHINESE HERBALISM

Leslie Berger, <u>Los Angeles Times</u>, August 24, 1994, p. 1, "Learning to tell custom from abuse", refers to "angry looking red streaks on ... neck and temples" left by the "common Vietnamese practice of massaging away fevers and aches with a heated coin or piece of metal that draws blood to the surface of the skin. 'Everybody has it done. You feel good after'", explained a recent immigrant from Vietnam.

As with coining, yoga procedures, massage, and even exercise in general stimulate increased flow of blood to the tissues, where, presumably antibodies to blood-borne antigens might hence form in increased quantities.

As for Chinese herbalism, what is the operative action? At first one might be inclined to think that the action is a protective one, that beneficial substances in the herbs provide a therapeutic action. However, we are reminded that epidemics may transcend barriers of both time and space: pathogenic strains recur periodically after gaps of years; and as Rosenow has shown, harmful pathogens are carried through the air and have even been collected at high altitudes in an airplane. This provides a possible explanation as to how pathogenic strains may spread over great distances, even without the aid of modern long-distance travel.

Thus an herb or herbs imported from China or elsewhere, at some time in the past, might have grown in an environment which afforded exposure to a pathogenic organism (or some close relative) that is currently causing a disease condition. In such a case the beneficial action of the herb might be related to the action of a therapeutic vaccine; i.e., the herb may have captured a component of the causative organism, which when ingested evokes an "active" immune response. Maybe. As noted by B. Wuethrich in Science 268, 1850 (30 June 1995), some of the same bacteria may cause infections in both plants and animals.


Berger, Leslie, Los Angeles Times, August 24, 1994, p. 1, "Learning to tell custom from abuse"


Mann 1973, Acupuncture


Smith, Kent, Homeopathy Medicine for Today's Living, Glendale, CA 1982


Wuethrich, B., in Science 268, 1850 (30 June 1995)

Chapter 9: MEDLINE UPDATES - AUTOHEMOTHERAPY/AUTOVACCINE

AUTOMED: Coming to terms with MEDLINE

Far from being out-dated or outmoded, both autohemotherapy and autogenous vaccine-therapy are, in practice if not in name, active and vital components of modern medical theory and practice.

Table 9-1 exhibits numbers of citations accessed through MEDLINE with keywords "autologous or autogenous", "autohemotherapy", "autogenous vaccine therapy" and other seemingly related terms. At the outset, note the striking increase in recent years in numbers of references to "autologous" or "autogenous" methods in general.

AUTOHEMOTHERAPY, AUTO- BLOOD, ETC:

In MEDLINE, the keyword "autohemotherapy" yields a meager 22 entries (1965-1995). It is noted that most of these refer to something other than the "classical" intramuscular or subcutaneous form.

Nonetheless, the substance of "classical" autohemotherapy appears to be embodied in many other articles accessible through MEDLINE using combinations of the following terms as keywords or subjects:

autologous autoblood blood hemotherapy intramuscular serum subcutaneous therapy

Examples of such articles are discussed below in "CLASSICAL (EXTRAVASCULAR) AUTOHEMOTHERAPY BY OTHER NAMES". Moreover, the field of bone-marrow transplantation is clearly in the process of auto-transforming into autohemotherapy (see MARROW).

As seen in Table 9-1, MEDLINE treats subject areas "PASSIVE IMMUNIZATION" and "SERUM THERAPY" as virtually synonymous, with several thousand citations since 1966. Of 221 such "autologous" citations during the period 1966-1993, a mere eleven involve "intramuscular" or "subcutaneous" or "intradermal" methods, and only one specifically refers to "autohemotherapy".

AUTOGENOUS VACCINE THERAPY, ETC.:

In contrast, as evident in Table 9-1, MEDLINE treats subject areas "ACTIVE IMMUNIZATION" and "VACCINE-THERAPY" as distinctly different. ACTIVE IMMUNIZATION has been a continuing MEDLINE

subject area, whereas VACCINE-THERAPY first became a MEDLINE
subject area in 1989.  Only a few "autologous" citations listed
in either of the two subject areas are common to both, indicating
that the field of vaccine-therapy is much larger than indicated
by numbers of articles in the so-named relatively-new subject
area.  Moreover, the very initiation within MEDLINE of a
"vaccine-therapy" subject area for the first time in 1989 would
seem to reflect a growing awareness and interest in the subject.

AUTOHEMOTHERAPY ON-LINE (MEDLINE)

Of 22 items accessed through MEDLINE (1965-1995 incl.) with the
keyword "autohemotherapy, all but 6 appear to involve forms other
than "classical" extravascular autohemotherapy; i.e., at least 8
seem to involve intravenous reinjection, 2 involve local
treatment, and 4 involve intraocular injections.  Insofar as
these articles are readily accessible through MEDLINE, citations
are not given here.

Some diseases discussed in those articles are listed below.
Codes have been assigned to aid in a search for further
information; e.g., "93G1" refers to the first article listed in
MEDLINE for 1993 using the keyword "autohemotherapy", 93G2 the
second 1993 article, etc.


--AIDS  92G2
--apoplexy, photosensitized oxidation autohemo- 93G3
--chronic fatigue syndrome  71G1
--common cold  71G1
--conjunctival bands, local autohemo- 71G1
--cysts, care and treatment according to Partsch  73G1
--eye burns, subconjunctival autohemotherapy of  92G1
--eye, chemical and thermal burns  79G1 [81F2]
--eye burns caused by alkalies  65G1
--headache, peridural autohemo after lumbar puncture  86G1
--herpes simplex  71G1
--herpes zoster  71G1
--inflammatory diseases, chronic, maxillofacial 74G1
--labialis and genitalis  71G1
--osteochondrosis, spinal  74G2
--papillomavirus  71G1
--psoriasis - pyrotherapy, autohemotherapy and laked blood  66G1
--respiratory diseases  71G1
--viral hepatitis  71G1
--viral diseases, immunodeficiencies, ozonization  92G2
--vulvae, essential pruritus-, kraurosis-, local 69G1

--vulvar irritation, idiopathic, local autohemo-  67G1


CLASSICAL (EXTRAVASCULAR) AUTOHEMOTHERAPY BY OTHER NAMES
  Examples of articles which may be intimately related to
"classical" (extravascular) autohemotherapy, which may be
accessed in MEDLINE using keywords other than "autohemotherapy",
are listed below.  Some of these involve the manipulation and
reinjection of autologous blood components, which raises the
question as to whether whole blood might have served as well.
Disease conditions mentioned in these articles include:


--Ascites:  Chiyoda S and T Morikawa, 1993
--B-Cell Lymphoma:  Kwak, L.W., et al. 1992
--Breast Cancer:   Bensinger, W, et al., 1993
--Cold: Donskov SI et al 1992; Khodanova RN et al 1989
--Drug Allergy:  Khodanova, RN, et al 1989
--Hemocytopenias:  Mascarin M,
--Leg Edema:  Chiyoda S and T Morikawa, 1993
--Lumbar Osteochondrosis:  Sokov EL, 1988
--Malignancies:  Bensinger, W, et al., 1993
--Non-Hodgkins Lymphoma: Bensinger, W, et al., 1993
--Peritonitis:  Manucharov NK, et al., 1992
--Rheumatoid Arthritis:  van Laar, JM, et al.
--Systemic Lupus Eryth.: Chiyoda & Morikawa 1993
--Testicular Carcinoma:  Bensinger, W, 1993
--Thrombocytopenic Purpura:  Vizcaino G, 1992
--Wilms Tumor:  Bensinger, W, et al., 1993


  EXAMPLES OF AUTOHEMO-ALIASES


  Bensinger, W, et al., Blood, 1993 Jun 1, 81 (11):3158-63,
"Autologous transplantation with peripheral blood mononuclear
cells collected after administration of recombinant granulocyte
stimulating factor." [MEDLINE kw: AUTOLOGOUS BLOOD SUBCUTANEOUS].
  Abstr: Bensinger et al., 1993, collected, cryopreserved,
  thawed and reinfused autologous peripheral blood mononuclear
  cells, along with other procedures, in 12 patients with
  malignancies (including breast cancer, non-Hodgkins lymphoma,
  testicular carcinoma and Wilms tumor), concluding that this
  led to more rapid recovery after myeloablative chemotherapy.


  Chiyoda S and T Morikawa, Japanese Journal of Clinical
Hematology, 1993 Jan, 34(1):39-43, "Reinfusion of concentrated

autogenous ascitic fluid in a patient with selective IgA deficiency." [MEDLINE keywords: AUTOGENOUS SERUM THERAPY]

Abstract: Concentrated autogenous ascitic fluid and prednisolone was administered to a patient with leg edema and ascites, with common cold-like symptoms, and diagnostic findings suggesting systemic lupus erythematosus. "His ascitic fluid disappeared and complements and albumin in his serum normalized. He has continued in good condition and is being treated as an outpatient."[Medline] (Note that the original autoserotherapy method of Gilbert of Geneva in 1894 involved the subcutaneous reinjection of autogenous serous fluid in pleural effusions.)

Donskov SI, et al., "A rise in activity of natural cold isolymphocytotoxins after hemostimulation". Human Immunology, 1982 Jul, 4(4):325-333. [MEDLINE kw: AUTOLOGOUS BLOOD THERAPY INTRAMUSCULAR]

Khodanova, RN, Seslavina LS, Golubeva NN, Zuyeva VA, Kutkova ON, Maltseva VV, Nikitina TI, Journal of Hygiene, Epidemiology, Microbiology and Immunology, 1989, 33(4):463-9, "Pattern of changes in clinico-immunological indicators of patients with drug allergy during treatment with autologous blood."
[MEDLINE kw: AUTOLOGOUS BLOOD: INTRADERMALLY/SUBCUTANEOUSLY]

Abstract: "An efficient method for the treatment of drug allergy was proposed and practically implemented. The method consists in autologous venous blood being lysed with sterile distilled water at a ratio of 5:1 and injected subcutaneously and partially intradermally into the reflexogenic zones of the back 2-3 cm from the spinal column. During the first week of treatment, increasing doses were injected (3 to 10 ml), whereas during the second week the doses decreased from 10 to 3 ml. Following treatment the patients felt better and featured enhanced working ability as well as markedly declined susceptibility to common colds. ..." [This is extra-vascular autohemotherapy.]

Kwak, L.W., et al., New England J. of Medicine, 1992 Oct 22, 327(17):1209-15.
[MEDLINE keywords: AUTOLOGOUS BLOOD:INTRAMUSCULAR OR SUBCUTANEOUS]

Abstract: Kwak, L.W., et al., 1992, 1209-15, discusses the use of autogenous immunoglobulin to treat B-cell lymphoma. The only toxicity encountered was mild reaction at the site of intramuscular injection. Sustained immunologic responses were induced in 7 of 9 patients; tumors of both of two patients with measurable disease receded. These results "provide the background for large-scale trials of active specific immunotherapy of this disease." [Medline] [While this article was originally accessed with the keywords "autologous blood", MEDLINE refers to "active" immunization and the article itself refers to treating nine lymphoma patients with vaccines made from their own cancers.  In "both of the patients with measurable disease", the cancer tissue completely disappeared. [see "A STRIKING CANCER CONNECTION ..." below; CANCER file]

Manucharov NK, et al., "The detoxifying and immunocorrective properties of some sorption treatment methods in suppurative-septic poisoning in experimental diffuse peritonitis." Biulleten Eksperimentalnoi Biologii i Meditsiny, 1992 Oct, 114(10):395-8. (Rus)  [MEDLINE keywords: AUTOBLOOD THERAPY]

Mascarin M, Trovo MG, Ventura A, "Anti-Rh(D): an efficacious therapeutic alternative in autoimmune hemocytopenias." Pediatria Medica E Chirurgica, 1993 Jul-Aug, 15(4):349-52. (ITA)

[MEDLINE keywords: AUTO# BLOOD INTRAMUSCULAR#]

Abstr.:  Mode of action:  "hypothesis most widely accepted is the blockade of Fc-receptors in the reticuloendothelial system."  [Note this is where antibodies are formed, as per Florence Sabin 1939]

Sokov EL, "Intramuscular and intraosseous block in the combined treatment of the neurological manifestations of lumbar osteochondrosis." Zh Nevropatol Psikhiatr, 1988, 88(4):57-61. (Russ)  [MEDLINE keywords: AUTOLOGOUS BLOOD THERAPY INTRAMUSCULAR]

van Laar, JM, et al., Journal of Autoimmunity, 1993 Apr., 6(2):159-67, "Effects of inoculation with attenuated autologous T cells in patients with rheumatoid arthritis".

[MEDLINE keywords: AUTOLOGOUS: SERUM THERAPY OR BLOOD SUBCUTANEOUS]

Abstr:  The authors isolated and subcutaneously reinjected autologous T lymphocytes from synovial tissue or fluid in 13 rheumatoid arthritis patients.  "On the average the patients showed a slight decrease in disease activity which was most marked at 8 weeks after the injection."  The authors concluded that the procedure was non-toxic and apparently beneficial. "The data suggest that the potential of T cell vaccination should be further explored in diseases with defined antigen reactivity." [Medline]

Vizcaino G, Diez-Ewald M; Arteaga-Vizcaino M, Torres E, "Use of anti-D (Rh) IgG or intramuscular polyvalent human immunoglobulin in the treatment of chronic autoimmune thrombocytopenic purpura". Invenstigacion Clinica, 1992, 33 (4):165-74.(SP)  [MEDLINE keywords: AUTO# BLOOD INTRAMUSCULAR#]

Abstract:  "... there were no adverse effects with the treatment.  In conclusion the intramuscular injection of immunoglobulins... produces an increase in the platelet count in some patients with CATP, several of them can obtain prolonged remissions, particularly children ... . This treatment is safe, ambulatory, easy to administer, and relatively inexpensive."[excerpts; MEDLINE]


EXAMPLE ALTERNATE KEYWORD CATEGORY: AUTOBLOOD THERAPY


As shown in Table 9-1, entering the MEDLINE command "FIND KW AUTOBLOOD THERAPY" yields 23 citations, including Manucharov above.  Manucharov uses the phrase "sorption", and it is further noted that this or "hemosorption" or "haemosorption" are found in 8 of the 23 citations.  All of these eight also involve ultraviolet irradiation of autoblood.  Two examples:


 - Nikninson RA, et al. [khirurgiia, 1994 Nov(11):22-6] discuss treatment of acute peritonitis, suggesting "along with the traditional infusion and antibacterial therapy in peritonitis, UVI of autoblood and intravenous laser irradiation of the blood in stages IIA and IIB are applied.  This should be followed by hemosorption which contributes to the active excretion of toxins from the organism. ... In the group of 369 patients who underwent operation 112 (29.5%) died."

 - Marusanov VE, et al., <u>Vestnik Khirurgii Imeni I.I. Grekova</u>, 1991 Apr, 146(4):104-9, note "Using the UV irradiation of autoblood in patients with clinically marked alterations of the peripheral blood circulation increases toxemia at the expense of release of toxic products from the "disclosed" system of microcirculation.  HS (Hemosorption) with the simultaneous taking the blood from the subclavian vein and abdominal aorta with using "Actilen" and return of the mixed blood into the peripheral artery interrupts and relieves the course of SPOI (syndrome of polyorganic insufficiency)."


Of the total 23 "KW AUTOBLOOD THERAPY" citations, 14 involve ultraviolet irradiation (all 14 are Russian).  For the most part the UV irradiation was presumed to be beneficial, whereas as noted by Marusanov et al (immediately above) this apparently is not always the case.  Hence, while "one swallow doth not a summer make", we have further grounds to question as to whether the irradiation may be superfluous (or sometimes even harmful), insofar as simple autotransfusion has been found to be immunologically beneficial [see AUTOTRANSFUSION AS AUTOHEMOTHERAPY, below].

In all, 19 of the 23 citations are Russian, 2 Japanese, 1 German, 1 American.  For the previous 5-year period, 19 of 20 citations are Russian and the 20th German.

A comparable overview of "AUTOLOGOUS BLOOD THERAPY" has not been attempted in that it contains a much larger number of citations (more than 1000). However, it is noted that less than 10% of these are Russian, the majority being in English.

## MARROW TODAY, BLOOD TOMORROW

Not specifically highlighted in Table 9-1, but to some extent overlapping with the many articles referred to therein which involve autologous blood therapy, is a rapidly expanding type of therapy which alone enables the statement to be made that the field of autologous blood therapy is poised to explosively grow. Such a prediction can be confidently made, thanks to the decision by the journal Bone Marrow Transplantation to adopt the new name of Blood and Bone Marrow Transplantation. This is due to the recognition of increased use of components taken from circulating blood rather than from bone marrow, for use in so-called bone-marrow transplantation procedures.

At the same time there has been a sustained trend toward the use of autologous methods, from 11.6% of all bone marrow transplants during the period 1966-1974, to 26.4% for the period 1990-1993.

This popular, growing and evolving use of autologous blood in therapy; whatever it's called, however explained, and totally independent of this current work and the rich tradition of autohemotherapy which it seeks to portray; seems to indicate that autohemotherapy is on schedule to become a dominant force in medicine by the early 21st century. [see MARROW file for projection and discussion]

## AUTOTRANSFUSION AS AUTOHEMOTHERAPY

Balazian VA, et al, "The effect of autologous blood transfusions on immunity in operated on neurosurgical patients", Zhurnal Voprosy Neirokhirurgii Imeni N. N. Burdenko, 1990 Jul-Aug (4):23-5. As compared to the use of donor blood, the authors found "Autohemo-transfusion proved to be more effective in preventing immuno-deficient states in the postoperative period, which was documented by increase of the absolute number of T-lymphocytes, stabilization of the content of immunoglobulin of the main classes, and decrease in the number of circulating immune complexes as compared to the initial values. The immunocorrective properties of donor blood yield noticeably to those of autologous blood."

## VACCINE-THERAPY UPDATE

## REINVENTING THE WHEEL - 1994

Science magazine in modern times (1994) has touted vaccine-

therapy as a desired <u>new</u> direction, citing prospects in therapy
of herpes simplex, leprosy and hepatitis. [J. Cohen (<u>Science</u>
264, 22 Apr. 94, 503-5; Merigan, T. in <u>ibid.</u>] Such a
characterization reflects little regard for the great amount of
useful work that has already been accomplished (for prime example
the work of E.C. Rosenow); and brings to mind Osler's admonition
that: "one who knows only current information about Medicine
does not even know that." [Sir William Osler, per McManus, J .F.
A., <u>The Fundamental Ideas of Medicine - A Brief History of</u>
<u>Medicine</u>, Charles C. Thomas, Springfield, Ill. 1963, p.6]
Certainly we are making progress in genuinely new ways - all the
more reason to integrate truly "new" facts with historical ones.

It is in any case encouraging that the concept of vaccine-
therapy is enjoying renewed attention, as in the above-referenced
and other contemporary <u>Science</u> and <u>Nature</u>, etc. articles on the
subject [e.g. Cohen, J., <u>Science</u> 265 (1994); P. Parham, <u>Nature</u>
368, 495-6 (1994); D.S. Burke, <u>Vaccine</u> 11, (1993) 883-94].


EXAMPLE: AUTOVACCINE FOR MS, DIABETES, ARTHRITIS - 1992

Numerous autovaccine items accessible through MEDLINE may be
identified through the use of the keywords/subjects listed in
Table 9-1. For example, Schwartz R, 1992, p. 1237, refers to
"reports of vaccination against experimental allergic
encephalomyelitis with clonotypic T-cell-receptor peptides, and a
preliminary report suggests the feasibility of key-cell
vaccination in MS." As per Altman 1992, Schwartz advocated such
an approach for treating a variety of diseases, "particularly
autoimmune disorders like MS, diabetes and rheumatoid arthritis."

The designation of "vaccine" implies the use of a properly
specific antigenic substance, which in the case of blood-borne
diseases will be carried in the circulating blood by definition;
thus autoblood used in autohemotherapy will presumably contain
the specific organism.

Even more preferable would be the use of specific autovaccines
prepared in accord with Rosenow's instructions, insofar as this
allows for controlling concentration of vaccine dosage. Note
Rosenow's successes with focus removal/autovaccines in these
conditions, in which he repeatedly fulfilled the Henle-Koch
requisites for establishing causation. (see *REFERENCE MANUAL*
*ROSENOW ET AL*)


A STRIKING CANCER CONNECTION - WHAT DOES IT MEAN?

Given the generic intravenous nature of serum therapy v. the
extravascular nature of vaccine therapy [see VASCULAR for
detailed discussion], autohemotherapy might be seen as a hybrid -
an extravascular form of serum therapy. From 1966-1993, of 221
total citations in MEDLINE subject "serum therapy", keyword
"autologous"; a mere 11 involve "intramuscular or subcutaneous or
intradermal" methods; of which only one refers to

autohemotherapy.  Three of the 11 have "melanoma" in the title.

As shown on the last line of Table 9-1, and in Table 9-2, of 215 total "vaccine therapy" citations in MEDLINE 1990-1993, 25 are "autologous" or "autogenous" (most are "autologous").  On closer inspection, these were found to have a most striking connection, i.e., as shown in Table 9-2, 23 of 25 also involve keywords "cancer" or "tumor".  In contrast, approaching the total 215 from another perspective, 103 or nearly half involve "cancer" or "tumor".  Thus only about one-fourth of these disease-qualified citations also have an "autologous" component, whereas most of the "autologous" citations relate to cancer therapy.

Within the subject area "serum therapy" for the period 1990-1993, 13 of 33 "autologous" citations similarly involve one of the two keywords "cancer" or "tumor".  Correlations are even stronger for the previous MEDLINE reporting period, from 1985 to 1989: 72 of 115 "serum therapy"/"autologous" citations involve "cancer" or "tumor".

What is to be made of these curious connections, relating to both "vaccine therapy" and "serum therapy"?

One might surmise this to reflect a tendency to employ, for the most serious diseases, the presumably more consuming and expensive procedures associated with the development of personalized "autologous" responses.  For less serious conditions, such levels of commitment might be considered unwarranted.  Should this be the case, it seems a shame that "autologous" therapy, now seemingly reserved for the most desperately ill, is being denied the masses; particularly when its safest, most proven and least expensive form (AUTOBLOOD-VACCINE) is so readily available - only a syringe away.

This is not intended to discourage efforts to develop even more effective methods.  However, (1) safe and inexpensive "classical" autohemotherapy can be initiated immediately in all cases, serious or not, and can be working toward improvement of the patient while manipulations or further investigations required by more sophisticated methods are performed, and (2) some detrimental side-effects of experimental methods, now in use on humans, might be kept to a minimum or confined to laboratory animals.  For example, one citation accessed under subject "vaccine therapy" [Sato K, et al., 1993] discusses "autoimmune hypothyroidism induced by lymphokine-activated killer (LAK) cell therapy", which LAK therapy is among "autologous" methods discussed in citations in MEDLINE subject "serum therapy" [e.g., Favrot MC, et al, 1990; Chuganju Y, et al., 1987].  (See MEDLINE for actual citations).

It is noted within the history of approaches to cancer treatment, that the autologous connection is as old as the field itself.  [See Chapter 10: AUTOLOGOUS THERAPY FOR CANCER]

TABLE 9-1:   MELVYL MEDLINE 1966 to 1994 (inclusive)

| | | Numbers of articles by years | | | | |
|---|---|---|---|---|---|---|
| | Years: | 1966 -'74 | 1975 -'79 | 1980 -'84 | 1985 -'89 | 1990 -'94 |
| keyword: | autologous or autogenous | 11158 | 8537 | 6046 | 7769 | 10236 |
| SUBJECT: | AUTOLOGOUS | 10722 | 6894 | 2504 | 2549 | 4588 |

BLOOD/HEMO/SERO

keywords:

| | 1966 -'74 | 1975 -'79 | 1980 -'84 | 1985 -'89 | 1990 -'94 |
|---|---|---|---|---|---|
| autohemotherapy | 9 | 1 | 0 | 3 | 7 |
| autoblood + therapy | 2 | 2 | 4 | 20 | 23 |
| autologous + blood + therapy | 248 | 362 | 397 | 778 | 1485 |
| "          "    + subcutaneous | 10 | 34 | 23 | 21 | 59 |
| "          "    + intramuscular | 6 | 6 | 4 | 4 | 8 |
| "     + hemosorption | 0 | 0 | 1 | 5 | 9 |
| "     + hemotherapy | 0 | 0 | 7 | 9 | 33 |
| "     + serum + therapy | 13 | 69 | 107 | 149 | 218 |

SUBJECT:

| | 1966 -'74 | 1975 -'79 | 1980 -'84 | 1985 -'89 | 1990 -'94 |
|---|---|---|---|---|---|
| SERUM THERAPY | 1728 | 1575 | 2236 | 3883 | 2160 |
| + keyword: autologous/autogenous | 26 | 17 | 29 | 116 | 35 |
| PASSIVE IMMUNIZATION | 1712 | 1570 | 2227 | 3873 | 2156 |
| + keyword: autologous/autogenous | 26 | 17 | 29 | 116 | 35 |

VACCINE

keywords:

| | 1966 -'74 | 1975 -'79 | 1980 -'84 | 1985 -'89 | 1990 -'94 |
|---|---|---|---|---|---|
| autogenous + vaccin# | 25 | 14 | 6 | 10 | 9 |
| autovaccin# | 29 | 13 | 15 | 12 | 19 |
| autologous + vaccin# | 14 | 59 | 48 | 78 | 209 |

SUBJECT:

| | 1966 -'74 | 1975 -'79 | 1980 -'84 | 1985 -'89 | 1990 -'94 |
|---|---|---|---|---|---|
| VACCINE THERAPY | 0 | 0 | 0 | 5 | 276 |
| + keyword: autologous/autogenous | - | - | - | 1 | 28 |
| ACTIVE IMMUNIZATION | 6664 | 3140 | 3023 | 3119 | 4075 |
| + keyword: autologous/autogenous | 7 | 11 | 8 | 16 | 29 |

Note: # = extension; listings include all words with root.

Table 9-2: THE AUTO/VACCINE/SERO CANCER-TUMOR CONNECTION

| | Years: | 1966 -'74 | 1975 -'79 | 1980 -'84 | 1985 -'89 | 1990 -'93 |
|---|---|---|---|---|---|---|

A. "Autologous" subject area, qualified
   by keyword: cancer, tumor or lymph#

| | 1966 -'74 | 1975 -'79 | 1980 -'84 | 1985 -'89 | 1990 -'93 |
|---|---|---|---|---|---|
| subject area: vaccine therapy | 0 | 0 | 0 | 5 | 276 |
| + keyword: autologous/autogenous | - | - | - | 1 | 28 |
|    and kw: cancer or tumor | - | - | - | 1 | 26 |
| | | | | | |
| subject area: active immunization | 6664 | 3140 | 3023 | 3119 | 4075 |
| + keyword: autologous/autogenous | 7 | 11 | 8 | 16 | 29 |
|    and kw: cancer or tumor | 1 | 1 | 0 | 7 | 11 |
| | | | | | |
| subject area: serum therapy | 1728 | 1575 | 2236 | 3883 | 2160 |
| + keyword: autologous/autogenous | 26 | 17 | 29 | 115 | 35 |
|    and kw: cancer or tumor | 2 | 2 | 10 | 72 | 14 |
| | | | | | |
| subject area: passive immunization | 1712 | 1570 | 2227 | 3873 | 2156 |
| + keyword: autologous/autogenous | 26 | 17 | 29 | 115 | 35 |
|    and kw: cancer or tumor | 2 | 2 | 10 | 72 | 14 |

B. Subject area (total), qualified
   by keyword: cancer, tumor or lymph#

| | 1966 -'74 | 1975 -'79 | 1980 -'84 | 1985 -'89 | 1990 -'93 |
|---|---|---|---|---|---|
| subject area: vaccine therapy | 0 | 0 | 0 | 5 | 276 |
|    and kw: cancer or tumor | - | - | - | 5 | 131 |
| subject area: serum therapy | 1728 | 1575 | 2236 | 3883 | 2160 |
|    and kw: cancer or tumor | 113 | 171 | 174 | 482 | 176 |

Chapter 10: AUTOLOGOUS THERAPY FOR CANCER


CANCER - MONEY HONEY


P. Parham [Nature 368, 495-6, 7 Apr. 94, "Politically incorrect viruses"] asserts "The cure and prevention of cancer by vaccination are the sustaining dreams of tumour immunology ... [but] the practice has yet to work in humans.  ... Almost by definition, the tumours that trouble humans are those against which there is inadequate immune response."

Parham discusses four tumour viruses - hepatitis B virus (HBV), human papilloma virus, human T lymphocyte virus 1 and Epstein-Barr virus (EBV), and concludes in view of "inevitably expensive and long-term clinical trials" which will be required for vaccine development, "the support of governments will be most urgently needed.

Notwithstanding Parham's dismal assessment, efforts at vaccine-therapy have to some extent been reported as successful.]


AUTOLOGOUS THERAPY FOR CANCER
 - A brief history

In a review of attempts to treat cancer patients by active immunization, Southam's very first (1902) and two of his next three citations are specifically noted as "autologous" (the source of vaccine in the other is not stated).  Southam's discussions of these attempts fall into two time periods, 1902-1922 and 1951-60, and include the following items:


Autologous therapy for cancer - 1902-1922

--1902 - injection of "two advanced cancer patients with a filtrate of their own tumor tissue.  There was no apparent change in their downhill course, but some enlarged glands appeared to shrink."

--1909 - "objective regression in one patient with cancer of the neck following autologous cancer vaccine injections ..."

--1910 - "treatment of seventeen patients with phenolized autogenous tumor homogenates.  No therapeutic effect was noted."

--1912 - "formalinized or phenolized (and occasionally fresh) autologous cancer tissue [was used]to vaccinate (subcutaneously) 39 patients ... none showed any objective improvement."

--1913 - "disappearance of uterine cancer after vaccine injections in one patient, who was still well 6 months after treatment."

--1914 - "patient with mammary carcinoma simplex and axillary and supraclavicular nodes had objective regression of ... lesions after IV and subcutanteous injections of an autogenous tissue [vaccine]." --1922 - "freshly excised and minced cancer tissue [was exposed] to x-ray at a dosage (2 rads) ... [and] then implanted in the rectus sheath ... . In no case was there any alteration of the course of disease that could not be attributed to antecedent treatment ... ."


Autologous therapy for cancer - 1951-1961:

--1951 - "autologous cancer tissue fragments [were] frozen at -20 degrees C for 5-23 days [and implanted] into 3 patients with breast cancer. One patient had a surgical cure ... another was followed for only a month ... and the third died of unknown cause ... ."

--1959 - of 29 advanced cancer patients injected with autologous cancer vaccines [preparation varied, including whole-cell suspensions, cell extracts, and cell fragments, administered intradermally or intramuscularly in Freund-type adjuvants], "there was objective evidence of tumor regression in three", however none satisfy criteria establishing that this was due to the vaccination.

--1960 - "repeated intramuscular injections of autologous cancer vaccines in Freund's adjuvant [were given] to nine male patients with advanced carcinomas and sarcomas. Their vaccines were whole tissue minces repeatedly frozen and thawed to kill the cells.. ... about 2 weeks after initial IM injection of the vaccine, there was inflammation followed by softening and shrinkage of subcutaneous tumors in all (? three) patients who had such lesions."

--1960 - gamma globulin from serum of 3 of these patients who had developed autoantibodies was prepared and injected into or around their tumor nodules, followed by "a significant shrinkage... .


Autologous therapy for cancer - as of 1961

Regarding the very possibility of therapy for cancer, Southam's 1961 assessment was not too hopeful overall, in that "the patient who has now *got* cancer must be an individual who has failed to respond to the stimulus of his own cancer. ... On the other hand, one can argue that ... a potentially effective antigen had somehow been prevented from acting -- perhaps because of ... failure of the antigen to reach the antibody-producing cells." [We are here reminded of Sir Almroth Wright's discussions of differences in bodily response from injection into the tissues vs. injection into the circulation.]

In the case of active immunity, Southam identified both humoral and cellular specific approaches as synonomous with "autologous cancer vaccines", but did not discuss them further. Regarding passive immunity, the author noted this requires "both the recognition and the production of yet-to-be-discovered humoral substances and introduces the problems of quantity production, doubtful efficacy in advanced disease, and toxic reactions."

As regards cancer prevention, Southam dismissed any possible role for passive immunity, saying that only in the mechanisms of specific active immunity was there "any real probability of cancer prophylaxis." (In the case of cancer therapy, these mechanisms corresponded to approaches identified by Southam as synonomous with "autologous vaccines"; in the case of cancer prevention, the assumption would be that there is no autologous-cancerous substance from which to make a vaccine.)

Southam concluded that "if neoplastic cells in the human population should be characterized by a finite number of cancer-specific antigens, and if these antigens are accessible to the action of antibodies, the possibility for prophylaxis does exist." However, he offered "if such antigens are unique in every individual there is clearly no possibility for prophylactic immunization".

[ON THE OTHER HAND, IF A CANCER-SPECIFIC ANTIGEN IS IN THE BLOOD PRIOR TO THE ADVANCE OF A CANCER, THEN AUTOHEMOTHERAPY (IM) MIGHT SERVE A USEFUL PROPHYLACTIC PURPOSE].


Autologous therapy for cancer - 1961-1970

In their final chapter, "Tumors of man", on the subject of "active immunization", Harris and Sinkovics refer to a number of autologous efforts over the prior decade, without specific reference to the fact that a large portion of their citations are autologous. These include production of vaccine from autologous tumor cell extracts in carcinomas and melanoma whereby "Four patients showed objective improvement after administration of the autovaccine"; and autologous leukemia cell extracts used for immunization after chemotherapy, whereby "patients receiving autovaccine appear to remain in remission for a more prolonged time." The authors also noted that "immunization against autologous tissue occurs upon freezing", as indicated by organ- and species-specific antibodies in rabbit serum four days after the freezing of their prostrate gland; in one human patient with malignant melanoma of the leg and one with basal cell carcinoma, temporary regression of the tumors and antibody response resulted. Additionally, "freeze-thawed, heat inactivated, and filtered extracts of condyloma acuminatum tissue was used as an autovaccine in 21 patients. The benign tumors dried up after the administration of 3 to 4 weekly injections of the autovaccine."

On the subject of "passive immunization" the authors are not encouraging, specifically highlighting complications of fatal glomerulonephritis and "production of tumor-enhancing antibodies".

With respect to "adoptive immunization", whereby "a tumor-bearing host may adopt lymphoid cells from a donor immunized to the tumor, the authors allow for a broad intrepretation so as to include treatment with the patient's own lymphoid cells - which are exposed to the tumor in vitro, mass-produced and reinjected. No results of this specific totally autologous method are detailed. However the authors do refer to several instances using other persons or animals as donors, including reduction of pleural effusion in two of 12 patients with neoplastic pleural effusions or ascites who were treated with spleen cells of rabbits immunized with the patients' neoplastic cells. [We may note that pleural effusions were successfully treated by Gilbert's simple autoserotherapy method 100 years ago, and by numerous practitioners since (far better than the 2 out of 12 in this rabbit study].

### Autologous therapy for cancer - as of 1970

In their 1970 discussions of the future of cancer therapy and prevention, Harris and Sinkovics emphasized the "autologous" component in discussions of the future of cancer therapy, without specific discussion of the merits of autologous vs. allogenic approaches.

In their concluding section, they briefly mentioned clinical work directed at "nonspecifically stimulating the host lymphocytes", but offer "It appears more promising to activate autologous lymphocytes by exposure to tumor antigens and to reinfuse these lymphocytes into the tumor-bearing patient. ... The approaches fit for further pursuit are those promising active immunization without the production of tumor-enhancing antibodies and methods of adoptive immunization with avoidance of both chronic homolgous disease and the necessity of prolonged extensive immunosuppressive treatment."

[None of these drawbacks would be involved with a strictly autologous approach, e.g., mascerated autologous cancer tissue in fresh autoblood, injected intramuscularly, biweekly; such an augmented autoblood-IM method would force exposure of any cancer antigen in cancer tissue or blood to lymphocytes within the autoblood and in the target tissues.]

### Autologous therapy for cancer - 1970-1994

In a summary discussion of human cancer vaccines of historical importance from the early 1970s to 1994, Sinkovics, Horvath and Szabo-Szabari cite an assortment of autologous and allogenic techniques; however, their concluding substantive section bears the title "Autologous human cancer vaccines we prepare", and is comprised of discussions of the authors' own efforts with autologous vaccines for melanoma, kidney carcinoma and bronchioloalveolar carcinomas.

For a comprehensive look at citations on cancer therapy since 1966, autologous or other, the reader is referred to the keyword "CANCER", etc., within MEDLINE subject areas VACCINE-THERAPY, ACTIVE IMMUNIZATION, and SERUM-THERAPY or PASSIVE IMMUNIZATION (as in Table 9-2).  Please note that within respective subjects "vaccine therapy" and "active immunization", keyword "autologous" citations for the most part are non-duplicative; this may be taken as an indication that some desired citations may have evaded inclusion in otherwise-presumed-comprehensive subject areas.


Friend, USA TODAY, Dec. 1988, discusses development of a vaccine against malignant melanoma, a deadly skin cancer, prospects of vaccine against other cancers, and hope for new melanoma cases.


Bibliography - Autologous Therapy for Cancer:


--Southam, C.M., "Applications of Immunology to Clinical Cancer; Past Attempts and Future Possibilities", Cancer Research 21 (1961), 1302-1317.

--Harris JE and JG Sinkovics, The immunology of malignant disease, C.V. Mosby Co., St. Louis, 1970.

--Sinkovics, J, Horvath J, and Szabo-Szabari M, "Human cancer vaccines", Leukemia, Apr. 1994, 8 Suppl.1:S194-7.


CANCER: AUTOTHERAPEUTICAL MISCELLANY


CELLCOR 1991

John Rennie in Scientific American 264, 120 (June 1991) discussed controversy over claims of a Newton Mass. firm, Cellcor Therapies, that its $22,000 autolymphocyte therapy can double the average survival time of some kidney cancer patients.  The method involves extraction, treatment and reinfusion of lymphocytes.


AUTOLYMPHYCYTES USEFULLY AUGMENT ULCER DRUG THERAPY 1990

Prevention 42, 18-20 , October 1990, discussed an April 28, 1990 report in Lancet on the research of M. Osband, which combined the "standard" cimetidine (ulcer) drug therapy with autolymphocyte therapy, indicating patients receiving this combined treatment lived at least 2.5 times longer than a control group receiving the drug only.


AUTOVACCINE FOR MELANOMA  1990

Berd D, et al, J of Clin. Oncolog, 1990 Nov, 8(11):1858-67, "Treatment of metastatic melanoma with an autologous tumor-cell vaccine" clinical and immunologic results in 64 patients", intradermally administered a vaccine made of autologous, enzymatically dissociated, cryopreserved, irradiated (25 Gy) tumor cells mixed with bacillus "Calmette-Guerin".  The authors asserted "This demonstration that an immune response to melanoma-associated antigens can be elicited in cancer-bearing patients provides some basis for optimism about the prospects for developing active immunotherapy that has practical therapeutic value."

UCLA 1995

Ben Gilmore, " UCLA treatment brings health, hope for kidney cancer victims", Daily Bruin News, Jan. 25, 1995, p. 8, 14, discusses a method pioneered by Dr. S. Rosenberg at the National Cancer Institute and developed for 5 years by UCLA doctors. The treatment involves removal of the cancerous tissue, extracting from it "tumor-infiltrating lymphocytes (TILs)", culturing these for about 55 days, and reinjecting them intravenously in the patient. The UCLA Kidney Cancer center has reported that 44% of patients have showed partial or complete responses, which "does not mean complete remission" cautioned one researcher. The UCLA study, which involved 25 patients, is being expanded to 200 patients in a national study. There are some side effects. According to one UCLA researcher, "It's a rough treatment, no doubt about it .... It's chronic and prolonged. Patients experience fever, chills, fatigue, nausea and diarrhea. ... The treatment is not yet FDA-approved. "Ironically, the component of the treatment which causes the adverse side-effects, interleukin II, is already FDA-approved .... Interleukin II, a growth factor which causes the TIL cells to multiply and become better cancer fighters, is included in the intravenous treatment."

CANCER - SOME CITATIONS IN AUTOMED BIBLIOGRAPHIES

A total 23 citations referring to cancer are found in AUTOMED bibliographies included in this series of volumes: three, at quarter-century-plus intervals from 1902, from the Rosenow Bibliography are listed below (from APPENDIX A2 in *REFERENCE MANUAL ROSENOW ET AL)*; eight, from 1929, are in the Auto-Vaccine Bibliography (APPENDIX D of this current volume; and twelve, from as early as 1913, are "autohemotherapy" or "autoserotherapy" items in the Autohemotherapy Bibliography (APPENDIX C of this current volume).

Autohemotherapy/autoserotherapy for cancer (see citations below, in APPENDIX C: AUTOHEMOTHERAPY BIBLIOGRAPHY):

--24A3 [autoserum], 27B13, 29A5, 29A18 [irrad.autoser], 53C3

--anaphylaxis in - 26A2

--breast - 13H1 [autoserotherapy]

--malignant tumors - 30B11 [irradiated autoblood]   --rectum - 16H4 [autoserum]

--uterus - 29B19 (changes in blood)

--washed auto-erythrocytes, vagaries - 34A22


Autogenous vaccine-therapy for cancer:

--cancer: 66P2 Snegotska O.  Folia Clin Int (Barc) 15:303-8, Jun 65 (Sp)

--canine lymphoma:77P1 Julliard GJ et al., Int J Radiat Oncol Biol Phys 1(5-6):497-503, March-Apr. 1976

--gastric cancer: 48J2 [C. Finkelstein] Gastroenterologia 73:45-55, '48

--mouse carcinoma, implanted: 29K11 (M. 63), [T. Lumsden]  Lancet 2: 814-816, Oct. 19, '29

--osteogenic sarcoma: 72F2 Marcove, R.C., et al., Surg. Forum 22:434-5, 1971; 74P1 Southam CM, Et al. Proc Natl Cancer Conf 7:91-100,1973; 75P1 Marcove RC. Beitr Pathol 153(1):65-72, Oct 74

--tumors: 79P1 Peters LC, et al. Cancer Res.39(4):1353-60, Apr 79

--uterine cervix cancer: 35J7 [T. Messerschmidt] Fortschr.d. Therap. 11:156-159, March '35


Rosenow, on cancer:

--agglutination titers, leukemia & carcinoma [Am. Practitioner and Digest of Treatment, 9(5), 1958, 755-761.]

--brain tumor, syphilis of central nervous system: [J. Infect. Dis. 52:167-184, 1933. (With LB Jensen)]

--urinary stone, tumor:  [Am. Jour. Med. Sc. 123:634-642, 1902.]


The writer is sufficiently encouraged by Rosenow's cancer work, however scanty, to (1) call attention once more to the role of the oral focus in initiating the disease process in the first place, arguing for removal of the oral focus in all cases of advance disease unless all hope is absolutely lost and stirring up the oral focal nest would likely only hasten the patient's demise; and (2) beyond this to suggest either (a) cultivation of a central-tumor-extract in accord with Rosenow's streptococcus-growing-recipe and preparation of Rosenow's antigen and antibody, possibly with autoblood as menstruum so as to assure inclusion of any/all hematogenous factors; or (b), failing this, a direct-tumor-extract-in-autoblood-menstruum intramuscular cocktail.  At least this is what the writer would choose to do for himself if confronted with the situation.


ORAL FOCUS IN DISEASE-CANCER CASCADE

In that there is a known progression from oral focal infection to systemic diseases such as stomach ulcers, and further a progression from such systemic disease to cancerous conditions, such as stomach cancer, the role of oral foci as kicking off the cascade to cancer seems clear.  One might suggest that the progression to cancer indicates attainment of some advanced and independent status for the secondary focus (e.g. the stomach lesion).  Clearly at such a point removal of the initiating oral focus alone will not cure the now-aggressively-independent secondary infection, except that this in conjunction with autogenous vaccine and removal of cancerous tissue, when and as possible, would seem to be indicated.  However, there is a ray of hope in such an assessment in that up to this point the lesion has not taken off on its own; hence up to this point the removal of any and all implicated oral foci, in conjunction with autovaccine, may be capable of curtailing or even reversing the involved disease processes without surgical intervention.  That at least is the logical theoretical position that follows from this characterization.

APPENDIX A: AUTOHEMOTHERAPY CHRONOLOGY


INTRODUCTORY


The term "autoserotherapy" enjoyed two distinct and somewhat overlapping identities, referred to herein and discussed below as "autoserotherapy #1" and "autoserotherapy #2",  The former, with specific reference to "Gilbert of Geneva", 1894, involved the subcutaneous reinjection of autogenous serous fluid in pleural effusions; and the latter, generally traced to Spiethoff 1913 but with prior precedents, involved the reinjection of venous blood-serum.  Initially the unqualified term "autoserotherapy" indicated Gilbert's method, but between 1913 and 1919 it underwent a transformation, referring less to Gilbert and moreso to reinjection of autogenous blood-serum.  Subsequent reference to the Gilbert method generally invoked his name.


AUTOSEROTHERAPY-#1: THE PIONEERING WORK OF "GILBERT OF GENEVA"


Beginning in 1891, Gilbert of Geneva [1894H1] treated pleuritic patients with "hypodermic injections of their own exudate ... the method was based on researches made in 1890 and 1891 by Debove and Rémond on the presence of tuberculin in the peritoneal exudate of tuberculosis subjects." [Austin, 11E2].  It is noted particularly that the Gilbert method was discussed for pleurisy in the following below-discussed items: 1894H1, 11E2, 11E4, 14H1, 16A1, 15H1, 16A1, 11E1, 31A7.  It is also noted that the Gilbert method continues to be utilized, as seemingly apparent in the work of Chiyoda and Morikawa 1993, listed and abstracted below.

Items discussing Gilbert's method are integrated below within this CHRONOLOGY, with specific reference to "GILBERT".


NOTES ON SERUM THERAPY; BACKGROUND FOR AUTOSEROTHERAPY #2


Apart from the direction of Gilbert's work, a tradition of serum therapy evolved from the work of Kitasato Shibasaburo and Emil von Behring's work in the 1890s; this work progressed despite Sir Almroth Wright's protestations that the reported beneficial action of this "serum therapy" appeared to be that of autogenous vaccine-therapy. [see VACCINE/WRIGHT]

Whatever the mechanism, by 1910 reportedly "millions of lives had been saved from death by diphtheria or tetanus by the judicious uses of immune sera from the blood of horses." Serum therapy treatment was found to provide temporary immunity. [Chase, 302].

Over the years, variations on the serum therapy theme have been employed in a wide range of diseases.  For example serum therapy is known to have been employed in the case of malaria since 1900 [P.E. Russell, MAN'S MASTERY OF MALARIA (1955), p. 106]. And in 1924 Calvin Coolidge Jr. received an infusion of blood from a donor who had been innoculated with killed bacteria from cultures, in the hopes of transferring passive immunity from an already too-massive staphylococcus albus bacteria infection, as part of an exhaustive and unsuccessful effort to save his life. [Lehrer, 277-8]

The tradition of serum therapy continues to the present time, as seen in the continuing existence of the well populated subject area of "serum therapy" in the NIH MEDLINE index [see MEDLINE UPDATES].

BIBLIOGRAPHY FOR "NOTES ON SERUM THERAPY"

P.E. Russell, MAN'S MASTERY OF MALARIA (1955), p. 106

Allan Chase, MAGIC SHOTS, William Morrow, 1982

Steven Lehrer, EXPLORERS OF THE BODY, Doubleday, 1979.

G. Marks and W.K. Beatty, EPIDEMICS.


AUTOSEROTHERAPY-#2:LITERATURE (VENOUS BLOOD)


"Autoserotherapy #2" evolved within the general framework of "serum therapy", (the reinjection of autogenous blood-serum) seems to have been given particular impetus by the 1913 works of Spiethoff (autoserum) [13E6, 13E7]. However, long before Spiethoff, as early as 1901, Jez [01H1] had reported the subcutaneous reinjection of autogenous blood-serum drawn from a vein in the treatment of erysipelas, and in 1905 Browning [] had discussed theoretical considerations based on Jez's experiments. Although Elfstrom had attempted the use of venous blood-serum as early as 1898, Jez apparently was the first to succeed.

Autoserotherapy (blood serum) items have been also integrated into this CHRONOLOGY, and do in any case involve blood. Although the field of autohemotherapy clearly had evolved from autoserotherapy (with blood serum), before long "autohemotherapy" virtually sqeezed out "autoserotherapy" from the "serum therapy" category of the INDEX MEDICUS. It is also noted that some of the articles with "autohemotherapy" in their titles are not actually discussing whole blood but rather are concerned with blood serum. This particularly applies to instances of intravenous reinjection.


THE RISE OF "CLASSICAL" AUTOHEMOTHERAPY

## Origins of Autohemotherapy

As has been noted in the case of the ancient practice of bloodletting (see Chapter 3, BLOODLETTING ...) that no definite date can be assigned to its origination, so it is with autohemotherapy.  If indeed to some extent the reported beneficial action of bloodletting may be attributed to resorption of some of the blood being let, then autohemotherapy is as old as bloodletting; or alternatively, bloodletting may be viewed as the earliest form of controlled autohemotherapy.  Thus it is to be expected that the roots of the "modern" (early 20th century) autohemotherapy movement might be at least somewhat muddled, as seen in the case of Elfstrom's 1898 efforts, and also for example in the case of Bier [05H1 per Tillman 35B14].


RAVAUT'S "AUTOHEMATOTHERAPY" MARKS BIRTH OF AUTOHEMOTHERAPY

Notwithstanding these efforts and the prior works of Elfstrom in 1898, Jez in 1901 and Bier in 1905 mentioned above, the main body of literature on the subject of the history of "autohemotherapy" generally refers to a 1913 article by Ravaut [13H2] as initiator of the field of autohemotherapy.  Ironically, Ravaut's title referred not to autohemotherapy, but rather to "autohematotherapy".

Immediately following Spiethoff's initial discussion of the use of "eigenserum" or autoserum, Ravaut reported on the use of a simplified procedure comprised of immediate reinjection of whole blood.  Spiethoff echoed with reference to his prior use of both autoblood <u>and</u> autoserum therapy, but credit for the whole blood method stuck to Ravaut.  The distinct body of literature that blossomed up through the 1920s and 1930s generally acknowledged the role of Ravaut as founder of the field of "autohemotherapy", which literature constitutes the heart of this volume.


START CHRONOLOGY


We will begin this chronology with Elfstrom's 1898 use of subcutaneously-reinjected leech-drawn blood, revisiting Gilbert's 1894 autoserotherapy through the writings of later writers, and Spiethoff and Ravaut in sequence..


1894H1:  Gilbert, Gaz. d. hospitaux, Paris, 1894, Vol. LXVIII. (as per 14H6.


1898H1:  Elfstrom, Carl E. and Axel V. Grafstrom, Heated Blood in Croupous Pneumonia, N.Y.Med. J. 26 Aug. 1898:307-9; 15 Oct. 1898:556; 30 Sept. 1899:486-7.


ELFSTROM'S PREHISTORIC (1898H1) USE OF SUBCUTANEOUS AUTOBLOOD

Although the Gilbert methodology was well known by the late 1890s, Carl E. Elfstrom of Brooklyn U.S.A. reportedly did not base his work on Gilbert, but rather in 1898 [1898H1] described how his "mind's eye" conceived of autogenous blood therapy. His method was based on the work of G. & F. Klemperer in 1891, who had "succeeded in conferring immunity upon susceptible animals by inoculating them with filtered cultures of the micrococcus" [pneumoniae crouposa] and found that the potency of the filtrates was increased upon heating (40-42 degrees C for 3-4 days or 60 degrees for 1-2 hours). Elfstrom reasoned that if heating might increase the potency of such filtrates, it might also increase the potency of those elements in the blood that confer immunity: "Does not lobar pneumonia, for instance, with its high temperature, limited time, and crisis, prove the plausibility of such a theory? ... Let some blood be taken from a patient suffering from an infectious disease, such as pneumonia, typhoid fever, diphtheria, yellow fever, etc., and heated to a temperature of 60 degrees for two hours, and let it be injected subcutaneously into the patient's body. Why, then, should not the immunity hereby be hastened, that is, the duration of the disease shortened?"

## AUTOBLOOD FOR CROUPOUS PNEUMONIA, SUBCUTANEOUS - 1898H1

Elfstrom's first reported case, croupous pneumonia complicated by otitis media, in a 30 year old woman: "Temperature 104 to 105 Deg. F; great prostration. I saw the patient the 7th day of the disease, and applied 2 leaches on the breast. When well-filled they were taken off, and by means of salt the blood was squeezed in a clean tumbler and mixed with a salt solution (9-tenths %) in a proportion of 1 to 6. This mixture was put in a test tube, which was finally placed in water and heated to 60 degrees for 2 hours. The blood was now subcutaneously injected into the breast of the patient. ... within a week the patient was restored to health."

A second case involved a 3-1/2 year old child with "croupous pneumonia unilateral, as a sequela of scarlatina and complicated by meningitis. High temperature. Comatose condition and twitching of both arms." Here Elfstrom withdrew venous blood, defibrinated it, mixed it with salt solution, heated it, and reinjected it. The child remained comatose and died 2 days later.

In two subsequent cases, both children, but neither comatose, Elfstrom used one leech on the arm and both patients recovered.

"Not seeing any advantage in taking blood directly from a vein, I now always employ leeches ... ." Elfstrom had also decided to use only one leech in each case, and that the temperature of heat be 176 degrees F. In pneumonia he had only used one injection each, but in other diseases, e.g. phthisis, he had not achieved "very brilliant" results even with repeated injections at intervals of 5-14 days, and had decided to repeat injections each 3rd day.

In subsequent reports, Elfstrom and Grafstrom restricted his comment to croupous pneumonia, in all reporting on 9 cases, of which 2 died. "As these latter already before the injections gave unmistakable signs of meningitis ... the percentage of cure ... up to the present, has been 100 percent."

05H1: Bier, A., Die Entzünndung. Arch. klin. Chir. Bd. 176, S 529.

LUNG INFLAMMATION - 05H1 per 35B14

Reportedly independent of prior efforts, Bier had injected autoblood in 1905 to treat lung inflammation.

11E1:  Lemann, I.I., Auto-serotherapy in the treatment of collections of fluids in serous cavities. N. ORL. M. & S. J., 1910-11, lxiii, 327-333.

SAFETY OF THE GILBERT METHOD - Lemann [11E1]:  "The procedure which I am about to present to you is, because of its simplicity and harmlessness, worthy of more attention and investigation than it has received. ... Fede reports ... no reaction, local or general took place, except in one case of tuberculosis. In this the prostration and rise in temperature promptly subsided."

11E2:  Austin, C.K., Reports on Autoserotherapy. INTERNAT. CLIN., PHILA., 1910, 20. s., iii, 24-32.

SAFETY OF THE GILBERT METHOD - Austin [11E2]:  "The treatment ... is dangerous neither during or after its application .... [Gilbert] does not hesitate to state that he looks upon the treatment as efficacious in the majority of cases, and without any risk whatever."

11E4:  Lemann, I.I., Autoserotherapy; the therapeutic use of the patients own serous exudates and transudates. INTERSTATE M. J., ST. LOUIS, 1911, xvii, 288-297.

GILBERT'S AUTOSEROTHERAPY -   Lemann [11E4]

Lemann [11E4] relates "The almost unanimous verdict of all those who have employed it, is that the method is entirely without danger and usually without systemic reaction. ... " Lemann p. 296-7 summarizes results of his and 28 other investigators, involving a total of 309 cases, mostly tuberculous pleurisies, of which 232 were considered successes, and 75 were listed as failures.

12E4:  Landmann, G., Ueber authämotherapie. VERHANDL. D.

GESELLSCH. DEUTSCH. NATURF. U. AERZTE, KÖNIGSB., LEIPZ., 1911, lxxxii, 2. Teil, 67-69.

AUTHÄMOTHERAPIE FOR TUBERCULOSIS - 12E4

AUTHÄMOTHERAPIE FOR INOPERABLE CANCER - 12E4

The term "autohemotherapy" was first used in the INDEX MEDICUS in reference to G. Landmann-Darmstadt's 1911 article, which article was actually entitled "Über authämotherapie" [12E4]). Landmann-Darmstadt had advocated the subcutaneous reinjection of autologous blood-serum for tuberculosis and inoperable cancer, referring to the prior work of Gilbert in the case of pleuritis. Also in 1911 C. Oliva [Zeitschr. fur Klin. Med., Berlin (1911), 289-297] had discussed the "physical chemical changes in the blood after bloodletting and subcutaneous injection." This included "kryoskopie", "viskosität", "electrische leitfähigkeit", "oberflächenspannung", and "refraktometrie".


13E6: Spiethoff, B. Zur therapeutischen Verwendung des Eigenserums. MÜNCHEN MED. WCHNSCHR., 1913, lx, 521.

AUTOSEROTHERAPY: DERMATOSES - 13E6

In 1913 Spiethoff [13E6] discussed the therapeutical attributes of homologous and heterogenous serum, and other organic fluids, as background to a description of the reinjection of autogenous serum to treat various dermatoses. His technic involved the withdrawal of from 50-100 cc from the "kubitalvene", centrifuged it electrically for 3 minutes, heated the serum for 1/2 hour at 55-56 degrees C, and reinjected 10-25cc into the vein. This procedure was repeated 2-3 times weekly for a total of 6 times.


AUTOSEROTHERAPY: INTRAVENOUS AT INCEPTION - 13E6

It is noted that Spiethoff's initial autoserotherapy technic involved intravenous reinjection of blood-serum [13E6], as did other enthusiastic proponents including Vorschutz. Robertson [16H6] attempted both intravenous and subcutaneous reinjection, noting a preference for the former [e.g., Robertson 16H6, ]. Fox [14H2] used subcutaneous and IV injections interchangeably, without stating a preference for one or the other; Kaiser [17H1] used IM reinjections, and intraspinal in chorea; Thomas [41A6] and Marks [42B1] used subcutaneous autoserum; Woo [37A1] subcutaneously reinjected autogenous blister-serum.


13E7: Spiethoff, B. Zur Behandlung mit Eigenserum und Eigenblut. MED. KLIN., BERL., 1913, ix, 949.

SPIETHOFF'S RELUCTANCE TO GRANT PRIORITY TO RAVAUT - 13E7

Spiethoff [13E7] followed up Ravaut's publication (13H2, below) with reference to "the very remarkable communication of Prätorius" on the successful use of autogenous blood and simplicity and neatness of his method, despite Spiethoff's own preference for use of autoserotherapy.  "The publication of Paul Ravaut on the same method [as Prätorius, at least according to Spiethoff] has induced me to briefly describe an independently discovered method".  Spiethoff described the withdrawal of autoblood and reinjection intravascularly, suggesting the action is the same as that of autoserum.

13H1:  Lewin, "Autoserotherapy in Cancer", Therapie der Gegenwart (June 1913) per N.Y. Med. J., May 30, 1914, 1091.

### GILBERT METHOD FOR CANCER - 13H1

Lewin [13H1] per NYMJ [May 30, 1914, 1091] reported on 2 cases of breast cancer "with repeated recurrences notwithstanding operative treatment, in which the subcutaneous reinjection of 2.5 drams (10cc) of ascitic fluid obtained from the patients themselves resulted in apparent cure in both instances.  The measure is recommended as an adjuvant to other treatment in cases of cancer with ascites."

13H2:  Ravaut, M. Paul, "Essai sur L'Autohématothérapie dans Quelques Dermatoses", Ann. De Derm. er Syph. 4:292-6, May 1913.

### RAVAUT'S CLASSIC 1913 ARTICLE - 13H2
### AUTOHEMOTHERAPY: HERPES, TOXIC DERMATOSES OF PREGNANCY - 13H2

In his "classic" 1913 article, Ravaut refers to Mayer and Linser, 1910, who reported successful treatment of herpes gestations by injections of a serum from the blood of a pregnant woman, and to reports by them and several others of similar treatment of "toxic dermatoses" of pregnancy, including urticaria, pemphigus, dermatitis herpiformis, strophulus, prurigo, eczema and pruritus and various hemorrhagic diseases of the skin; Spiethoff, who was apparently the first in the series of investigators cited by Ravaut to use the serum obtained from the patient himself (autogenous), and who also in certain cases continued to advocate bloodletting; Hueck on Duhring's disease, psoriasis, eczema, urticaria and pruritus.  [13H2; see also Jones and Alden, 37B3; Wein, 25E7]

Ravaut refers to his "more simple" method of reinjection as "autohématothérapie", and pointed out that there was less risk of infection than might be encountered as a result of manipulation of autogenous serum, or due to someone else's infected blood. Ravaut concluded that it was more useful to inject the total blood to insure the inclusion of all blood elements that might play a useful role.

Ravaut emphasized that it seemed preferable to inject the total blood prior to allowing it to coagulate so that the substances or microbial bodies will, when resorbed by the organism, provoke a useful reaction.  Ravaut reported on the treatment of 3 acne, 3 psoriasis and seven other various skin disease cases.

13E11:  Mattei, C.  Modifications leucocytaires au cours de l'auto-hémato-thérapie.  COMPT. REND. SOC. DE BIOL., PAR., 1913, lxxv, 228.


AUTOHEMOTHERAPY - EFFECT ON BLOOD - 13E11

Shortly after the publication of Ravaut's article, Mattei [13E11] reported on studies of the effects of autohemotherapy on leukocytes.  It is noted for all 3 of 3 cases in which 4-day-later status was indicated, increases were indicated for "Globules blancs" and "Moyens mono."


13H2:  Ravaut, M. Paul, "Essai sur L'Autohématothérapie dans Quelques Dermatoses", Ann. De Derm. er Syph. 4:292-6, May 1913.


AUTOHEMOTHERAPY COMPELS PRODUCTION OF ANTIBODY - 13H2

Ravaut suggested that the reabsorption of blood injected under the skin compels the organism to produce a greater quantity of antibodies.


14H1:  Fisher, Henry M., "Autoserotherapy in Fibrinoserous Pleurisy ...", N.Y. Med. J., May 23, 1914, 1037-8.


GILBERT'S AUTOSEROTHERAPY - Fisher [14H1] discusses Schnütigen's report of success with 14 of 15 cases, with complete resorption of fluid within two weeks.  According to Fisher, Schnütigen insisted that "there is not the same danger of the formation of thick fibrinous exudation in the pleura in these autoinjected cases as when paracentesis has been performed."

As per Fisher, Gilbert had recommended the use of small amounts, 1-2cc at intervals of one or 2 days, and a total of 6 inoculations; some subsequent operators had used 5cc or more.


14H2:  Fox, Howard, "Autogenous serum in the treatment of psoriasis", J.A.M.A. LXIII(25):2190-4, Dec. 19, 1914


AUTOSERO: PSORIASIS - 14H2

In 1914 Fox [14H2] described the use of autogenous serum in the treatment of 28 psoriasis patients, 17 females and 11 males, from ages 11 to 54.  Different forms of the disease were represented, including "the guttae, mummular and diffuse" of varying grades of severity.


AUTOSEROTHERAPY METHOD  - 14H2

Fox's technic consisted of drawing 50cc of blood from the cubital vein, centrifuge it at 1800 rpm, and when the serum was thoroughly separated from corpuscles and fibrin, drawing it off in a glass syringe and injecting it "without delay, either intravenously or intramuscularly. The amount of serum obtained varied between 15 and 25 cc. The entire procedure was completed in under a half-hour. Generally at least 3 injections were given, at intervals of from 3-5 days, each followed by local application of a 10% chrysarobin ointment. [It is noted that Fox used both intravenous and intramuscular reinjection.]

## AUTOSEROTHERAPY RESULTS - 14H2

"The results of the treatment in general were very satisfactory and in some of the cases decidedly brilliant." One psoriasis patient characterized the results as "perfectly marvelous", another "like magic"; particularly pleased was "a man who was relieved of his psoriasis for the first time in 24 years."

## AUTOSEROTHERAPY SAFETY, WITH VENOUS BLOOD - 14H2

"No ill effects from the serum treatment were observed except in one case in which the 3rd injection was followed by a rather violent urticaria lasting a week. Urticarial rashes were also observed by Linser in several cases, generally lasting from 12 to 24 hours [non-autogenous injections]. In the case of autogenous serum injections, it is hardly conceivable that any serious ill effects could result when proper aseptic precautions were observed.

## AUTOSEROTHERAPY AS VENESECTION? - 14H2

"The idea naturally presents itself that the beneficial action might be solely due to the bloodletting. That this therapeutic measure may lessen the intensity of some inflammatory skin diseases there can be no doubt; that the results obtained were due, however, to the injections of the serum and not merely to the venipuncture has been shown by comparative tests with the two methods of treatment."

14H3: Gottheil, Wm. S. & David L. Satenstein, "The Autoserum Treatment in Dermatology", J.A.M.A. LXIII:1190-1194, 3 October 1914.

## AUTOSEROTHERAPY: INITIAL SKEPTICISM OF ONE CONVERT - 14H3

Gottheil and Saterstein [14H3] relate "It was with considerable skepticism that we read the reports that have been published during the last year or two concerning the treatment of certain dermatoses with serum, autogenous or foreign; and the more so since these reports were in some cases of that very rosey hew which we have learned to know as the reflection of the subjective illumination of the observer.

AUTOSEROTHERAPY METHOD - 14H3

From 40-200 cc blood is removed, usually the larger amount, allowed to clot for about 10 minutes, broken up with a glass rod and centrifuged at about 5000 rpm for 30-40 minutes.  40-45% of the blood drawn is recovered as serum, and reinjected in a vein usually on the opposite side from that drawn.

AUTOSEROTHERAPY, SAFETY OF  - 14H3

"We have now given over 250 of these autoserum injections, without seeing, save in a single case, any contra-indications to their employment. ... The one exception was in a very bad case of gangrenous radiodermatitis in a case of leukemia in which the patient did marvelously well under the first four, but had a reaction, and chills followed by fever after the 5th and 6th .... [Nonetheless] the result here was not to be described as otherwise than astounding. ... The patient [previously] was apparently in a hopeless condition .... at present the patient is perfectly well and attending to his business ..."

AUTOSEROTHERAPY, RESULTS OF  - 14H3
AUTOSERO:  PSORIASIS  - 14H3
AUTOSERO:  URTICARIA  - 14H3
AUTOSERO:  ACNE  - 14H3
AUTOSERO:  LICHEN PLANUS  - 14H3
AUTOSERO:  FURUNCULOSIS - 14H3

Results in the other cases:  In 12 cases of severe and extensive psoriasis, following 4-6 injections at intervals of 5-7 days, "every lesion had disappeared," and cases of pustular acne, urticaria, lichen planus and furunculosis had all improved.

AUTOSERO: SUSPECTED MECHANISM - EXTERIORIZATION - 14H3

"Blood serum is an extremely complex material, and it is undoubtedly changed by its retention outside the body, by the coagulation and centrifugation."

AUTOSEROTHERAPY AS BLOODLETTING - 14H3

"Is it possible that the good results attained [by autoserum in psoriasis] are due to the bloodletting alone?  The thought has often struck me as it must have struck others, that the generations of acute observers and able clinicians who practiced bloodletting in so many affections cannot have been entirely wrong; they must have seen some good result in some cases at least.  And there is at least one case of psoriasis on record, to which our friend Dr. P. Brynberg Porter has called our attention, in which the late Weir Mitchell in his young days, being left in charge of a very bad case of psoriasis and not knowing what to do, put the patient to bed and bled her everyday, and cured her disease.  Bloodletting alone, however, has been tried, and has not given results.  We do not think that the benefits of this procedure can be ascribed to it."


15H1:  Pierce, E.A., "Autoserotherapy vs. Arthficial Pneumothorax in the Treatment of Pleurisy with Effusion", Northwest Medicine VII, n.s., Dec. 1915, 386.

GILBERT'S AUTOSEROTHERAPY - E.A. Pierce [15H1], per NYMJ, recommended and described the Gilbert method to treat pleurisy: "In favor of autoserotherapy are, that it is very simple, that it leads to absorption of the exudate in a short period of time in the majority of cases, and it entirely free from danger so long as we are careful to inject only perfectly clear serum removed from the chest.  The simplest technic is to use a large all glass syringe and a long needle.  The needle should be introduced into the chest near the upper border of a rib to avoid the danger of injuring the intercostal vessels, and at lease ten cc of fluid should be aspirated into the syringe.  If this fluid is clear the needle should be partly withdrawn and its point thrust further under the skin, and the contents of the syringe, not to exceed ten cc, are injected subcutaneously.  [It is noted that other writers have commonly reported the use of smaller doses, about 2cc per injection.]  If at the end of a few days the fluid in the chest has not begun to recede, or if it stops receding after an initial diminution, the procedure should be repeated.  There are no contraindications to the procedure."

E.A. Pierce [15H1] provided detailed instructions for application of the Gilbert method:  "Have the patient in a sitting position with the forearm of the affected side across the top of the head.  A glass syringe of suitable size, armed with a rather long needle of proper gauge is used. [... an all glass syringe of 10cc capacity, and fitted with a slip point 18 gauge leur needle is preferable ...]  Carefully select a site below the level of the fluid and, having sterilized the skin with tincture of iodine, insert the needle immediately above the upper border of the selected rib, thus avoiding the artery and nerve.  Having inserted the needle the desired distance, carefully withdraw the piston until 5-10cc of fluid are obtained.  Should no fluid be encountered, insert the needle further, withdraw it, or otherwise manipulate until the fluid is found.  Great care should be observed to avoid puncturing the diaphragm.  Having filled the syringe with the desired quantity of fluid, carefully inspect the same and, if it be found to be nonpurulent, withdraw the needle so that the point remains just under the skin. Then reinsert the needle under and parallel to the skin into the subcutaneous tissue and inject the contents of the syringe.  Then withdraw the needle and close the puncture with adhesive plaster or collodion."

E.A. Pierce provides this further clarification:  "Should the
fluid prove to be purulent, do not reinject but treat the case
surgically, or according to the method of Duncan by filtration
and ingestion."  [see also AUTOTHERAPY]


GILBERT'S AUTOSEROTHERAPY - SEROFIBRINOUS PLEURISY  15H1

JAMA [April 18, 1915] notes per EA Pierce [15H1] Pfender's
summary of reports of 565 cases of serofibrinous pleurisy in the
literature since 1894, of which 424 were cured and 31 benefited.

Continuing, "Fishberg says autoserotherapy appears to be worthy
of further trial.  Considering that it is absolutely devoid of
any danger, that there have never been observed the slightest
unfavorable effects on the patient, and that it can be performed
by anyone who can make an exploratory puncture, it ought to be
tried in every case of pleural effusion in which the fluid is not
purulent.  Indeed, inasmuch as in practically every case of
pleurisy showing signs of effusion exploratory puncture is to be
done with a view to determining the character of the fluid in the
pleural cavity, it is advisable, when the contents of the pleural
cavity are found to be serous, that the needle should not be
withdrawn completely but that, when its point is brought to the
subcutaneous tissue, it should be injected then and there.  The
quantity of the fluid to be injected subcutaneously need not be
very large; from 2 to 5 cc is quite enough."


SAFETY OF THE GILBERT METHOD  15H1

EA Pierce [15H1]:  "No contraindications have been noted and a
careful and extensive study of the literature fails to find
mention of any such."


16A1:  Huber, Autoserotherapy. N.Y. Med. J. 103:164, Jan. 22,
1916; ibid. 104:20, July 1, 1916.

GILBERT'S AUTOSEROTHERAPY - Huber [16A1] notes that the Gilbert
method involved the immediate subcutaneous reinjection of about
2cc of fluid from a pleural effusion "if the fluid is pale
yellow, transparent, or even somewhat hemorrhagic."  Huber
further noted that for cases "in which a cure follows the single
exploratory puncture and the withdrawal of a few cc of fluid -
may we not unintentionally have resorted to autoserotherapy?  A
small amount of fluid which is subsequently absorbed, escaping
into the tissues, through the small wound made by the exploring
needle, accomplishes the same purpose as though it had been
injected."


SAFETY OF THE GILBERT METHOD - Huber [16A1]:  "Carried out
under the usual aseptic precautions, no local or general ill

effects follow. Occasionally we meet with a case in which the
fluid is turbid and has a decided odor; under such conditions the
method is not to be resorted to."


16H3:  Gottheil, Wm. S., "The value of Autoserum Injections in
Skin Diseases", N.Y. Med. J. CIII:1209-1211, 24 June 1916.


   AUTOSEROTHERAPY: PSORIASIS - 16H3

   Gottheil in 1916 [16H3] reaffirmed his 1914 result, emphasizing
his success with 31 psoriasis cases, almost all of them
extensive, severe, recurrent and many recalcitrant: "In every
case the body was cleared in a remarkably short time, and with
mild local medication after the autoserum course."


   AUTOSEROTHERAPY: FREQUENCY OF INJECTION - 16H3

   Injections were given "at shorter intervals, say 3 days or so,
so as to abbreviate the preliminary treatment, and complete it in
2 or 3 weeks."


16H4:  Paget, O., Autoserum in Treatment of Cancer., Medical
Record, N. Y. LXXXIX (April 8, 1916, per abstr. in N.Y. Med. J.,
May 29, 1916, p. 997.

   AUTOSERO FOR CANCER, WITH FLUID FROM ARTIFICIAL BLISTER - 16H4

   Owen Paget [16H4] stimulated the skin cells by a blister, and
then inoculated the fluid from the blister into a man with
inoperable carcinoma of the rectum.  A "marked improvement"
followed, with the patient gaining weight and his tumor greatly
diminishing in size and hardness."


16H5:  Trimble, Wm. B. and John J. Rothwell, "Treatment of
Psoriasis with Autogenous Serum", J. Cutaneous Dis., Sept. 1916,
per abstr. in N. Y. M. J., 1 April 1916, 660-1.

   AUTOSEROTHERAPY, FAILURE - 16H5

   Trimble and Rothwell [16H5] per NYMJ, concluded "that
autogenous serum alone, so far as a curative effect on psoriasis
goes, is absolutely a failure [and] that the serum in combination
with chrysarobin ointment seems also worthless. ... The apparent
improvement reported by earlier observers was probably not due to
the use of serum, but to the enthusiasm of the patients in
carrying on a new method of treatment."


16H6:  Robertson, W.E., "Intravenous serobacterin therapeutics",
N.Y.M.J. 103 (April 22, 1916), 777-780.

   AUTOSEROTHERAPY:  IV v IM  16H6

   Robertson [16H6] expressed a preference for IV injections:

"Studies in anaphylaxis have shown the vastly greater
susceptibility of an animal to intravenous injections than to
those given subcutaneously or intramuscularly. ... It seem
possible that ... when we inject subcutaneously, or especially
intramuscularly, prompt reactions and beneficial results follow
only in cases in which by chance we happen to enter a vein."


17A1:  Spiethoff, B., Venesection plus autoserotherapy.  Med.
Klin. 12: 1223, Nov. 19, 1916; cont. 12: 1252, Nov. 26, 1916.


SERUM THERAPY BENEFIT NOT DUE TO "PASSIVE" MECHANISM - 17A1

Spiethoff [17A1] per JAMA [68 (1917),316] contrasted the
equally favorable results obtained with autogenous serum with
those of alien serotherapy, pointing out that "The benefit does
not depend on supplying certain lacking elements but on a broader
principle which includes the individual's own serum."


VENESECTION IS VACCINE THERAPY  17A1

AUTOSERUM IS VACCINE THERAPY - 17A1

Spiethoff [17A1] per JAMA [68 (1917),408] offers that "The
benefit from venesection and the reinjection of serum is best
explained by stimulation of the production of antibodies and
their mobilization."


AUTOSEROTHERAPY, SAFETY OF  - 17A1

Spiethoff [17A1] noted that he had "never witnessed with this
form of serotherapy [autogenous] anything like the phenomena of
hypersusceptibility sometimes noted with foreign serum, but there
is usually a transient general and a focal reaction."


AUTOSERUM, RESULTS OF  - 17A1

AUTOSERUM FOR URTICARIA  - 17A1

AUTOSERUM FOR ECZEMA  - 17A1

AUTOSERUM FOR PEMPHIGUS  - 17A1

AUTOSERUM FOR SCALP DISEASE  - 17A1

AUTOSERUM FOR GANGRENOUS ULCERS  - 17A1

AUTOSERUM FOR PRURITUS  - 17A1

Spiethoff [17A1] relates promising experiences in cases of
urticaria, eczema, pemphigus, scalp disease, gangrenous ulcers,
and particular good results with pruritus.


17H1:  Kaiser, A.D., "Serum and Blood Therapy", N.Y.M.J. Sept.
29, 1917, 595-6.

AUTOSEROTHERAPY, I.M., AS "VACCINE" - 17H1

AUTOSERO:  BRONCHIAL ASTHMA, I.M.  - 17H1

Kaiser [17H1]  "During the past 2 years the so-called autoserotherapy has been practised.  This method consists of withdrawing from the patient several ounces of blood and separating serum and cellular elements.  The serum is then injected intramuscularly and in chorea intraspinously. ... In injecting the serum of the patient's blood in bronchial asthma it is assumed that the foreign proteins responsible for the asthma are contained in the serum and by frequent injections produce an immunity to this irritating protein.   Excellent results have been reported."


AUTOSEROTHERAPY FOR POLIO, INTRASPINAL - 17H1

"Perhaps the most successful results in the treatment of anterior poliomyelitis were with the use of convalescent serum. In this disease the serum was injected into the spinal canal."


Kaiser [17H1] on autohemotherapy

AUTOHEMOTHERAPY FOR HEMOPHILIA, PURPURA - 17H1

"In diseases where the coagulability of the blood is delayed, as in purpura and hemophilia, injections of whole blood either intramuscularly or intravenously may be beneficial." 17H1


PERNICIOUS ANEMIA, BENEFIT OF REPEATED SMALL TRANSFUSIONS - 17H1

"the uses of whole blood in primary and secondary anemia are well known.  Repeated small transfusions in pernicious anemia are of greater benefit than fewer transfusions of large amount."


AUTOHEMOTHERAPY (IM OR IV) FOR SEPTICEMIA - 17H1

"In any severe infection where the body is being overwhelmed by the infection and no specific serum or convalescent blood is at hand, whole blood either by intramuscular or intravenous injection is advocated.  ... I would recommend its use especially in cases of septicemia."


CONVALESCENT BLOOD, IM   17H1

Kaiser recommended "the use of convalescent blood in infections where there is no specific serum and where the etiological factor is unknown.  In using convalescent blood whole blood is preferable.  The blood can be collected and by the use of sodium citrate may be preserved for hours.  It is usually injected deep into the muscles."


SAFETY OF SERUM OR BLOOD INJECTIONS, I.M. V. I.V. 17H1

I.M. V. I.V., SAFETY OF SERUM OR BLOOD INJECTIONS  17H1

"In selecting the route for serum or blood injection, one must be guided by the individual case.  Generally speaking, the intramuscular route is the safer."

21A1:  Escomel, E., Autoserotherapy of infections. Ann. de Fac. de Med., Montevideo 5: 604, Nov. 1920 - Feb. 1921; ab. J.A.M.A. 76: 1375, May 14, 1921.

AUTOSERUM, HEATED, FOR VENEREAL DISEASES - 21A1

Escomel [21A1] reported remarkably favorable results with heated autoserum, injecting small quantities of 1 to 10 cc, heated to 56 or 58 degrees C.  Benefits in 2 cases of acute gonorrhea and secondary syphilis are cited.

21A2:  Sen, D.N., Auto-haemic or auto-serum therapy, Indian M. Gaz. 56: 94, March 1921.

AUTOSEROTHERAPY SAFETY - 21A2

Escomel 1921 notes "autoserotherapy is free from all the drawbacks of other forms, and is applicable in all infections of known and unknown nature."

23A7:  Quenay, A., Autoserotherapy in gonorrhea, J. D'Urol. 16:234-235, Sept. 1923; ab. J.A.M.A. 81:2152, Dec. 22, 1923.

AUTOSERUM FOR GONORRHEA, FAVORABLE RESULT - 23A7

Quenay [23A7] obtained favorable results in treating complications of gonorrhea with 2-4cc of autoserum, but no action at all in a case of urethritis.

23E1:  Rogers, Loyal Dexter, AUTO-HEMIC THERAPY; administering a remedy made from the patient's blood without drugs or bacteria. 3.ed. Chicago,  1922, Auto-hemic Therap. Found. inc., 332 p., 8&.

AUTOHEMIC SERUM: CURE LAZINESS, UGLINESS, FRIGITIDY  23E1

"'Autohemic Serum', A Cure for Laziness, Ugliness, Frigidity and Many Other Things", so read the title of an item in JAMA 74 (July 14, 1920, p. 477-8), referring to "charlatan" Dr. L. D. Rogers of Chicago and his "auto-hemic" serum. [see 23E1]

"What is auto-hemic therapy? ... According to a very lurid poster it is described as 'The Missing Link in Medicine', possibly referring to the ease with which one may make monkeys out of certain physicians.  More specifically, although still vaguely, we learn: 'It consists of giving the patient a solution made by attenuating, hemolyzing, incubating and potentizing a few drops of his or her own blood. ...'"

Dr. Rogers' first publisher was "Ideal Life Extension Press", which name contains a concept still capable today of selling millions of books and magazines.


AUTOBLOOD, USE IN SURGERY/LAKED AUTOBLOOD  - 23E6

Descarpentries, 1923 [23E6], reported on the favorable use of subcutaneous injections of "laked" autoblood in surgical cases, phlegmons, etc., citing the value in terms of improvement of torpid cases, preventing postoperative complications, localizing suppration, and promoting healing.


23H1:  Moberg, "Autohyämotherapie bei Hautkrankheiten", Svensk Läkaresällsk. förhandl. 1923, H.6, S. 289. [per Deutsche Med. Woch. S.49 (1923), 1314]

   IV v. IM  Ormsby in Wright  23H1

Ormsby O, in Wright C S [23H1], discussion, reported less satisfactory results with intramuscular than with IV serum. Wright responded that his experience was virtually the same with both, whereas with the IV method there may be more reaction, which might account for occasional better results [and greater danger].


AUTOHEMO: SKIN DISEASES - DECREASING DOSE TECHNIC  - 23H1

Moberg [23H1] employed autohemotherapy with decreasing doses, 20cc at first and later 10cc, in pemphigus, dermatitis herpiformis, urticaria, eczema, and prurigo.  In most cases of eczema some improvement was observed. [Such an approach is compatible with the concept of passive immunization, hence compatible with Rosenow's skin-reaction demonstrations of both active and passive processes, albeit not in accord with either predominant autohemotherapy methodology or vaccine therapy as per Wright.]


24A3:  Zerner, H., Autoserum treatment of cancer, Med. Klinik 20: 212-213, Feb. 17, 1924; ab. J.A.M.A. 82:1088, March 29, 1924.

   AUTOSERUM FOR CANCER, REPORTED LIMITATION OF  - 24A3

Zerner [24A3] found autoserum treatment useful only as an adjuvant to operations or irradiation in the treatment of cancer.


24A10:  Vorschütz, J. & B. Tenckhoff, Treatment with own blood, Deutsche Ztschr. f. Chir. 183:364-379, 1924; cont. 184:200-207, 1924; ab. J.A.M.A. 82:1087, March 29, 1924, and 82:1740, May 24, 1924.


AUTOHEMO: POSTOPERATIVE LUNG INFECTION - 24A10

Vorschütz and Tenckhoff [24A10]  In the case of postoperative lung infections, the authors reported "astonishing success": "Intramuscular injections of from 30-80cc of own blood were given as soon as high fever appeared.  The symptoms are overcome with surprising rapidity if the treatment is given the first day of the illness."

24E1:  Moutier, F. and Rachet, J., Incidents et accidents de l'autohemotherapie.  PRESSE MED., PAR., 1922/3, xxxi, 708; ab. J.A.M.A. 81:1476, Oct. 27, 1923.
   AUTOHEMOTHERAPY TECHNIC - 24E1
   Moutier and Rachet [24E1] would withdraw from 2 to 20 cc of blood, depending on the pathological condition, from the vein in the bend of the elbow, and reinjected it immediately into the gluteal muscle, not allowing the blood time to clot.

   AUTOHEMO, MECHANISM OF ACTION AS DESENSITIZATION  24E1
   Moutier and Rachet, 1923 [24E1], per JAMA, "... autohemotherapy seems to be a kind of desensitization..."

24E3:  Nicolas, Gate and Dupasquier.  Sur certaines reactions cliniques dans l'autohemotherapie (purpura).  COMPT. REND SOC. DE BIOL., PAR., 1923, lxxxviii, 211.
   AUTOHEMO: MECHANISM OF ACTION LIKENED TO HEMOCLASTIC SHOCK - 24E3
   Nicolas and Gaté [24E3], per JAMA, "Autohemotherapy does not act like a vaccine; the effect is more like a hemoclastic shock."

   AUTOHEMO: METHOD, DOSAGE, FREQUENCY, LENGTH OF SERIES - 24E3
   Nicolas, et al [24E3], withdrew blood from a vein, 10cc from an adult and 2cc from a child, and reinjected immediately subcutaneously or into the gluteal muscles.  This was repeated every second or third day, for a total of 15 or 20 injections, in order to prevent recurrences.

   AUTOHEMO RESULTS - FURUNCULOSIS; STAPH. SEPTICEMIA - 24E3
   Nicolas et al [24E3], per JAMA, report having had no failures in 2 years experience with autohemotherapy, note the almost constant success of autohemotherapy in typical furunculosis, emphasizing their having obtained prompt relief of pain and subsidence of the chronic staphylococcus septicemia.

24E8:  Vorschutz, J., and Tenckhoff, B., Von der Behandlung mit Eigenblut. I. DEUTSCHE ZTSCHR. F. CHIR., LEIPZ., 1923-4, cixxxiii, 364-379

AUTOHEMO: PROPHYLACTISM/CURE FOR ALL DISEASES - 24E8

Vorschütz and Tenckhoff 1924 [24E8] report having used both intramuscular whole-blood injections and intravenous defibrinated blood injections, as reported in JAMA, expressing confidence that it will help in every infectious disease, chronic or acute.  Autogenous or convalescents' blood treatment is advocated as offering all the advantages of serotherapy and autogenous vaccines, even for prophylactic treatment.

25A26:  Vorschütz, J., Treatment with own blood; 208 cases. Arch. f. klin. Chir.  133:509-516, 1924 (in German).

AUTOHEMO RESULTS  25A26

AUTOHEMO FOR: CARBUNCLE - 25A26

AUTOHEMO FOR: FURUNCULOSIS - 25A26

AUTOHEMO FOR: BUBO AXILLARIS - 25A26

AUTOHEMO FOR: SEPSIS - 25A26

AUTOHEMO FOR: WOUND INFECTION - 25A26

AUTOHEMO FOR: NEURALGIA - 25A26

AUTOHEMO FOR: ECZEMA - 25A26

AUTOHEMO FOR: GONORRHEA - 25A26

John Vorschutz, 1924 [25A26], p. 509-10, reported healing or improvement in 154 of 195 cases, including carbuncle, furunculosis, bubo axillaris, sepsis, wound infection, eczema, neuralgia, gonorrhea, and many others.

25E7:  Wein, M.A., Salutzki, L.E., and Konigsberg, L.M., Die Autohämotherapie bei einigen kutanen und venerischen krankheiten. DERMAT. WCHNSCHR., LEIPZ. U. HAMB., 1924, lxxix, 1629-1637.

AUTOHEMOTHERAPY FOR: FURUNCULOSIS - 25E7

AUTOHEMOTHERAPY FOR: ANTHRAX - 25E7

AUTOHEMOTHERAPY FOR: MASTITIS - 25E7

AUTOHEMOTHERAPY FOR: ECZEMA - 25E7

AUTOHEMOTHERAPY FOR: SKROPHULUS - 25E7

AUTOHEMOTHERAPY FOR: PRURIGO ERYTHEMA - 25E7

AUTOHEMOTHERAPY FOR: SLEEPING SICKNESS - 25E7

AUTOHEMOTHERAPY FOR: TYPHUS - 25E7

AUTOHEMOTHERAPY FOR: INFLUENZA - 25E7

AUTOHEMOTHERAPY FOR: SCARLET FEVER - 25E7

AUTOHEMOTHERAPY FOR: MEASLES - 25E7

AUTOHEMOTHERAPY FOR: VD - 25E7

AUTOHEMOTHERAPY FOR: INTERNAL DISEASES - 25E7

AUTOHEMOTHERAPY FOR: INFECTIOUS DISEASES - 25E7

AUTOHEMOTHERAPY FOR: INFANTILE ATROPHY - 25E7

AUTOHEMOTHERAPY FOR: CANCER - 25E7

AUTOHEMOTHERAPY FOR: SURGERY - 25E7

According to Wien et al [25E7] some of the other earlier investigators included Naswitis, who had reported good results with frozen and rethawed blood only; Dold, who reported good results with unaltered autoblood in the case of eczema; and Fauvet who also reported favorable results in cases of furunculosis, anthrax, mastitis, eczema, skrophulus, and prurigo erythema.

As summarized by Wein et al [25E7], who incidentally does not credit Ravaut with priority, numerous authors figured into the development of hemotherapy in the early 20th century, with reports of applications in cases of infectious diseases, influenza, typhus recurrens, Flecktyphus, internal illness, scarlet fever, measles, and even sleeping sickness, gynecology, surgery, infantile atrophy, cancerous illnesses, and venereal diseases - gonorrhea and syphilis. According to Wien as of 1925, a veritable "blitz" of articles on the use of autohemotherapy in dermatology had been published during the preceding decade.


25H1: Shamberg, JF and H Brown, "Effects of various agents - ultraviolet light, vaccines, turpentine, neoarsphenamin and autoblood injections - on the enzymes of blood and skin", Archives Int. Med. 35 (May, 1925), 537.

AUTOHEMOTHERAPY, EFFECTS ON THE BLOOD - 25H1

Schamberg and Brown [25H1] withdrew 20cc of blood from the vein, and immediately reinjected it into the gluteal muscles, in 5 patients (3 psoriasis and 2 generalized pruritus) in order to assess the effect of these injections on the serum enzymes. The summary result: "The intramuscular injection of freshly drawn autoblood appears to stimulate an increase in the lipolytic and proteolytic activity of the blood serum."


26A2: Zerner, Anaphylaxis in autohemotherapy of cancer. Ztschr. f. Krebsforsch. 23:9-11, 1926.


27B13: in cancerous diseases, [S. V. Kaufman] Klin.Med, 5: 433-437, 27


27H1: O'Leary, Arch. Dermat. and Syph.:15:470, April 1927

AUTOSERUM FOR LICHEN PLANUS, FAVORABLE EXPERIENCE - 27H1

O'Leary [27H1] reported: "A few cases of lichen planus reacted favorably to autogenous serum after they had failed to respond to the mercury and arsenic."

29A5: in cancer, [F. Blumenthal] Med. Welt 2: 1819' Dec. 8, '28

29A18: value of autoserum irradiated with radium for treatment of cancer' [H. Peters] Ztschr.f.Krebsforsch. 28: 186—190, '28

29B19: various changes of blood in autohemotherapy in cancer of uterus and vomiting during pregnancy, [T. I. Dikoff] Klin.j.saratov.Univ.  5: 449-461, April '28

30B11: general treatment of malignant tumors with special regard to injections of patient's own blood which has been treated with roentgen rays, [S. von Dziembowski] Fortschr.d.Med. 48: 567-571, July 11, '30

30B13: in chronic malaria; cases, [M. Padoan & M. Frizziero] Riv.di malariol. 9: 135-149, March-April '30

AUTOHEMOTHERAPY FOR MALARIA - 30B13

Padoan and Frizziero [30B13] routinely used series of 12 injections of 10cc each in treating chronic malaria patients.

p. 135:  The authors place the origin of autohemotherapy in a very early time, invoking reference to the works of Galen.

p. 136:  "Autohemotherapy constitutes, in our experience, the single and exclusive practical treatment [for malaria].

p. 148:  Autohemotherapy of chronic malaria is a treatment of certain effectiveness, always to be suggested... .
["L'autoemoterapia nell malaria chronica sará quindi una curá collaterale di sicura efficacia, sempre consigliabile ed eseguibile in tutti quei casi in sui facile ne riesca la practica."]

31A7- effects of Gilbert's autoserotherapy on blood picture in serofibrinous pleurisy; 6 cases, [M. A. Sisti]  Diagnosis  10: 237-250, Aug. '30

GILBERT METHOD - SEROFIBRINOUS PLEURISY  31A7

The Gilbert method was generally well-received from the mid-1890s to the 1930s.  For example, in 1930 Sisti referred to "effects of Gilbert's autoserotherapy on the blood picture in serofibrinous pleurisy; 6 cases [31A7].  And without reference to these early efforts, we find reference to a apparently related methodology in the current literature.

31H1:  Wright, Carroll S., "Nonspecific Therapy in Dermatology, a 5-year Study", Archives of Dermatology and Syphilis 23:118-131 (Jan. 1931)

## AUTOHEMOTHERAPY AS NON-SPECIFIC - 31H1

C.S. Wright 1931 [31H1] reported results of a 5-year study of so-called "non-specific therapy" in dermatology including autohemotherapy, milk preparations, non-specific vaccine therapy, and turpentine.  "The method employed by Dr. Schaumberg and myself consists in withdrawing from 20 to 30cc of blood and reinjecting it immediately into the deep muscles of the buttocks. ... it is one of the mildest forms of non-specific therapy, and yet it exerts an action in some conditions which cannot be accomplished by any other form of nonspecific therapy."

[It is noted that Wright uses the term "autohemic" without reference to Rogers, a particularly notorious practitioner of such. (see 23E1 above)]

Wright [31H1], p. 120, "In 1913 Luithlen showed by the results of unusual experimentation that inflammatory reaction of the skin to external irritants could be favorably influenced by injections of homologous, autogenous, or foreign serum or blood."

Wright [31H1], p. 120, notes that Spiethoff 1913 concluded that autoserum injections "resulted in a reduction of the sensitiveness of the skin to endogenous irritation."

Wright [31H1] p. 120, "Hilario, 1914, claimed that autoserum injections alone would result in the spontaneous involution of certain dermatoses, especially those of actinic nervous origin; that they acted as a antipruritic agent, and that following their use, the resistance of psoriasis to drugs was reduced."


## AUTOSEROTHERAPY CRITICIZED  [31H1]

"Trimble and Rothwell (1915) and Willock (1915) believed autoserotherapy to be of no value either alone or as an adjunct to local therapy.  In an informal discussion of the subject, Schamberg, Gilchrist and Wile (1915) expressed the opinions that little or no benefit was to be derived from this form of treatment."


## AUTOSEROTHERAPY CRITIC CONVERTED TO ADVOCATE AUTOHEMIC - 31H1

"It is of interest that Dr. Schamberg has since become a warm advocate of the value of autohemic therapy as an adjunct to the local therapy of psoriasis."[31H1]


## AUTOHEMOTHERAPY FOR PSORIASIS, SUCCESSFUL IN - 31H1

Wright 1931 [31H1], 121, summarizes results of autohemotherapy in psoriasis, reporting improvement in over 80% of 247 cases with three "autohemic" injections.  Improvement was marked in 68 cases, moderate in 86 and slight in 45; 40 cases showed no improvement and 8 worsened.  Wright, p. 123, notes that "remarkable results" will occasionally be observed.  Favorable results were also obtained in over 70% of 49 cases of urticaria treated by autohemotherapy.


AUTOHEMO FOR URTICARIA, OFTEN STRIKING SUCCESSFUL - 31H1

[31H1] p. 122, "The results in urticaria following the use of injections of autogenous blood are often striking and leave no doubt as to the occasional value of procedure...


AUTOHEMO FOR ANGIONEURITIC EDEMA - 31H1

[31H1] p. 123, "Basing his therapy on the theory that urticarial lesions are antiphlactic, Schulman [1924] used autohemotherapy with good results and advised continuation of the treatment for several weeks after the cessation of all symptoms. Good results in urticaria and angioneuritic edema are also reported by Achard and Flandin, 1920. They believed that reinjection of a patient's own blood or serum brings about a desensitization."


AUTOHEMO FOR PEMPHIGUS - 31H1

AUTOHEMO FOR DERMATITIS HERPIFORMIS - 31H1

AUTOHEMO FOR PRURIGO - 31H1

[31H1] p. 123, "Ullmann and Hueck, 1924, used autohemotherapy with good results in the treatment of pemphigus, dermatitis herpiformis, and prurigo. ...

Ravaut [1913] observed good results in the treatment of pruriginous dermatoses. ...


AUTOHEMO FOR PRURIGO - 31H1

AUTOHEMO FOR LICHEN CHRONICUS - 31H1

AUTOHEMO FOR ECZEMA - 31H1

AUTOHEMO FOR WARTS - 31H1

"Nicholas, Gaté and DuPasquier [1924] found autohemotherapy to be of value in the treatment of prurigo, lichen chronicus (Vidal), eczema and dermatitis herpeformis. ..."

Wein etal [25E7], reported favorable results in 47 cases of eczema after an average of 6 or 7 injections, and

Sezary, 1928, reported the disappearance of warts after a few intramuscular autoblood injections.


32A1: autohemotherapy, [N. Burgess]  Brit.J.Dermat.  44: 124-131, March '32

AUTOHEMO EXPLANATION; PROCESS OF ELIMINATION - 32A1

Burgess 1932 [32A1], 131:  In his investigation of the underlying mechanism of action of autohemotherapy, Burgess first proposed that certain possibilities be eliminated:

"(1) The action of whole-blood injections does not depend on the production of a leucocytosis. (2) ... no relation between whole-blood injections and the haemoclastic reaction was discovered. (3) Whole blood injections had no effect on the sedimentation rate of the red corpuscles as estimated by the method of Zeckwer and Goodell. (4) ... No constant effect on the production of proteose by a single whole-blood injection could be demonstrated."

32H1: Low, Cranston R., "The Uses of Non-Specific Protein Therapy", Brit. M.J., Sept. 24, 1932, 577-80

AUTOHEMO FOR PEMPHIGUS: ASTONISHING RESULTS - 32H1

Low 1932 [32H1], 578: "Autoserotherapy has given astonishing results in a few cases [of chronic pemphigus]. Praetorius reports complete cure in a case of 2-years' duration .... Breda treated 3 cases [with autohemotherapy], and in all the eruption disappeared completely."

AUTOHEMO FOR STREPTOCOCCAL INFECTIONS - 32H1

Low 1932 [32H1], p. 579, "Hoff and Heesch used autoblood [in streptococcal infections], and Pines reports recovery in a very bad case in an infant after injections of the father's blood."

AUTOHEMO FOR ULCERS - 32H1

AUTOHEMO FOR GLANDS - 32H1

Low 1932 [32H1], 580, "Treubel, and Bussalai and Devoto saw rapid healing of ulcers and glands with autohemotherapy.

AUTOHEMO FOR GONOCOCCAL INFECTIONS - 32H1

Low 1932 [32H1], "Spiethoff recommends autoserum for gonorrheal prostatitis, and Bussalai and Devoto and Mariani report equally good results with autohemotherapy in all forms of gonococcal infection."

AUTOSERUM SAFETY - 32H1

AUTOHEMO SAFETY - 32H1

Low 1932 [32H1], 580, "In autoserum and autoblood injections, there is no risk such as is always present when foreign serums are used."

MALARIAL THERAPY - 32H1

PYROTHERAPY (HEAT) - 32H1

Low 1932 [32H1], p. 580, "Within recent years malarial therapy has been very extensively used in the treatment of neurosyphilis,

and especially in tabes and G.P.I.  The results have, on the
whole, been very satisfactory .... The Malarial treatment,
however, has certain disadvantages. ... Once the attacks are
established, their severity cannot always be controlled.  In
addition, there has been a certain mortality from this treatment.
 For these reasons other easier and safer methods of producing a
temperature reaction have been experimented with."  These include
milk injections combined with arsenic in neurosyphilis,
tuberculin injections combined with mercurial treatment, typhoid
and other bacterial vaccines, and hot baths.

### ACCIDENTAL CURE AS AUTOHEMOTHERAPY - 32H1

 Low, 1932 [32H1], 579, "Beume reports a case of syphilis which
did not clear up with several courses of neosalvarsan, mercury
and bismuth.  this man had an accident which resulted in
extensive hemorrhage into and around the knee and ankle joints.
The syphilitic eruption rapidly disappeared and the Wasserman
reaction became negative, even although no further drug treatment
was being given.  This must be looked upon as a case of autohaemotherapy."

33B10-further observations (in skin diseases of allergic origin),
[N. Burgess] Brit.J.Dermat. 45: 333-340, Aug.-Sept. '33
### AUTOHEMOTHERAPY EXPLAINED AS DESENSITIZATION - 33B10

 In a follow-up article, Burgess 1933 [33B10], p. 339. offered:

 "In the present state of our knowledge it would be unwise to be
dogmatic concerning the interpretation of skin-reactions, but
this work tends to suggest that the blood in these cases contains
antigens, and that the injection of the patient's blood or serum
leads to desensitization."  Burgess cites a study in which 15
patients had given positive skin reactions before treatment.
Eleven of these were benefitted by autohemotherapy, and "after
treatment and relief negative reactions were obtained.  Those
cases which were not relieved continued to give positive
reactions."

 Burgess, 1933 [33B10], 336, "It was found that only 16% of
normal controls gave positive reactions to their proteoses, while
67% of those suffering from the skin diseases under consideration
[primarily urticaria, psoriasis and eczema] gave positive
reactions."

### AUTOHEMOTHERAPY: PSORIASIS OF PARTICULAR INTEREST - 33B10

 Burgess, 1933 [33B10], 337, notes that the cases of psoriasis
are of particular interest: "all the acute cases gave positive
skin-reactions, 3 out of 5 cases of sub-acute psoriasis gave
positive reactions, while 3 out of 4 cases of chronic psoriasis
gave negative reactions to their own proteoses. ... the best
results of treatment with autohemotherapy were obtained in acute

cases, and the greatest number of failures were among the chronic cases."


  AUTOHEMO FOR VARICOSE DERMATITIS - 33B10
  Burgess 1933 [33B10], "Consistently good results were obtained in cases of varicose dermatitis of the leg in which a generalized sensitization eruption had occurred; all the cases treated were known to be cured with the exception of three who ceased to attend."


  AUTOHEMOTHERAPY RESULTS, VARIOUS DISEASES - 33B10
  AUTOHEMO FOR PSORIASIS - 33B10
  AUTOHEMO FOR VARICOSE DERMATITIS - 33B10
  AUTOHEMO FOR ECZEMA - 33B10
  AUTOHEMO FOR URTICARIA - 33B10
  AUTOHEMO FOR TOXIC ERYTHEMA - 33B10
  AUTOHEMO FOR PRURIGO - 33B10
  AUTOHEMO FOR FURUNCULOSIS - 33B10
  Burgess 1933 [33B10] results - 39 successes of 58 total cases:

```
-psoriasis -            10/15
-varicose dermatitis - 15/18
-eczema                  4/10
-urticaria               2/ 5
-toxic erythema          3/ 3
-prurigo                 2/ 3
-furunculosis            3/ 3
-pruritus                0/ 1
   TOTAL                39/58
```


34A13-ovarian hemocrinotherapy in scleroderma, [A. Sézary & A. Horowitz]  Bull.Soc.franç.de dermat.et syph.  41: 68-71, Jan. '34


AUTOHEMOCRINOTHERAPY FOR SCLERODERMA - 34A13:
  (a partial translation)
BULL., (FRAN".) SOC. DE DERMAT. ET SYPH. 41: 68-71. Jan.1934:
The treatment of scleroderma by ovarian hemocrino-therapy
by MM. A. Sezary and A. Horowitz

    "We know little of treatments effective for scleroderma. Therefore we believe it would be of interest to you that we communicate the results we have obtained with hemocrinotherapy. Under that name, M. Filderman designates the therapy which consists of injecting into the muscles a glandular extract mixed with the patient's blood.

"Our attention had been directed to this method by the positive effect obtained by Mr. Filderman with a woman suffering from generalized scleroderma, who we had observed in 1929 and who left the hospital after a few days, confined to her own care. The result given by the ovarian hemocrinotherapy had been very good (See The Medical Society of Paris Bulletin, June 29, 1929, No. 12).

"Subsequently we utilized this treatment with diverse fortunes with more cases of scleroderma.

"We would like today to relate to you a case of complete recovery, and sum up the results obtained in 5 other cases.

"Madame H. ... 46 years old, we consulted on June 24, 1933, for a 'plaque' of typical morphology ... .

    ...

"We suspended thyroid treatment and prescribed ovarian hemocrinotherapy in a series of 12 injections of 'Choay' ovarian extract (2 cm3 for the first six, 5 cc for the last six) mixed with 20 cc of blood drawn from the vein of the patient.  We repeated the injections 3 times a week.

"The first series, accomplished in July, gave no result.

"The second series, accomplished in September, was of the contrary effect.  By the 6th injection, the 'plaque de morphe' disappeared in a few days.

    "On November 29, we examined the patient.  There was hardly a trace of lesion.  The consistency of the skin had grown normal. On inspection only a small zone of atrophic "lenticulaire" in the root of the nose and a small "zone d;prime mais non infiltr;e" on the border of the hair.  The grain of the skin had become normal.
 ...

"Before interpreting this good succcess, we report briefly that which we have obtained in 5 other cases (the detailed observations are published elsewhere).

    ...

[Here are described briefly the 5 other cases]

    ...

"As is seen, the results obtained were not consistently as good as in the case of M. Filderman and that of our first observation.  Note however that in our six cases, a complete recovery was obtained in one, a marked and lasting improvement in two, and a temporary improvement in one.  The method failed in two cases, where the patients, it is true, did not receive but a single series of injections (recall that in our first observation, the recovery did not occur until during the second series).  ..."

34A22—vagaries of cancer and deductions therefrom (use of washed autogenous erythrocytes), [H. Gray] Internat.J.Med.& Surg. 46: 578-583, Dec. '33

35A1 autogenous, [Vorschütz] Ztschr.f.ärztl.Fortbild. 31: 703-706, Dec. 15, '34

AUTOBLOOD AS OLD AS MEDICINE 35A1

In 1934 [35A1], p. 703, Vorschütz declared "Autoblood treatment is as old as medicine. The author discusses the possibility that reinjected autoblood comprises both passive and active immunization.

35A14: intramuscular autohemotherapy, new treatment for cerebral hemorrhage; 7 cases; preliminary report, [R Colella & G Pizzillo] Ztschr.f.d.ges.Neurol.u. Psychiat. 152: 337-344, '35: also, Med.argent. 14:1-5, Jan. 35; also, Riv.di pat.nerv. 45:116-127, Jan.-Feb. 35, also, Forze san. 4: 212-219, Feb. 10, 36; also, Wien.med.Wchnschr. 85: 341-344, March 23 '35; also, Presse med. 43: 574-576, April 10, '35

AUTOHEMO FOR CEREBRAL HEMORRHAGE - 35A14

AUTOHEMO FOR HIGH BLOOD PRESSURE PROPHYLAXIS - 35A14

Colella and Pizzillo, 1935 [35A14], p. 344, reported results in seven cases of cerebral hemorrhage. They conclude: "Autohemotherapy helps with cerebral hemorrhage, during and after the attack. It is absolutely indicated as preventive treatment in cases of established hereditary disposition to high blood pressure."

AUTOHEMO EXPLANATION NOT IMPORTANT W/FAVORABLE RESULT - 35A14

"... the theories about autohemotherapy are numerous ... ... However, the explanation is not important ... if the therapy gives a favorable result. This favorable result is present without doubt in this new treatment of cerebral hemorrhage ... to which we have wished to direct attention." [35A14]

35B14: autohemotherapy ot pneumonia: 10 years of experience. [G. Tillmann] München.med.Wchnschr. 82:1604-1607 Oct. 4, 35

AUTOHEMOTHERAPY FOR LUNG INFLAMMATION - 35B14

Tillman [35B14] reported on ten years' experience with autoblood treatment in lung inflammation, asserting that autoblood deserves the very first place of treatment methods for treating uncomplicated lung congestion.

37A11: autoserum treatment for opium addicts observation on 1,000 cases, [A. W. Woo] Chinese M.J. 51: 8.0-90, Jan. '37

AUTOSERUM FOR OPIUM ADDICTION, FROM ARTIFICIAL BLISTER - 37A11

In 1937 Woo [37A11] reported on 1000 cases of opium addiction, treated over a period of 4 months with subcutaneous auto-serum injections.  The serum is taken from an artificially produced blister (induced by application of Cantharides plaster) and immediately injected subcutaneously, usually in the arm, after it has been cleaned with 1 oz. of picric acid.  More than 1/3 of the total 1000 patients were reported as having been completely cured or taking 90% less opium; more than 3/4 of the total 1000 patients were reported as taking 50% less opium or better.  Of the remainder, it is noted:  "We feel certain that many more have been completely cured after treatment but have not returned to report themselves. ... Every case reported which was not completely freed from the habit, smoked much less than formerly...."

For those regarded as cures, the average size and number of injections was about 2.6 cc per injection over a course of seven injections.

Woo reported that "we find that whole blood taken from the vein and reinjected into the patient does not give the best result..."

Woo's results of 1000 cases:

    161 completely cured
    179 taking 90% less opium
    187   "     75%  "     "
    237   "     50%  "     "
    236 little or no improvement, or did not return


37B3: autohemotherapy in dermatology especially in psoriasis and herpes zoster) , [J. W. Jones & M. S. Alden] South.M.J. 30: 735-737, July '37

AUTOHEMO FOR PSORIASIS IS OFTEN SPECTACULAR - 37B3

AUTOHEMO FOR HERPES SIMPLEX OFTEN SPECTACULAR - 37B3

AUTOHEMO FOR HERPES ZOSTER OFTEN SPECTACULAR - 37B3

Jones and Alden, 1937 [37B3]  "The one disease in which we particularly would like to commend the use of autohemotherapy is herpes zoster.  In fact we have been so favorably impressed with the results obtained that it has become routine in the office in the treatment of this disease. ... no case has ever failed to respond."  The authors assert that the use of autohemotherapy in psoriasis, herpes simplex and herpes zoster "has often been spectacular."


AUTOHEMO TECHNIC  37B3

Jones and Alden [37B3], p. 736, "8-10cc of fresh blood are withdrawn from the cubital vein and immediately injected into the

gluteal muscle at weekly intervals, using along with it mild
local applications."  In contrast to more complex methods, "The
simpler method most commonly used at the present time is
intramuscular injections of the freshly withdrawn blood before it
has had time to clot, a method first introduced by Ravaut in
1913."


AUTOHEMO SAFETY  37B3

Jones and Alden, 1937 [37B3], "Moutier and Rachet (1923) say
that they have had no serious by-effects in 400 injections of the
patient's own blood in 70 cases."


AUTOHEMO EXPLANATION  37B3

Jones and Alden [37B3], 736, note "there has never been a
completely satisfactory explanation of the mechanism of
autohemotherapy."


37B12 -different types of rheumatism and their treatment with
sulfur, sunlight, vitamins and autohemotherapy. [J. Le Calvé]
Presse Med. 45: 1409-1410, Oct. 6, 37

AUTOHEMO: RHEUMATIC PAINS AND ENDOCARDITIS - 37B12

JAMA 111 (1938), p. 661, refers to Le Calve's [37B12]
successful use in rheumatic conditions and to cure symptoms of
endocarditis.


37B25 -ultraviolet irradiation and autohemotherapy in syphilis;
treatment of persistent serologic positive and latent syphilis,
[H. L. Baer] Pennsylvania M.J. 40: 943-948 Aug., '37

AUTOHEMOTHERAPY AND IRRADIATION - SYPHILLIS  37B25

Baer [37B25] reported observations on 27 cases of syphillis, of
which ten "showed a complete reversal of their serologic
findings."  Baer noted, however, subjective improvement in the
general condition of all patients, regardless of serologic
findings, including weight gain and "increase in vital energy".

Based on a method pioneered a decade earlier by Rajka and
Radnai, Baer exposed the entire body to ultraviolet radiation
biweekly, over 15 weeks, and followed the first and last ten
treatments with 15cc intramuscular autohemotherapy, one-half hour
after irradiation.


AUTOHEMO SAFETY  37B25

AUTOHEMO RECOMMENDED WHERE FEVER THERAPY IS CONTRAINDICATED
37B25

AUTOHEMO FOR CARDIAC, NEUROSYPHILITIC  37B25

Baer asserted "As a rule there are no technical difficulties, no shock symptoms, and no discomforts noted by the patients with this form of therapy. ... This treatment is quite simple, inexpensive, and safe, and the patient remains ambulatory.  This form of therapy is safe for the cardiac and neurosyphilitic and may be employed where fever therapy is contraindicated."

PYOTHERAPY  37B25

MALARIA THERAPY  37B25

Baer p. 944,  discusses mechanical methods intended to produce a sustained elevation of temperature, whose "advocates claim results equally as good as the malarial treatment without the attending mortality risk of 10 to 20%".

Editorial, JAMA 111 (1938), p. 343

 AUTOHEMO:  AMA ENDORSEMENT - PSORIASIS:  JAMA 111 (1938), p. 343

 "INJECTIONS OF WHOLE BLOOD IN PSORIASIS

*To the editor*:  -Please give me any information available concerning the use of whole blood in the treatment of psoriasis.  Some current articles are reporting good results from taking the blood of an affected individual and injecting it immediately intramuscularly.  Bliss L. Finlayson, M.D., Price, Utah.

 ANSWER. -There have been several articles in recent years reporting improvement in psoriasis from intramuscular injection of whole blood.  Jones and Alden (South. M.J. 30:735 [July] 1937) [37B3] have contributed a valuable article discussing its use in other diseases as well.  From 5 to 10 cc. of blood is withdrawn from a vein in the arm and reinjected into the gluteal muscles. Usually from eight to ten injections are given. There is little discomfort from its use.  The method is certainly worth a trial in obstinate cases of psoriasis."

38A6 -autohemotherapy in pulmonary tuberculosis, [E. B. Freilich and G. C. Coe] Illinois M. J. 73:154-157, Feb. '38

 AUTOHEMO FOR PULMONARY TB; TECHNIC  38A6

Freilich and Coe, 1938 [38A6], p. 154, "Fifteen patients were selected with unquestionable pulmonary tuberculosis of the moderately or far advanced types, who were not making progress but who were also not moribund. ... Eight females and 7 males were studied for 14 weeks and each received three treatments per week averaging 52 injections of 10 to 15cc of whole fresh blood taken from the arm under sterile conditions and injected directly into the buttocks, with the blood remaining in the syringe for an average time of 50 seconds."

## AUTOHEMO FOR PULMONARY TB, SUBJECTIVE IMPROVEMENT ONLY - 38A6

The authors [38A6] concluded: "While there was abundant evidence of subjective improvement, objectively, very little was accomplished."

## AUTOHEMOTHERAPY SAFETY - 38A6

Freilich and Coe, 1938 [38A6], 155, "No toxic effects, local or general, were evidenced in any of the [15 pulmonary TB] patients during the 14 weeks of the experiment, although five of the men had an associated arteriosclerosis and one was a mild diabetic."

## AUTOHEMO THEORY - EXTERIORIZATION OF BLOOD  38A6

Freilich and Coe [38A6] 156, offered the opinion that "The blood, after being removed from the body, in the short time that elapses before reinjection, goes through some change, as yet unknown, and becomes a heterogenous foreign body.  ... It must ... be stressed that the substances which give the blood the characteristics typical of the heterogenous protein are not present in the circulating blood but are formed during the 'exteriorization' of the blood."

38A16 -intravenous autohemotherapy with hemolyzed blood; technic and leukopoietic response; Preliminary report [S.R. Dean & H.C. Solomon] J Lab & Clin Med. 23:775-786, May 38

### AUTOHEMO:  ANTICOAGULANTS DENOUNCED  38A16

Dean [38A16, 784] in his article on intravenous autohemotherapy, notes that "Descarpentries emphatically denounces the use of anticoagulants, claiming that any substance that disturbs the physiologic functions of the blood to the point of preventing coagulation, must equally disturb other functions whose aim it is to defend the organism against infection."

### AUTOHEMO, IV WITH HEMOLYSED BLOOD, AND MALARIA THERAPY 38A16

Dean 1938 [38A16] , The realization that artificially induced malaria infection might bring about benefit in some cases of neuro-syphilis had fostered "the modern vogue of treating neurosyphilis with mechanical hyperpyrexia" (induction of fever).

Dean 1938 [38A16], 775-6, sought to improve on this by duplicating another aspect of the "mechanism of malaria", blood destruction, to be used in conjunction with artificial induction of fever.  While his is thought to be the first attempt to combine the two components of induced fever and hemolyzed autoblood, he discusses some earlier works from 1923 to 1926 involving hemolyzed autoblood: Descarpentries (1923, 1926) had lysed 10cc of blood in 20cc distilled water, agitated the mixture with marbles, and injected the resultant clear fluid subcutaneously; Zimmerman, 1923, added 2cc of water to 20 cc autoblood and immediately reinjected it intramuscularly or intravenously; and Brunner and Breuer, 1924, placed 14cc water in a 20cc syringe, aspirated venous blood into the same syringe to capacity, and immediately reinjected the mixture without drawing the needle out of the vein.

[38A16] p. 776, "Descarpentries employs distilled water and blood in a proportion of 2:1, lysing 10cc uncitrated blood in 20cc distilled water; he then agitates the mixture in a flask containing several marbles, about which the clumps of fibrin adhere; finally he injects the clear fluid subcutaneously in divided doses - a momentarily painful, but according to him, a very beneficial procedure in various septic conditions."

[38A16] p.778, Notwithstanding Descarpentries' admonitions to the contrary, Dean mixed 1 part sodium citrate and 9 parts blood (10-50cc), shaken for 5 minutes, added 15 parts of distilled water, agitated again for 5 minutes, and reinjected intravenously (26-150cc total)


38B2 -autohemotherapy; case of purpura rheumatica with new method of treatment [L.Saxon] Illinois MJ 74:191-193. Aug. '38


AUTOHEMO: PREDICTION OF LOWER MORTALITY WHEN POPULAR   38B2

Saxon [38B2] "In our opinion autohemotherapy should be used much more than it has been, and the therapy of several diseases with a high mortality will be favorably influenced when this simple method will become more popular, and the basis of its use and dosage will be more thoroughly understood."


AUTOHEMO TECHNIC   38B2

Saxon [38B2]   "The procedure consists of withdrawing varying amounts of blood from the vein and either injecting the whole blood quickly before it coagulates, into the muscles, or allowing it to stand for several hours until the serum separates from the solid particles, and then only utilizing the blood-serum.  Some men have also subjected the venous blood after its withdrawal to further treatment (for example, ultra-violet irradiation) and others have reinjected the blood serum again intravenously."


AUTOHEMO FOR PURPURA RHEUMATISM   38B2

Saxon [38B2, p. 191] notes that purpura rheumatica usually begins with an attack of pharyngitis or tonsillitis; and that Henoch's type has often been diagnosed as appendicitis or cholecystitis. Saxon also mentions Werlhoff's disease (hemorrhagic purpura) which involves a marked decrease in blood-platelets.  Saxon reports on a grave case of purpura rheumatica that had "assumed all the earmarks of a septicemia", and was complicated by acute endocarditis.  After two injections of autoblood, the disease appeared to have been cured.

## AUTOHEMOTHERAPY AND VENESECTION   38B2

Saxon [38B2] "Where large amounts of blood are withdrawn, we are reminded of the time-honored method of 'bloodletting' or 'venesection' .... The effect of this method in the pneumonias is gaining new support; we know that by removing the venous engorgement in the circulation of the lungs, we can prevent the development of pulmonary edema; we relieve the work of the heart, which is under a considerable stress in pneumonia, and this may therefore be a lifesaving measure.  The effect of venesection in chronic bronchitis is specifically mentioned by Osler, and several authors have advocated the use of bloodletting in desperate cases of eclampsia.

## AUTOHEMO DOSAGE: LARGE IN INFECTIOUS CONDITIONS   38B2

p. 193  "In infectious conditions, as those of the respiratory organs, and in septic conditions, the dosage should be larger, and the intervals longer. ... Thus in pneumonia, where the method of Tillmann  [IV reinfusion] was used, doses as high as 100cc repeated at an interval of 2 days, has been found very effective; for most other conditions 5-10cc [IM] are sufficient...."

## AUTOHEMOTHERAPY THEORY: NOT PROTEIN SHOCK THERAPY   38B2

Saxon [38B2]  "It has been contended that it [autohemotherapy] is a form of protein shock therapy, but according to F. Scheuer this idea must be discarded, as the blood, after being reinjected, is absorbed very rapidly within an hour - that is, much more quickly than with foreign proteins."

39A3 -autohemotherapy; new method of treating hyperemesis gravidarum [L Sax151on & J. E. Stoll] Illinois MJ 75:352-355, April '39

## AUTOHEMO: HYPEREMESIS GRAVIDARUM (MORNING SICKNESS)   39A3

Saxon and Stolle [39A3, p. 355]  The authors have used autohemotherapy "in about 75 cases of hyperemesis, and have yet failed to see a case that did not respond."  The authors provide examples of successful autohemotherapy treatment in the first, second and third trimesters.  The technic involved 3-10 injections of 2-10 cc  at intervals of 2-7 days, including one case receiving 10 injections of 10 cc at weekly intervals.

"We assume that in toxemias of pregnancy a certain toxin is elaborated and absorbed in the blood streams of the pregnant woman.  The effect of these small amounts of blood injected into the tissues is in the nature of a desensitizing process; we ... get similar results in other allergic conditions such as urticaria and asthma."

## AUTOHEMO FOR TOXEMIAS IN GENERAL   39A3

Saxon and Stolle [39A3, p. 352] "We believe that we have found a method that is applicable to all types of toxemias, even to beginning eclampsia, a method which is practical, safe, economical and available at the home as well as in the hospital."

41A6: herpes simplex; case of unusually extensive, recurrent type, apparently cured after autoserotherapy, [C.C. Thomas] Arch Dermat & Syph. 43:817-821, May '41

## AUTOHEMOTHERAPY, DOSAGE FORMULA FOR   41A6
## AUTOHEMO:   URTICARIA   41A6
## AUTOHEMO:   BRONCHIAL ASTHMA   41A6

Kondo [41B6] described how "ten bronchial asthma and seven urticaria patients were treated by intramuscular injection of their own blood.  At intervals of 3-7 or more days, 10-20cc of blood (maximum, .40cc per 1 kg. of body weight) was injected into the Gluteus maximus.  On the 3rd day after the first injection patients generally became aware of an improvement and felt better after each succeeding injection."  One of the 10 asthma and 3 of the urticaria patients stopped treatment after the initial injection; all remaining patients were cured (2-3 injections for urticaria; 3-5 for bronchial asthma).

## AUTOSERUM FOR HERPES SIMPLEX, SUBCUTANEOUS - 41A6

Thomas [41A6] reported on a case of herpes simplex recurring at different sites on the body over a period of 12 years, involving during that time the arms, shoulders, flanks, buttocks, thighs and external genitalia.  Apparent cure was obtained by subcutaneous injections of autoserum.

When material from a typical 3-day-old lesion was inoculated into the cornea of a rabbit, it developed typical symptoms of keratitis and encephalitis, taken by Thomas as a demonstration of the presence of herpes virus.  However, repeated attempts at autoinoculation with the contents of the herpetic vesicles both by intracutaneous injection and after scarification of the skin were unsuccessful.  Culture of the vesicle contents and use of the Gram stain revealed no organisms.

"It was then decided to attempt desensitization by injections of autoserum according to the method of Gerber, as described by Urbach in connection with the treatment of menstrual dermatoses."  Blood was drawn at the height of an attack of herpes, and serum separated by centrifugation and stored in sterile ampule vials with tricresol as preservative.  Twice weekly .2cc intracutaneous injections, at the same site for 4 successive injections, over 10 weeks with 3 different batches of autoserum, were employed.

During the first month of treatment, 3 outbreaks of lesions
occurred, one in the second and third, an attack of grip in the
fourth, and a final mild herpes attack in the fifth; patient was
free of lesions for the subsequent one-year period. [It is noted
that Rosenow had referred to the increased presence of antigen
during disease exacerbations, which would thus provide the
rationale for autohemotherapy as clearly comprising
autovaccinetherapy at such a time.]

42B1: Marks, M.M., Lymphopathia venereum, autoserum as specific
antigen, South.M.J. 35:1092-1097, Dec. 1942.

AUTOSERUM: LYMPHOPATHIA VENEREUM, SUBCUT. UP TO 20 MONTHS -
42B1

Marks [42B1] in a study of 53 cases of lymphopathia venereum,
found autoserum injections to be a "therapeutically useful source
of specific human antigen". He developed a routine of treatment
wherein 10-15 cc of blood was take from the median basilic vein
and the serum removed by centrifuge or after clotting. The serum
was injected under the skin of the abdominal wall, with treatment
given at 4-day intervals, totalling 12 injections per series,
with 2 weeks rest between series, over periods ranging from 6 to
20 months.

47A3: Ross, B., and P.J. Richeson, Intensive autohemotherapy of
acne. U.S.Nav.M.Bull. 47:154-155, Jan.-Feb., 1947.

AUTOHEMO: ACNE  47A3

Ross and Richeson [47A3] obtained improvement in 10 of 10 cases
of acne after 10 injections; notably after only 5 injections, one
case had gotten worse and 6 others had not improved.

A feature of their technic: "No local applications were
permitted during the course of treatment. ... The method adopted
was the usual method of autohemotherapy, consisting of
withdrawing blood from a cubital vein, and immediately
reinjecting it in the buttock. The planned course consisted of 2
injections a week for a total of 10 injections. The first
injection was a test dose of 5 cc of whole blood, and all
subsequent doses were 10cc."

49B1: Poth, D.O., Autohemotherapy of herpes zoster; results in
154 cases. Arch. Dermat. & Syph. 69:636-638, Oct. 1949.
AUTHEMO: HERPES ZOSTER  49B1

Poth [49B1], points out that "Most textbooks do not mention
this type of treatment", citing 2 contemporary books (1938-43)
with no mention of autohemotherapy, and one which made one

mention of it.

Poth reports having cured 137 of 141 cases of herpes zoster with autohemotherapy. 27 received one injection; 21, two; 77, three; and 16 received four injections. "These 141 patients averaged 2.5 injections and obtained complete relief of pain in 5.22 days, although severe pain had usually subsided before the 2nd or 3rd injection was given. ...

"Injections (10-15cc) were given every third day until relief of pain was reported by the patient."

49H1:  Saxon, Leo, "Treatment of herpes zoster with special reference to autohemotherapy", J. Am. Inst. Homeop. Oct. 1949, 213.

AUTOHEMO:  HERPES ZOSTER, POLIO AND RABIES  49H1

Saxon [49H1] discusses the utility of autohemotherapy in various conditions, with particular focus on herpes zoster, which condition "belongs to the significant group of neuro-tropic virus diseases, the others being acute anterior poliomyelitis and rabies." Aside from this implication by association that autohemotherapy might be useful in rabies and polio, Saxon does not refer to having attempted it in either.

AUTOHEMO:  IRRADIATION NOT NECESSARY  49H1

Saxon [49H1] asserted that it was not necessary to subject autoblood, after withdrawal, to the action of ultraviolet light, as had been practiced by the Hahnemann school of Philadelphia. Saxon's 10 years' experience led him to "claim that the curative effect in this therapy is the blood serum, which contains all the protective bodies - whatever they may be ..." and not any changes in the plasma that might be attributed to ultraviolet rays.

VACCINETHERAPY, DANGERS OF OVERDOSAGE WITH   49H1

Saxon [49H1] "... the failure of vaccine therapy ... in my opinion is due to over-dosage and upsetting the delicate immunological balance."

49H2:  Mease, "Modified Autohemic Therapy", J.Florida M.A.,, SSSVI July 1949, 22-25.

AUTOHEMIC THERAPY - TAKE TWO  49H2

A method of blood manipulation and reinjection termed "auto-hemic" therapy was proposed in 1949 by Mease [49H2, p. 23]. While this may have been derived from Rogers' method of the same name from the 20s [23E1], it is noted that Wright also used the term without reference to Rogers [31H1]. Of Mease's method, Dr. Robert J. Campbell [49H2, p. 24] noted "The results that Dr. Mease has obtained are interesting, but I do not believe that the shaking and incubation procedures are necessary to achieve such

results, because many investigators have found that injection of
fresh whole blood can be followed by similar beneficial results
in selected patients.


## AUTOHEMO, WHY LOST  49H2

J. Robert Campbell in Mease, 1949 [49H2], "... I could not help
comparing the beneficial effects of histamine in various diseases
and in the treatment of various symptoms with the results
frequently derived in the case of autohemotherapy."


## AUTOHEMOTHERAPY; ACTION LIKENED TO HISTAMINE  49H2

Dr Campbell commented on having used autohemotherapy early in
his practice, and how he had likened its effects to that of
histamine.  Dr. Campbell warned against dangers of the method
proposed by Mease: "The incubation procedures used by Dr. Mease
must enable some change to occur which makes the blood derivative
more liable to produce sloughing than does fresh whole blood."

It may be offered, as other writers have noted, that any
alteration of the blood introduces some form of risk that is
nonexistent in the case of use of whole blood.


51C7:  Sauer, G.C., and Simm, F., "Evidence of adreno-cortical
stimulation by autohemotherapy." JOURNAL OF INVESTIGATIVE
DERMATOLOGY, 16:3 (March 1951), p. 177-192. [56822]


## AUTOHEMO THEORY - ADRENAL CORTEX  51C7

Sauer, 1951 [51C7] studied hematologic changes following
autohemotherapy, in 20 patients of which were hospitalized
dermatology patients, and suggested that the mechanism of action
may be stimulation of the adrenal cortex.  Frandsen and Samsoe-
Jensen, however, in a subsequent study of 16 dermatology
patients, found no evidence of adreno-cortical stimulation.


51C11:  Reddick, R. H., "Autohemotherapy in chronic mental
disorders; a preliminary report.", JOURNAL OF THE AMERICAN
INSTITUTE OF HOMEOPATHY 43:10 (Dec. 1950), p. 263-9. [34410]


## AUTOHEMO:  MENTAL ILLNESS  51C11

Reddick 1950 [51C11], p. 264, "25 female patients ranging in
age from 27 to 70 were studied for a period of 6 months.  All
were chronically psychotic and had displayed mental abnormalities
for periods of from 3 to 32 years ... "  These patients received
from 2 to 25 treatments total, initially 5cc, then increased to
10cc.  In most instances a few drops of 25% citric acid was
"introduced through the needle into the syringe before the blood
was withdrawn."

## AUTOHEMO THEORY 51C11

Reddick [51C11, 266-7] discussed the numerous theories of several (27) investigators purporting to explain the action of autohemotherapy.

## AUTOHEMO, IMPETUS FOR USE IN MENTAL ILLNESS  51C11

[51C11] p. 264, Reddick asserted "Scattered reports in the literature concerning the efficacy of autohemotherapy in neurotropic virus diseases, such as herpes zoster which may, incidentally, result in psychotic manifestations) prompted the author to investigate the effects of this procedure upon a group of chronic mental patients. ... I have yet to find any prior report indicating that it has ever been used before in the therapy of the psychoses."

[It may be noted, however, that the QCIM lists no less than 19 articles between 1927 and 1939 dealing with autohemotherapy in psychiatry, mental illness, etc.]

## BLOOD AND MIND IN HISTORY  51C11

Reddick [51C11] p.264 cites Hippocrates as having stated that one of the causes of psychiatric disorders was an alteration of the blood physiology of the brain.  Subsequently, Celsus and Aretaeus the Cappadocian, Galen in the 2nd century, and Paracelsus and Alexis of Piemont several centuries later all "attempted to correlate mental pathology and abnormal conditions of the blood.

## BENEFICIAL EFFECT OF OTHER DISEASES ON MENTAL ILLNESS  51C11

Reddick [51C11], p. 263 notes "it has frequently been observed that intercurrent diseases have a beneficial effect on mental illness."

53B7:  Heimark, J.J. & R.L. Parsons, Spinal injection of blood to lower blood pressure in essential hypertensive patients; 2 cases, Minnesota Med. 36:738-739, July 1953

## AUTOHEMO FOR HYPERTENSION; INTRASPINAL - 53B7

Noting that "many hypertensive patients who sustain a severe cerebro-vascular accident and survive, eventually develop a normal blood pressure", Heimark and Parsons, 1953 [53B7], tried "beating the hypertensive cerebro-vascular accident to the draw, so to speak."  The authors reviewed many known facts concerning blood in the spinal fluid: The presence of blood in the cerebro-spinal fluid after accidents; occasional accidental entry of blood into the spinal canal during spinal punctures; the fact that "Medical as well as neurological textbooks describe no pathology, nor entity, nor syndrome that is attributed to a bloody spinal fluid 'per se'; and further, discussions "with able clinicians, neurologists and a neuro-pathologist" all of whom "could not recall any residual pathology produced by blood in the spinal canal 'per se'. With this background, two patients were each given four intraspinal injections of whole blood: 1, 1, 2, and 4cc; the second patient received a fifth injection of 5cc. In all cases the blood was withdrawn from the arm and rapidly injected.

"The followup in Case 1 was not too satisfactory. On July 30, 1952, when the patient reported to the office, her blood pressure was 200/106. On Sept. 30, 1952, it was 190/96. No further readings have been recorded. she volunteered the information she felt so different that she believed it was not necessary to report further."

In the case of the second patient, her blood pressure readings were not appreciably lowered, except that there was "very marked reduction in the nervous tension as well as increased calm so very noticeable in her behavior. ...

"the one observation that really stimulated us to report these two cases was the very noticeable calm and absence of tension in both of the patients following the treatment."


53C3: Peters, H., Therapeutic venous and muscular stimulation as supportive treatment in carcinosis; pyrogenated serotherapy and autohemotherapy, PRAKTISCHE ARZT (Wien) 6:63 (15 August 1952), p. 447-8. [51647]


55C2: Reddick, R.H., "Autohemotherapy in psychiatry.", MARYLAND STATE MEDICAL JOURNAL (Baltimore), p. 22-31. [47013]

Reddick [55C2], p. 22, discusses beneficial effects from the use of autohemotherapy having been reported, over the previous three decades, in several diseases.


### AUTOHEMO TECHNIC  55C2

"The initial treatment consisted of the removal of 5cc of blood from one of the median basilic veins under aseptic conditions, followed by immediate deep intramuscular reinjection into the upper outer quadrant of the buttock of the opposite side. A few drops of 4% sodium citrate solution were introduced through the needle into the syringe before the blood was withdrawn; the average length of time which the blood remained in the syringe was fifty-five seconds." [55C2] p. 23


### AUTOHEMO: MENTAL ILLNESS RESULTS  55C2

Reddick [55C2] reported on 2 series of psychiatric trials, involving 25 patients each.

Of the first grouping of 25 [see 1950 above], "nineteen patients or 76% of those treated displayed a social recovery, inasmuch as they were able to leave the hospital and to resume their former activities.  Of the 6 patients still requiring hospitalization at the conclusion of the treatment period [6 months], three were much better; and one remained unchanged.

His second group of 25 was studied in conjunction with a control group of ten, and here 23 of the 25 displayed a social recovery (in contrast to none of the ten in the control group, who had been treated with saline in place of autoblood).  Of the remaining 2 patients still hospitalized after 6 months, one has received only eleven treatments to date and had already been released on 4 trial visits, one lasting 10 days, to the custody of her daughter.  A more permanent release was "anticipated in the near future."  the final patient was a 63-year-old woman who had sustained a cerebro-vascular accident 8 years before, had been hospitalized in 7 private institutions prior to current public institutionalization, and had been diagnosed as 'chronic brain syndrome associated with cerebral arteriosclerosis, with psychotic reaction'.  In addition she suffered from systemic syphilis.,

"Her condition is now improved and she is scheduled for staff presentation in the near future for the purpose of discussing the advisability of granting her a trial visit to the custody of her husband."

Reddick presents one case of a 34-year-old woman with "very poor prognosis because of the long duration of her illness", who despite 3 courses of electroshock therapy and other attempted therapy was "still deeply psychotic."  After an initial 5cc dose and subsequent weekly 10cc injections over a period of 16 weeks, "her degree of improvement was so marked that she was described as displaying a complete social remission."  However, it was noted that this patient had "exhibited a generalized cutaneous eruption of innumerable small pustular lesions" following each IM reinjection, most of which ruptured spontaneously within a day or so.  [It is suggested that this may have been due to the use of the citric acid anti-coagulant, insofar as such reaction was not generally encountered in the literature.]

## AUTOHEMOTHERAPY IS SPECIFIC    55C2

"No therapy can possibly be more specific than the resistance of the individual patient to his own disease processes..."

## AUTOHEMO SAFETY   55C2

Reddick [55C2] credits autohemotherapy with the "advantage of being a safe and effective means of bringing into play the helpful portions of the body's defenses without exposing the patient to the possibility of unnecessary incidental damage. ... Autohemotherapy helps the sick person to heal himself."

57C3:  Ansfield, F.J., and J. L. Rens, "Autohemotherapy; an
effective treatment for herpes zoster." WISCONSIN MEDICAL JOURNAL
(Madison) 55:12 (Dec. 1956), p. 1319-1320. [27579]

AUTOHEMO FOR HERPES ZOSTER - BACKGROUND/IMPETUS     57C3

Ansfield and Rens, 1956 [57C3], 1319, note "Van Blarrim and
Horax [JAMA 161 (1956):511-515] have recently described the
radical surgery, from lobotomy to chordotomy, that has been done
in an attempt to relieve the suffering from this agonizing
neuralgia. ...

"Among the newer methods of treatment of herpes zoster,
including the use of Chloromycetin or Aureomycin, is the use of
gamma globulin; a very interesting report describing the
effective treatment of 5 patients with this method was made by
Weintraub [JAMA 157 (1955):1611].  In 1942, J.W. Nixon-Davis,
M.D., of Chicago, informed one of us (JLR) that injecting a
patient's own blood intramuscularly was the treatment of choice
in dealing with herpes zoster."


AUTOHEMO FOR HERPES ZOSTER: SAFETY/EXPENSE  57C3

Ansfield and Rens [57C3], p. 1320, "There were no reactions
from autohemotherapy other than some local discomfort at the site
of the infection; and there is no expense to the patient for his
own blood ... "


AUTOHEMO TECHNIC   57C3

[57C3]  "... we have treated 54 cases of herpes zoster by
intramuscular injections of 15cc of the patient's own blood. ...
At the time the diagnosis [of herpes zoster] was made, 15cc of
blood was withdrawn from the antecubital vein of the patient and
injected deep into the gluteal muscle on one side.  the patient
was instructed to return in 48 hours.  If the pain had entirely
subsided no further treatment was given.  Eight patients were in
this category.  The response of the vesicles went hand in hand
with that of the subjective symptom of pain.  On the second
visit, if the patient still had pain, a second injection of 15cc
of his blood was given in the opposite gluteal muscle, and he was
instructed to return in 48 hours.  If the pain had subsided then,
no further treatment was given.  34 patients were cured after
this second injection.  After 2 such injections at 48 hour
intervals, 12 patients still had painful herpes zoster and were
given a third injection of 15cc of their blood and instructed to
return again in 48 hours.  In 10 of these 12 patients requiring a
third injection, the pain had subsided and the vesicles were
clearing rapidly,; but 2 patients failed to respond to all 3
injections.  One of these patients was given 2 injections of 1000
micrograms of vitamin B12, which apparently cleared the pain
promptly."  The final patient did not respond to vitamin B12, but

the pain gradually subsided over the next 3 months.

In summary, "The results were most gratifying in 52 cases, with the pain entirely controlled within 2 to 7 days. We feel that these results are unsurpassed and heartily urge that autohemotherapy be used routinely in treating herpes zoster."

## AUTOHEMO SAFETY/COST     57C3

[57C3] p. 1320, "There were no reactions from autohemotherapy other than some local discomfort at the site of the injection; and there is no expense to the patient for his own blood, in contradistinction to the high cost of gamma globulin or moderately high cost of broad-spectrum antibiotics."

60H1:  Schiff, Bencel L., "Autohemotherapy in the treatment of post-herpetic pain", Rhode Island Med.J. 43 (Feb. 1960), 104.

## AUTOHEMO: POST-HERPETIC NEURALGIA  60H1

Schiff, 1960 [60H1], p. 104, "Herpes zoster is a highly characteristic virus disease confined to man that attacks sensory nerve roots and shows itself on the skin as a grouped vesicular eruption in the dermatome of the infected nerve. ...

"The cause of herpes zoster is a virus that is believed to be identical with or closely related to that of chickenpox."  Schiff cites "epidemiological observations" of cases of herpes zoster appearing in adults exposed to children with varicella and cases of chickenpox appearing in children exposed to adults with herpes zoster.

Schiff concerned himself with "management of neuralgic pain following herpes zoster which, particularly in older people, may be so severe as to produce in them a state of utter despondency."

Noting that Ansfield and Rens in the course of their treatment of herpes zoster with autohemotherapy had also been able to control pain within 2-7 days, Schiff undertook to study the effects of autohemotherapy on the pain itself.

## AUTOHEMO METHOD  60H1

[60H1]  "The autohemotherapy consisted of the withdrawal of 10cc of whole blood from an antecubital vein followed by its immediate injection into the gluteal muscles. ... Injections were given ... once every three days [for a total of from 8-14 injections], but the interval between treatments was increased as the symptoms and signs abated."

## AUTOHEMO RESULTS  60H1

[60H1] "Disappearance of the pain was noted in 8 cases and 3 failed to respond."

The MEDLINE INDEX began in 1966, and lists some 22 items under the keyword "autohemotherapy between 1965 and 1995. Abstracts of three of the nine articles listed from 1990-5 are provided below, all of which involve intravascular reinjection. A full listing of 22 keyword:autohemotherapy items in MEDLINE has been incorporated into APPENDIX C: AUTOHEMOTHERAPY BIBLIOGRAPHY.

65F1:  Bacskulin J, & Bacskulin E, Further experiences with subconjunctival autohemotherapy in fresh and old corrosions. Amer. J. Ophthal. 59:674-80, Apr. 1965

AUTOHEMO, DANGER OF CITRATED BLOOD, SUBCONJUNCTIVAL - 65F1

Bacskulin and Bacskulin [65F1] reported good results with subconjunctival autohemotherapy in corrosions of the eye, injecting "1.5 to 2.0 cc of fresh blood into the perilimbal and fornix region as quickly as possible." However, they warned against the use of citrated blood:  "It is especially important that no citrated blood be used. After citrated blood, almost all cases show heavy vascularization with corneal leukoma, and often a pointed deformity of the lid.  In contrast, the control eye treated with fresh blood of the patient and the recommended additional therapy always shows satisfactory end results.

"This can be explained by the fact that, when calcium is combined with the acids of mucopolysaccharides and extracted by sodium citrate, a new complex (CaNaCitrate) is formed. ... However, because CaNaCitrate is almost water insoluble, it cannot diffuse out of the corneal tissue, and so remains in the corroded corneal parenchyma as a foreign body."

92G2:  Bocci V., Medical Hypotheses, 1992 Sep, 39(1):30-4., "Ozonization of blood for the therapy of viral diseases and immunodeficiencies. A Hypothesis."

VIRAL DISEASES  92G2

AIDS  92G2

HEPATITIS, VIRAL  92G2

HERPES SIMPLEX  92G2

HERPES ZOSTER  92G2

LABIALIS  92G2

GENITALIS  92G2

PAPILLOMAVIRUS  92G2

RESPIRATORY DISEASES  92G2

CFS  92G2

COMMON COLD  92G2

Bocci 1992 calls for investigation of his methodology by biologists and clinicians. "Once this is done, owing to the large range of medical applications and the simplicity of the procedure, autohemotherapy could become very valuable particularly in underdeveloped countries."[Medline] "If autohemotherapy can be understood on a scientific basis, it may become an acceptable practice in orthodox medicine".[Bocci]

Bocci lists a number of viral diseases that may benefit from so-called "major autohemotherapy" [intravenous reinjection, after exposure to ozone], including viral hepatitis; herpes simplex, zoster, labialis and genitalis; papillomavirus;

respiratory diseases; CFS; common cold; AIDS, etc. He makes no mention of exhaustive body of literature discussing extravascular autohemotherapy, which practice he briefly refers to as "minor" autohemotherapy.

Chiyoda S and T Morikawa, Japanese Journal of Clinical Hematology, 1993 Jan, 34(1):39-43, "Reinfusion of concentrated autogenous ascitic fluid in a patient with selective IgA deficiency."

GILBERT METHOD - LEG EDEMA AND ASCITES  Chiyoda and Morikawa 1993

As recently as 1993 [MEDLINE] Chiyoda S and T Morikawa discussed the reinfusion of concentrated autogenous ascitic fluid in the case of a patient with leg edema and ascites, with common cold-like symptoms, and diagnostic findings suggesting systemic lupus erythematosus. "His ascitic fluid disappeared and complements and albumin in his serum normalized. ...."

93G2: Bocci V, Luzzi E, Corradeschi F, Paulesu L, Di Stefano A., "Studies on the biological effects of ozone: 3. An attempt to define conditions for optimal induction of cytokines." Lymphokine and Cytokine Research, 1993 Apr., 12(2):121-6. Abstract Avail. (UI: 93312993)

CITRATED BLOOD V. HEPARIN & CACL2, AND OZONIZATION  93G2

Bocci et al 1993 [Lymphokine and Cytokine Research, 1993 Apr., 12(2):121-6] note that ozonization of the blood is normally carried out with citrated blood, but that this "may be at a loss when employed in viral diseases or in immunodeficiencies. Instead the authors indicated a preference for use of heparin, supplemented by CaCl2, as anticoagulant, which "favors production of cytokines by leukocytes with only a modest increase in hemolysis." In contrast, high levels of glucose, glutathione and ascorbic acid were said to decrease cytokine's yield through antioxidant action.

95G1: Hernandez F; Menendez S; Wong R.  "Decrease of blood cholesterol and stimulation of antioxidative response in cardiopathy patients treated with endovenous oxone therapy." Free Radical Biology and Medicine, 1995 Jul, 19(1):115-9.


CARDIAC INFARCTION PATIENTS  95G1

CHOLESTEROL IN CARDIOPATHY PATIENTS, AFTER AUTOHEMO  95G1

Hernandez 95 report that results with 22 patients who had had an infarction between 3 months and one year prior to study, who were subsequently treated with 15 sessions of intravenous ozone ("ozone by autohemotherapy").  The authors report "a statistically significant decrease in plasma total cholesterol and low density lipoprotein [and] high biologically significant increases in erythrocyte glutathione peroxidase and glucose 6-phosphate dehydrogenase activities ..."

APPENDIX B:   REPRINT: JONES & ALDEN 1937

## AUTOHEMOTHERAPY IN DERMATOLOGY

By Jack W. Jones, M.D. and Herbert S. Alden, M.D., Atlanta, Georgia

Chairman's Address, Section on Dermatology and Syphilology, Southern Medical Association, Thirtieth Annual Meeting, Baltimore, Maryland, Nov. 17-20, 1936.  Reprinted by permission from the SOUTHERN MEDICAL JOURNAL (Volume 30, No. 7, 735-7, 1937).

As practical physicians we are constantly taking up new methods of treatment, trying them out for varying periods of time, and if not immediately impressed with the results obtained, discarding them for methods more promising.  When one briefly reviews dermatological therapy he is surprised at the hectic history of any measure.  To be convinced of this, one has only to review his personal experience of the past ten or fifteen years.  In some instances he would be chagrined and often amused at the outlines of treatment followed in the past.

We are all experimenters at heart and for some reason, or apparently for no reason at all, chance upon a line of therapy. If it gives or promises results it is published or passed by word of mouth to colleagues, who immediately seize upon it and not being content with the original method, immediately try it out on similar conditions or upon those conditions for which there is no satisfactory treatment.  If this particular treatment is of sufficient value in any one disease to withstand its various criticisms, it will remain as a standard therapeutic procedure; otherwise, due to the many conflicting reports from all types of experimentation, it is slowly but surely discarded, and often becomes the stock in trade of the quack or charlatan, who exploits to the full any value there may be in the procedure.  If there is any virtue in it, many years later the same procedure is brought forth again in the same or in a little different guise and, going through the same process, is more carefully analyzed and confined more particularly to its peculiar value without expecting or finding it to be a panacea, it then receives its true place in our therapeutic armamentarium.

In December, 1910, Mayer and Linser[1,2,3,8] published a communication on the results of treatment of a case of herpes gestations by injections of a serum obtained from the blood of a pregnant woman.  Following this report, the treatment of other toxic dermatoses was reported by the same writers, then by Freund,[3] by Fetzer[5] Veiel,[6] Rubsamen,[7] Heuck,[9] and

Practorius.[10]   The conditions treated by this method included urticaria, pemphigus, dermatitis herpetiformis, strophulus and various hemorrhagic diseases of the skin.  Other writers, including Ullman, were less favorable in their comments. Spiethoff[13] apparently was the first to use the serum obtained from the patient himself.  He claimed good results in a number of dermatological conditions.  Gottheil and Satenstein11 were the first in this country to report on the treatment of dermatologic conditions with autohemotherapy.  Their report included patients with psoriases, radiodermatitis, furunculosis, dermic abscesses, chronic urticaria and lichen planus.  This was quickly followed by a report from Howard Fox,[12] whose work was limited almost entirely to the treatment of psoriasis.  These reports were followed by others in various dermatoses with moderately favorable results.  There were numerous communications for a time which might be termed enthusiastic, but a little later as the treatment was used for more and more conditions the tone of the reports began to change to a more pessimistic note.  All of these reports described the complicated method of removal of blood and a later intramuscular injection of the centrifuged serum.  the simpler

method most commonly used at the present time is intramuscular injection of the freshly withdrawn blood before it has had time to clot, a method first introduced by Ravaut[14] in 1913.  Various observers have pointed out that different clinical results may be obtained by the different methods used in the injection of blood, but Wright,[15] in 1930, was still enthusiastic concerning the simpler method of autohemotherapy as an adjunct in the treatment of psoriasis.


   There has never been a completely satisfactory explanation of the mechanism of the action of autohemotherapy.  Burgess,[16] in 1931, after a study of the various explanations offered, drew the following conclusions:


   (1) The action of whole blood injections does not depend upon the production of a leukocytosis.


   (2) The hemoclysis crisis is not a satisfactory test for allergy and bears no relation to the whole blood injections.


   (3) Whole blood injections had no effect on the sedimentation rate of the red corpuscles as estimated by the methods of Zechner and Godell.


   (4) Proteose was obtained from the urine of normal persons and from those suffering from various dermatoses.  No constant effect on the production of proteose by a single whole blood injection

could be demonstrated.

We first began the use of autohemotherapy as an adjunct in the treatment of psoriasis some six or eight years ago and use the following routine: eight to ten cubic centimeters of fresh blood are withdrawn from the cubital vein and immediately injected into the gluteal muscle at weekly intervals, using along with it mild local applications.  This method of treatment has served us extremely well as an aid in the intractable cases of psoriasis. We have been somewhat unfair to autohemotherapy in that we have reserved its use for the most difficult cases.  The average number of injections required for relief is approximately ten. This method of treatment in psoriasis has unquestionably given us good results in the attack, but it cannot be said that it is curative, although the intervals between attacks has seemed to be lengthened.

The following case is typical:

Mrs. Mc., aged 33, a physician's daughter, had not been clear of psoriasis since she was a small girl in spite of treatment under the direction of competent physicians with the usual drugs such as chrysarobin and ammoniated mercury.  The eruption was present particularly in the scalp and to a lesser degree on the trunk and extremities.  She was given autohemotherapy at weekly intervals for ten weeks, when her skin became normal in appearance.  The disease recurred in a few months' time and she again responded to the blood injections.  since she has not been regular with the treatment we have not been able to follow her case over a sufficient period of time to determine whether or not it can be controlled by the continuous injection method.

We feel that we can recommend autohemotherapy as a most useful adjunct in the treatment of psoriasis.

There have been numerous reports of the efficacy of autohemotherapy in vesicular and bullous diseases.  Our first attempt in this direction was a patient, Mrs. M., with recurring herpes simplex, who had been treated by several competent dermatologists with local applications, x-ray, calcium and the usual non-specific therapy with apparently no results, was started on autohemotherapy.  Her improvement was so spectacular that we have since used it in many such cases, and although apparently no case has ever failed to respond, there have been a number in which recurrences took place.

The one disease in which we should particularly like to commend the use of autohemotherapy is herpes zoster.  In fact, we have been so favorably impressed with the results obtained that it has become routine in the office in the treatment of this disease. the relief of pain and symptoms in the large majority of cases treated by this method have been most spectacular, many of the cases reporting relief in a few hours or within the first day. A patient who came in from a neighboring city seventy-five miles away, who had previously required morphine for relief of pain, reported entire relief of pain before she reached home in her car. In the treatment of herpes zoster it has been our custom to repeat the injection in two days if necessary. In most cases at the end of this period the patients do not feel that they need further treatment, as the symptoms have usually disappeared and the vesicles have dried.

Although we have used autohemotherapy in numerous other conditions, our results have been so uncertain as not to warrant report. However, we do feel that this procedure deserves favorable mention in that group of so-called non-specific desensitizing agents, such as calcium, sodium thiosulphate and x-ray. Its use in this role in atopic eczemas and toxic dermatoses such as urticaria and erythema muliforma at times seemed of marked benefit as an adjunct. But its use in psoriasis, herpes simplex and herpes zoster has often been spectacular.

- - - - - - - - - - - - - -

1. Mayer, A; and Linser, P.: Ein versuch schwangerschaftstoxikosen durch Einspritzungen von Schwanger-schaftserum zu heilen. Munchen Med. Wchnschr., 7:2757, 1910.

2. Mayer: Normales Schwangerenserum als Heilmittel gegen Schwangerschaftsdermatosen im besonderen und Schwangerschafts-toxikosen uberhaupt. Zentralbl f. Guiak, 35:350, 1911; Weiter Erfahrungen uper die Behandlung von Schwangerschaftstoxikosen mit Normalen Schwangerenserum. Ibid., 35:1299, 1911.

3. Freund, R.: Serimtherapie bei Schwangerschaftstoxikosen. Med. Klin. 7:371, 1911.

4. Linser, P.: Uber Hauterkrauk-nungen bei Schwangerschaft und deren Heilung.Dermat. Ztschr.,18:217, 1911.

5. Fetzer: Die Therapeutische Verendung von Normalen Schwangeren-serum Nebst versuch einer Erklarung auf experimenteller Grundige. Deutsch Gesellsch. f Gyuik. 14:712, 1911.

6. Veiel, F.: Ein Beitrag Zur Serumbehandlung der Schwangerschafts dermatosen. Munchen. Med. Wchnschr., 59:1911,

1912.

7.  Rubsamen, W.: Weiterer Beitrag zur
Schwangerschafterumtherapie der Schwangerschaftstoxikosen.
Deutsch. Med. Wchnschr., 39:931, 1913.

8.  Linser, P.: Uber Einige mit Serum gehielte Falle von
Urtikaria.  Med. Klin., 7:136, 1911.  Uber die Therapeutische
Verendung von normalem Menschlichen Serum ver Handl. d. Vong. f.
inn.  Med. 28:125, 1911.  Uber die therapeutische Ver Wending von
Normalen Menschlichen serum Haut- und innerlichen Kraukheiten.
Arch. Derm. u. Syph., 113:701,1912.

9.  Heuck, W.: Erfahrungen uber Behandlung Hautkranken mit
Menschen-serum.  Munchen. Med. Wschnschr., 59:2608, 1912.

10.  Practorius, G.: Pemphigus Malignus durch ein malige
Intravenose Blutinjektion gehilt.  Munchen. Med. Wchnschr.,
60:867, 1913.

11.  Gottheil, W.S.; and Satenstein, D.L.: The Autoserum
Treatment in Dermatology.  J.A.M.A., 63:1190, 1914.

12.  Fox, Howard:  Autogenous Serum in Treatment of Psoriasis.
J.A.M.A., 63:2190, 1914.

13.  Spiethoff, B.: Zur Therapeutischen Verwendung des
Eigenserums.  Munchen. Med. Wchnschr., 60:521, 1913.

14.  Ravaut: Ann. de Derm. & Syph., 4:292, 1913.

15.  Wright, C.S.: Arch. de Derm. & Syph., 23:118, 1931.

16.  Burgess: Brit. Jour. Derm. & Syph., 44:124, 1932.

APPENDIX C:  AUTOHEMOTHERAPY BIBLIOGRAPHY

Key: All listings indicate year, source, and sequential item (e.g., 35A3 is from 1935, source "A", third article.)

Sources: A,B = QUARTERLY CUMULATIVE INDEX MEDICUS, 1916-56 (American Medical Assn.); "Serotherapy"

C,D = CURRENT LIST; 1941-1959 (Army/Nat'l Lib. of Med.); "Serotherapy", plus "Hemotherapy" 1941 & "Autohemotherapy" 1947

E = INDEX MEDICUS, 1903-1927 (Carnegie Inst.); "Serotherapy"

F = Cumulated INDEX MEDICUS, 1960-1982 (A.M.A. & N.L.M.), "Serotherapy"

H = Miscellaneous, 1894-1940

1894H1:  Gilbert, Gaz. d. hospitaux, Paris, 1894, Vol. LXVIII. (as per 14H6.

1898H1:  Elfstrom, Carl E. and Axel V. Grafstrom, Heated Blood in Croupous Pneumonia, N.Y.Med. J. 26 Aug. 1898:307-9; 15 Oct. 1898:556; 30 Sept. 1899:486-7.

01H1:  Jez, Valentin, "Ueber die Behandlung des Erysipelas mit Serum von an Erysipel erkrankten Individuen." Wiener Medicinische Wochenschrift, 31 August 1901:1613-1621; abstr. J.A.M.A., Oct.-Dec. 1901: 1074.

05E1:  Browning, G.S., Auto-serotherapy.  MED. HERALD, ST. JOSEPH, 1905, n.s., xxiv, 419-425.

05H1: Bier, A., "Die Entzünndung. Arch. klin. Chir. Bd. 176, S 529.

06E1:  Landolfi, M., Autosieroterapia ed autosierodiagnosi.  GAZZ. INTERNAZ. DI MED., NAPOLI, 1905, vii, 267-71.

06E2:  Baccari, A., L'auto-sieroterapia nelle pleuriti siero-fibrinose e nelle peritoniti tubercolari a forma ascitica e le aggressine.  N. RIV. CLIN.-TERAP., NAPOLI, 1906, ix, 469-475.

09E1:  Hort, E. C., Auto-inoculation versus hetero-inoculation in the treatment of established infective disease, in pyrexial and in apyrexial conditions ..., PROC. ROY. SOC. MED., LOND., 1909, ii, Med. Sect., 177-228.

09H1:  Marcou, M., Autoserotherapy in pleural effusion, La Presse Médicale, 4 Sept., 1909:627-8.

10E1:  Busquet, P., Contribution á l'étude de l'autosérothérapie.  GAZ. HEBD. D. SC. MÉD HEBD. D. SC. MÉD DE BORDEAUX, 1910, xxxi, 169-173.

10E2:  Le Play, A., Autosérotherapie des épanchements séreux.  BULL. MÉD

PAR., 1910, xxiv, 707-710.

10E3:  Godlemski, E., Deux cas d'autosérothérapie ascitique. BULL. ET MEM. SOC. DE MÉD DE VAUCLUSE, AVIGNON, 1910, vi, 419-422.

11E1:  Lemann, I.I., Auto-serotherapy in the treatment of collections of fluids in serous cavities. N. ORL. M. & S. J., 1910-11, lxiii, 327-333.

11E2:  Austin, C.K., Reports on Autoserotherapy. INTERNAT. CLIN., PHILA., 1910, 20. s., iii, 24-32.

11E3:  Braga, A., and Copelli, M., Sierositi ed autosieroterapia. BOLL. D. SOC. MED. DI PARMA, 1910, 2.s., iii, 182-198.

11E4:  Lemann, I.I., Autoserotherapy; the therapeutic use of the patients own serous exudates and transudates. INTERSTATE M. J., ST. LOUIS, 1911, xvii, 288-297.

11E5:  Angel Elvira, Autosueroterapia. REV. DE MED. Y CIRUG. PRACT., MADRID, 1911, xc, 414-417.

11E6:  Riviere, C., The role of auto-inoculation in medicine; a plea for its rational extension. PROC. ROY. SOC. MED., LONDON, 1910-11, iv, Therap. & Pharmacol. Sect., 39-50.

11E7:  Chaumier, E., á propos de l'autosérithérapie des maladies

bactériennes.  GAZ. MÉD. DE PAR., 1911, lxxxii, 115-118.

11E8:  Garmagnano, C., Considerazioni sulla auto-sieroterapia.  GAZZ. D. OSP., MILANO, 1911, xxxii, 475.

11E9:  Synot, M.J., Auto-inoculation; its practical application in the treatment of various infections and as a substitute for bacterial vaccines. MED. REC., N.Y., 1911, lxxx, 125-127.

11E10:  Duncan, C.H., Auto-therapy.  N. AM. J. HOMEOPATHY, N.Y., 1911, clxv, 709-714.

11H1:  Oliva, C., Zeitschr.f.klin. Med., Berl. lxxiii (1911), 289-297, "Physikalisch-Chemische Veränderungen des Blutes nach Aderlass und subkutaner Infusion."

12E1:  Duncan, C.H., Autotherapy, LANCET-CLINIC, CINCIN., 1911, cvi, 472-481.

12E2:  Modinos, P., L'autosérothérapie dans les maladies infectieuses. PRESSE MÉD, PAR., 1911, xix, 1006.

12E3:  Fiori, L., Dell'autosieroterapia in generale con speciale riguardo ai risultati dell'autosieroterapia dell'idrocele. RIV. OSPEDAL., ROMA, 1912, ii, 2-12.

12E4: Landmann, G., Ueber authämotherapie. VERHANDL. D. GESELLSCH. DEUTSCH. NATURF. U. AERZTE, KÖNIGSB., LEIPZ., 1911, lxxxii, 2. Teil, 67-69.

12E5: Jousset, A., Recherches expérimentales sur l'autosérothérapie. ARCH. GÉN DE MÉD., PAR., 1912, v, 139-249.

12E6: Rosenthal, G., Note sur l'autosérothérapie a liquide filtré. REV. MÉD., PAR., 1912, xxii, 100.

12E7: Briand. Trois cas de pleurésie aérofibrineuse et deux d'hydrocéle, traités par l'autosérothérapie. ANN. D'HYG. ET DE MÉD, COLON., PAR., 1912, xv, 362.

12E8: Eisner, G. Experimentelle Untersuchungen Über Autoserotherapie. ZTSCHR. F. KLIN. MED., BERL., 1912, lxxvi, 34-44, 1 pl.

12E9: Indelli, A. Alcune note cliniche e critiche sulla cura alla Gilbert. FRACASTORO, VERONA, 1912, viii, 173-183.

13E1: Baccari, C. La tripsina nel-l'autosieroterapia. TOMMASI, NAPOLI, 1912, vii, 699-702.

13E2: Bonardi, E. L'auto-sieroterapia quale efficace mezzo di cura di alcuni trasudati (ascite da cirrosi epatica; idrocele). R. IST. LOMB. DI SC. E LETT. RENDIC., MILANO, 1912, 2. s., xlv, 366-374.

13E3: Caforio, L. L'autosieroterapia alla Gilbert. GIOR. INTERNAZ. D. SC. MED., NAPOLI, 1912, n.s., xxxiv, 927-935.

13E4: Duncan, C.H. Autotherapy; the natural autogenous toxine complex in the treatment of disease. N. YORK M. J., 1912, xcvi, 1217; 1278.

13E5: Rudolfi, A.F., Ob autoseroterapiij. VOYENNO-MED. J., ST. PETERSB., 1912, ccxxxiv, med.-spec. pt., 227-240.

13E6: Spiethoff, B. Zur therapeutischen Verwendung des Eigenserums. MÜNCHEN MED. WCHNSCHR., 1913, lx, 521.

13E7: Spiethoff, B. Zur Behandlung mit Eigenserum und Eigenblut. MED. KLIN., BERL., 1913, ix, 949.

13E8: Duncan, C.H. Autotherapy in purulent infections and the technic of its application. AM. PRACT., N.Y., 1913, xlvii, 461-472.

13E9: Smith, C.E., jr. The present status of autoserotherapy. ST. PAUL M. J., 1912, xv, 435-443.

13E10: Duncan, C.H. Autotherapy in surgery. AM. J. SURG., N.Y., 1913, xxvii, 381-385.

13E11: Mattei, C. Modifications leucocytaires au

cours de l'auto-hémato-thérapie. COMPT. REND. SOC. DE BIOL., PAR., 1913, lxxv, 228.

13H1:  Lewin, "Autoserotherapy in Cancer", Therapie der Gegenwart (June 1913) per N.Y. Med. J., May 30, 1914, 1091.

13H2:  Ravaut, M. Paul, "Essai sur L'Autohématothérapie dans Quelques Dermatoses", Ann. De Derm. er Syph. 4:292-6, May 1913.

14E1:  Antonio, A. L'autosieroterapia alla Gilbert. GAZZ. MED. ITAL., TORINA, 1913, lxii, 413.

14E2:  Battaglia, M.  Contributo clinico alla cura della pleurite sierosa e dell'orchite sierosa, con l'autosieroterapia.  GIOR. INTERNAT. D. SC. MED., NAPOLI, 1913, n. s., xxxv, 894-897.

14E3:  Duncan, C.H., Autotherapy of urine and sea plasma. THERAP. REC., LOUISVILLE, 1914, ix, 38-42.

14E4:  Duncan, C.H.  Autotherapy in the prevention and cure of purulent infections. PRACTITIONER, LOND., 1914, xcii, 551-566.

14E5:  Duncan, C.H., Autolactotherapy, a new system of therapeutics.  N. YORK M. J., 1914, c, 464-469.

14E6:  Pierce, E.A. Autoserotherapy.  NORTHWEST MED., Seattle, 1914, vi, 223-229.

14H1:  Fisher, Henry M., "Autoserotherapy in Fibrinoserous Pleurisy ...", N.Y. Med. J., May 23, 1914, 1037-8.

14H2:  Fox, Howard, "Autogenous serum in the treatment of psoriasis", J.A.M.A. LXIII(25):2190-4, Dec. 19, 1914

14H3:  Gottheil, Wm. S. & David L. Satenstein, "The Autoserum Treatment in Dermatology", J.A.M.A. LXIII:1190-1194, 3 October 1914.

14H4:  Duncan, C.H., "Autotherapy in Gynecology and Obstetrics", The Medical Times, May 1914, 146-8.

14H5:  Duncan, C.H., "Autoimmunization in Respiratory Infections", Medical Record, Sept. 5, 1914, 408-414.

15E1:  Duncan, C.H.  A few points in autotherapeutic technique.  MED. SENTINEL, PORTLAND OREG., 1915, xxiii, 1985-1993.

15E2:  Kreucher, P.H., Auto-sensitized autogenous vaccines. (Preliminary report.) SURG. CLIN., CHICAGO, 1914, iii, 1119-1122.

15E3:  Nesfield, V., The treatment of suppration by pus inoculations, and the treatment of pneumonia by subcutaneous injections of the patient's own blood.  INDIAN M. GAZ., CALCUTTA, 1914, xlix, 471-476.

15E4: Spiethoff, B., Zur Methode der Eigenblutbehandlung. MED. KLIN., BERL., 1915, xi, 38.

15E5: Robertson, W.E., Autoserotherapy, also the therapeutic use of inactivated pus and the value of tuberculins in serous cavities. BOSTON M. & S. J., 1915, clxxii, 559.

15E6: Palmer, E.E. & Secor, W.L., An improved and simplified technique for autoserotherapy. MED. REC., N.Y., 1915, lxxxviii, 108.

15E7: Duncan, C.H., A positive method of curing purulent infection, an appeal to the army surgeon. INTERSTATE M. J., ST. LOUIS, 1915, xxii, 996-1003.

15E8: Duncan, C.H., A positive method of curing purulent infection, an appeal to the army surgeon. AM. MED., BURLINGTON, VT. & N.Y., 1915, x, 772-775.

15H1: Pierce, E.A., "Autoserotherapy vs. Artificial Pneumothorax in the Treatment of Pleurisy with Effusion", Northwest Medicine VII, n.s., Dec. 1915, 386.

16A1: Huber, Autoserotherapy. N.Y. Med. J. 103:164, Jan. 22, 1916; ibid. 104:20, July 1, 1916.

16A2: Belliboni, Autoserotherapy, mode of action and indications for. Gazz. d.

Osp. 37:1058, Aug. 24, 1916.

16E1: Parham, J.C., Autotherapy. SOUTH. M. J., NASHVILLE, 1916, ix, 303-307.

16E2: Wohl, M.G., Autosensitized vaccines. MED. REC., N.Y., 1916, lxxxix, 770-772.

16E3: Huber, F., Autoserotherapy. N. YORK M.J., 1916, civ, 20.

16E4: Belliboni, E., Studio preparatorio per conoscere il meccanismo di azione e le indicazioni della autosieroterapia. GAZZ. D. OSP., MILANO, 1916, ii, 423.

16H1: Dumke, E.R., "Vaccine and serum therapy", N. W. Medicine XV(5):168-171, May 1916.

16H2: Duncan, Charles H., N.Y.M.J. 1916:342-3 (Poliomyelitis); 517 (Autotherapy); 901 (Ivy Poisoning)

16H3: Gottheil, Wm. S., "The value of Autoserum Injections in Skin Diseases", N.Y. Med. J. CIII:1209-1211, 24 June 1916.

16H4: Paget, O., Autoserum in Treatment of Cancer., Medical Record, N. Y. LXXXIX (April 8, 1916, per abstr. in N.Y. Med. J., May 29, 1916, p. 997.

16H5: Trimble, Wm. B. and John J. Rothwell, "Treatment of Psoriasis with Autogenous

Serum", J. Cutaneous Dis., Sept. 1916, per abstr. in N. Y. M. J., 1 April 1916, 660-1.

16H6:  Robertson, W.E., "Intravenous serobacterin therapeutics", N.Y.M.J. 103 (April 22, 1916), 777-780.

17A1:  Spiethoff, B., Venesection plus autoserotherapy.  Med. Klin. 12: 1223, Nov. 19, 1916; cont. 12: 1252, Nov. 26, 1916.

17E1:  Bronfenbrenner, J., and Schlesinger, M.J., Some suggestions for rational auto-serum-therapy.  PROC. SOC. EXPER. BIOL. & MED., N.Y., 1916, xiv, 61-63.

17E2:  Duncan, C.H., Autotherapy.  LONG ISLAND M. J., BROOKLYN, 1916, x, 325-333.

17E3:  Sinclair, H.H., Auto-sero-therapy in acute infections.  INTERNAT. J. SURG., N. Y., 1917, xxx, 114.

17E4:  Belin., Autopyothérapie. COMPT. REND. SOC. DE BIOL., PAR., 1916, lxxix, 1093-1095.

17H1:  Kaiser, A.D., "Serum and Blood Therapy", N.Y.M.J. Sept. 29, 1917, 595-6.

18E1:  Louis-Aguste.  Sur l'autosérothérapie des épanchements pleuraux et ascitiques. PROGRES MÉD., PAR., 1917, 3. s., xxxii, 182-185.

18E2:  Sweek, W.O., The autosensitized serobacterin. SOUTHWEST MED., EL PASO, 1917, i, No. 10, 21-25.

18E3:  Dewey, W.A., Isopathy, homeopathy and immunity.  J. AM. INST. HOMEOP., CLEVELAND, 1917-18, x, 660-675.

18E4:  Bazy, L., & Cuvillier, L., L'obtention d'auto-vaccins sensibilisés mono- ou polyvalents au moyen du sérum de Leclainche et Vallée.  PRESSE MÉD, PAR., 1918, xxvi, 219-221.

18E5:  Müller, R., Die Nachbarwirkung des Eigenserums und deren therapeutische Verwertung.  WIEN. KLIN. WCHNSCHR., 1917, xxx, 805-813.

18E6:  Martinez, Bk.D., Sueros hemopoiéticos.  SEMANA MÉD., BUENOS AIRES, 1918, xxv, 156.

19E1:  Duncan, Charles H., AUTOTHERAPY.  N.Y., 1918, C.H.Duncan, 376 p.

19E2:  Rosler, K., Die Autoserumbehandlung der akuten Infektionskrankheiten.  I. TEIL. MED. KLIN., BERL., 1916, xii, 944.

19H1:  Chalier, successful treatment of hemophilia with 11 IV injections of mother's serum, 25-40cc, Soc. Med. D. Hop. De Lyon 1919, per Voncken, Jules, "Homohemotherapy" J.A.M.A. 75:307-8, 31 July 1920.

20A1:  Achard, C. & C. Flandin, Autoserotherapy in hay fever, urticaria, etc.  Bull. et Mém.

Soc. Méd. d. Hôp. de Par. 44: 723, May 21, 1920; ab. J.A.M.A. 75:508, Aug. 14, 1920.

20A2:  Pehu & P. Durand, Phenomena with reinjection of serums. Ann. de Méd. 7:196, 1920; ab. J.A.M.A. 75:571, Aug. 21, 1920.

20E1:  Achard, C., and Flandin, C., Traitement de l'urticaire H répétition, de la maladie de Quincke et du rhume des foins par l'autoserothérapie désensibilatrice. BULL. ET MÉM. SOC. MÉD. D. HÔP. DE PAR., 1920, 3. s., xliv, 723-730.

21A1:  Escomel, E., Autoserotherapy of infections. Ann. de Fac. de Med., Montevideo 5: 604, Nov. 1920 - Feb. 1921; ab. J.A.M.A. 76: 1375, May 14, 1921.

21A2:  Sen, D.N., Auto-haemic or auto-serum therapy, Indian M. Gaz. 56: 94, March 1921.

21A3:  Sen, D.N., Addendum to auto-haemic or auto-serum therapy, Indian Med. Gaz. 56:326, Sept., 1921.

21A4:  Escomel, E., Integral autoserotherapy, Siglo Méd. 68:741, Aug. 6, 1921.

21E1:  Carbier (V). Les dangers de l'autoserotherapie. BULL. GEN. DE THERAPY. [etc.], PAR., 1920-21, clxxi, 104.

21E2:  Pehu (M) and Durand (P), Recherches cliniques sur les phenomenes observes dans les reinjections seriques. ANN. DE MED., PAR., 1920, vii. 196-225.

21E3:  Escomel (E.) La autoseroterapia integral de las microbiosis humanas. AN. FAC. DE MED., MONTEVIDEO, 1920-21, v. 604-617.

21E4:  Escomel (E.) La autoseroterapia integral de las microbiosis humanas. GAC. MED. DE CARACAS, 1921, xxviii, 86-90.

21E5:  Sen. (d.N.) Auto-haemic or auto-serum therapy. INDIAN M. GAZ., CALCUTTA, 1921, lvi, 94-96.

22A1:  Roch, M. & P. Gautier, Hemoclasis from autoserotherapy, Presse Méd. 30: 209-210, March 11, 1922; ab. J.A.M.A. 78:1348, April 29, 1922.

22A2:  Escomel, E., Integral serotherapy - using whole blood. An. de Fac. de Med., Montevideo 6:344-359, June 1921 (illus.)

22E1:  Escomel (E.) Curacion de las enfermedades por la autosero y la autoserovaccinoterapia integral. CRON. MED., LIMA, 1921, xxxviii, 240-246.

22E2:  Flandin (Ch.) & Tzanck (A) L'autoplasmotherapie desensibilisatrice. BULL. MED., PAR. 1921, xxxv, 725-728.

22E3:  Nourney. Ueber Eigenblutbehandlung. MÜNCHEN MED. WCHNSCHR., 1921, lxviii, 1521.

22E4:   Pansera (G.) Contributo clinico all'autosieroterapia da vesicacante. RIV. MED. MILANO, 1921, xxix, 119.

22E5:   Stewart (T.M.) Autotherapy. N. YORK M. J. [etc.], 1922, cxv, 135-137.

22E6:   Lauze, M., L'autohematotherapie dans les maladies infectieuses a forme trainante. BULL. ET MEM. SOC. MED. D. HOP. DE PAR., 1922, 3. s., xiv, 538-541.

22E7:   Raymond, F., L'autohemotherapie dans les maladies infectieuses a forme trainante. BUL. ET MEM. SOC. MED. D. HOP. DE PAR., 1922, 3. s., xlvi. 578.

22E8:   Boschetti, F., Presentando l'auto-sieroterapia. "Vita nuova" immunitaria? MED. ITAL., MILANO. 1922, iii, 21-32, 1 ch.

22E9:   Escomel, E., Algunos hechos nuevos en autoseroterapia integral. CRON. MED., LIMA. 1922, xxxix, 133-16.

22E10:  Gupta, K.M., Auto-haemic treatment. ANTISEPTIC. MADRAS, 1922, xix, 234-237.

23A1:   Moutier & J. Rachet, Autohemotherapy, Presse Méd. 31:708-9, Aug. 15, 1922; ab. J.A.M.A. 81:1476, Oct. 27, 1923.

23A2:   Nicholas, J., J. Gaté, & D. Dupasquier, Autohemotherapy

in dermatology, Médicine 4:147-149, Nov., 1922.

23A3:   Nicholas, J., J. Gaté, & D. Dupasquier, Autohemotherapy in dermatology, Lyon Chir. 20:553-561, Sept.-Oct. 1923; ab. J.A.M.A. 81:2211, Dec. 29, 1923.

23A4:   v.Torday, A., Wien. Klin. Wchnschr. 36:762-764, Oct. 25, 1923.

23A5:   Merklen, P. & F. Hirschberg, Autohemotherapy in local infections, Bull. et Mém. d. Hôp. de Par. 47: 1081-1086, July 6, 1923; ab. J.A.M.A. 81:1151, Sept. 29, 1923.

23A6:   Levi, E., Autohemotherapy in typhoid, Gazz. d. Osp. 44:591-595, June 24, 1923 (charts)

23A7:   Quenay, A., Autoserotherapy in gonorrhea, J. D'Urol. 16:234-235, Sept. 1923; ab. J.A.M.A. 81:2152, Dec. 22, 1923.

23A8:   Zimmerman, R., Hemolyzed own blood as nonspecific irritant, Zentralbl. f. Gynäk. 47:1504-1509, Sept. 22, 1923.

23A9:   Descarpentries, M., Injections of hemolyzed own blood., Arch. Franco-Belges de Chir. 26:63-69, Jan. 1923; ab. J.A.M.A. 80:1180, Apr. 21, 1923.

23E1:   Rogers, Loyal Dexter, AUTO-HEMIC THERAPY; administering a remedy made from the patient's blood without drugs or bacteria.  3.ed.

Chicago, 1922, Auto-hemic Therap. Found. inc., 332 p., 8&.

23E2: Descarpentries. Les injections de sang hemolyse du malade lui-meme en therapeutique chirurgicale. BULL. ET MEM. SOC. DE CHIR. DE PAR., 1922, xlviii, 852-854.

23E3: Spiethoff, B., Defibriniertes Eigenblut in der Reiztherapie. MÜNCHEN MED. WCHNSCHR., 1922, lxix, 1003.

23E4: Modinos, P., Quand et comment doit-on employer l'autoserotherapie. REV. GEN. DE CLIN. ET DE THERAP., PAR., 1922, xxxvi, 295.

23E5: Sfondrini, A., Autosieroterapia da vescicante. RIV. MED. MILANO, 1923, xxxi, 17-19.

23E6: Descarpentries. Les injections d'auto-sang hemolyse en chirurgie et en pathologie externe. CLINIQUE. PAR., 1923. xviii, 93-95.

23E7: Lyon, G., Auto et hetero-serotherapie, auto et hetero-hematotherapie. BULL. MED. PAR., 1923, xxxvii, 423-427.

23E8: Monziols & Pauron. A propos de la derniere communication de Nicolas, Gate, Dupasquier et Dumollard; autohemotherapie et choc hemoclasizue. COMPT. REND. SOC. DE BIOL., PAR., 1923, lxxxix., 249-251.

23E9: Mouriquand, G., and Buche, A., A propos de l'autohemotherapie. LYON MED., 1922, cxxxi, 111-113.

23E10: Castellino, P.G., Autosieroterapia nel reumatismo gonococcio ed in alcune dermatosi. FOLIA MED., NAPOLI, 1923, ix, 121-128.

23H1: Moberg, "Autohämotherapie bei Hautkrankheiten", Svensk Läkaresällsk. förhandl. 1923, H.6, S. 289. [per Deutsche Med. Woch. S.49 (1923), 1314]

24A1: Spillmann, L., Autohemotherapy in herpes zoster, Médicine 5: 130-131, November 1923.

24A2: Billington, S.G., Auto-haemo-therapy in bacterial infections. Lancet 1:431-435, March 1, 1924 (charts)

24A3: Zerner, H., Autoserum treatment of cancer, Med. Klinik 20: 212-213, Feb. 17, 1924; ab. J.A.M.A. 82:1088, March 29, 1924.

24A4: Steiner, Injections of own blood, Deutsche Med. Wchnschr. 50:438-439, April 4, 1924

24A5: Linhart, W., Own blood in treatment of furunculosis, Zentralblat. f. Chir. 51:1501-1502, July 12, 1924; abs. J.A.M.A. 83:653, Aug. 23, 1924.

24A6:  Goljanitski, J.A., Own blood in treatment of infected wounds, Zentralblatt f. Chir. 51:1566-1569, July 19, 1924; addendum 51:2019, Sept. 13, 1924; abs. J.A.M.A. 83:653, Aug. 23, 1924.

24A7:  Wolfson, G., Own blood treatment of infected wounds; comment on Gojanitzki's article, Zentralblatt f. Chir. 51:2194-2195, October 4, 1924.

24A8:  Nourney, Own blood treatment of carbuncle, Zentralblatt f. Chir. 50:1636-1637, Nov. 3, 1923 (illus.).

24A9:  Brünner, K., & F. Breuer, Protein therapy with hemolyzed own blood, Monatschr. f. Geburtsh. u. Gynäk.65:341-50, March 1924; ab. J.A.M.A. 82:1742, May 24, 1924.

24A10:  Vorschütz, J. & B. Tenckhoff, Treatment with own blood, Deutsche Ztschr. f. Chir. 183:364-379, 1924; cont. 184:200-207, 1924; ab. J.A.M.A. 82:1087, March 29, 1924, and 82:1740, May 24, 1924.

24E1:  Moutier, F. and Rachet, J., Incidents et accidents de l'autohemotherapie. PRESSE MED., PAR., 1922/3, xxxi, 708; ab. J.A.M.A. 81:1476, Oct. 27, 1923.

24E2:  Nicolas, Gate, et al., Autohemotherapie et choc hemoclasique. COMPT. REND. SOC. DE BIOL., PAR., 1923, lxxxviii, 1298-1300.

24E3:  Nicolas, Gate and Dupasquier.  Sur certaines reactions cliniques dans l'autohemotherapie (purpura). COMPT. REND SOC. DE BIOL., PAR., 1923, lxxxviii, 211.

24E4:  Zimmermann, R., Haemolysiertes Eigenblut also unspecifisches Reizmittel. ZENTRALBL. F. GYNAEK., LEIPZ., 1923, xvii, 1504-1509.

24E5:  Romanelli, E., L autolinfoterapia. GAZZA. MED. NAPOLET., 1923, vi, 179.

24E6:  Stewart, T.M., Fascinating developments of the auto-therapy; practical resume of technic and sphere of action.  AM. PHYSICIAN, PHILA., 1923, xxviii, 807-811.

24E7:  Mathieu, C., De l'emploi de la methode de Descarpentries (sang hemolyse) en chirurgie. REV. MED. DE L'EST, NANCY, 1923, li, 582-586.

24E8:  Vorschutz, J., and Tenckhoff, B., Von der Behandlung mit Eigenblut. I. DEUTSCHE ZTSCHR. F. CHIR., LEIPZ., 1923-4, cixxxiii, 364-379

24E9:  Bruenner, K., and Breuer, F., Ueber parenterale Eiweisstherapie mittels haemolysierten Eigenblutes. MONATSCHR. F. GEBURTSCH. U GYNAEK., BERL., 1923-4, lxc, 341-350.

24E10:  Diot, Les caprices de l'auto-hemo-therapie. SOC. DE

MED. MIL. FRANC., BULL. MENS., PAR., Par., 1924, xviii, 64-66.

24E11: Mino, P., and Garlasco, P., Riceche sul meccanismo della autoemoterapia. GAZZ. D. OSP., MILANO, 1924, xlv, 531-533.

24E12: Vorschutz, J., and Tenckhoff, B., Von der Behandlung mit Eigenblut. II. Erfolge bei akut entzundlichen Lungenerkrankungen. DEUTSCHE ZTSCHR. F. CHIR. LEIPZ., 1924, clxxxiv, 200-207.

25A1: Tenckhoff, B., Autohemotherapy, Deutsche med. Wchnschr. 50:1748-1752, Dec. 12, 1924; ab. J.A.M.A. 84:405, Jan. 31, 1925.

25A2: Koenigsfeld, H., Autoblood versus autoserum; comment on Tenckhoff's article. Deutsche med. Wchnschr. 51:1389-1391, Aug. 21, 1925.

25A3: Funck, C., Autohemotherapy in diabetes. Med. Klinik 21:506-507, April 3, 1925.

25A4: Mazzeo, A., Autohemotherapy in eczema of exudative diathesis. Pediatria 33:700-706, July 1, 1925; ab. J.A.M.A. 85:781, Sept. 5, 1925.

25A5: Richter, W. Autohemotherapy in erysipeloid, Deutsche med. Wchnschr. 51:562-563, April 3, 1925.

25A6: Lewy, W., Autohemotherapy in fracture of metatarsus, Med. Klinik 21:627, April 24, 1925 (Illus.)

25A7: Saïgràjeff, M.A., Autohemotherapy in gonorrhea. Ztschr. f. Urolog. 19:339-349, 1925; ab. J.A.M.A. 85:79, July 4, 1925.

25A8: Castellino, P., Autoserotherapy and autohemotherapy in dermatology, Riforma med. 41:97-98, Feb. 2, 1925; ab. J.A.M.A. 84:1088, April 4, 1925.

25A9: Iaccia, P., Autoserotherapy with cantharidin blister fluid. Pediatria 33:89-94, Jan. 15, 1925.

25A10: Rogge, Autoserum treatment. München med. Wchnschr. 72:1555-56, Sept. 11, 1925 (charts).

25A11: Tenckhoff, B., Comparison of effects of treatment with autotransfusion and X-rays. Deutsche med. Wchnschr. 51:1308-1310, Aug. 7, 1925.

25A12: Pometta, D., Danger of Gilbert's method of treatment of exudative pleurisy. Schweiz. med. Wchnschr. 55:1005-1006, Oct. 29, 1925; ab. J.A.M.A. 85:1922, Dec. 12, 1925.

25A13: Külbs, F., Diabetes and autohemotherapy. Klin.Wchnschr. 4:1725-1726, Sept. 3, 1925.

25A14: Ebers, N., Infiltration of tissue by injections of own blood. München. med. Wchnschr. 72:565-566, April 3, 1925.

25A15: Tenckhoff, Instruments for autohemotherapy. Deutsche med. Wchnschr. 51:400, March 5, 1925.

25A16: Weltgasser, J., Intracutaneous autohemotherapy. Med. Klinik 21:318-319, Feb. 27, 1925; ab. J.A.M.A. 84:1312, April 25, 1925.

25A17: Paulian, D., Intraspinal autoserotherapy in parkinsonism and encephalitis sequelae. Bull. et. mém. Soc. med. d. hòp. de Par. 49:203-204, Feb. 6, 1925.

25A18: Bussalai, L. & A. Devoto, Own blood in treatment of certain venereal disease complications. Gior. Ital. d. mal. ven. 65:1844-1849, December 1924.

25A19: Schlesinger, A., Own blood infiltration in treatment of furuncles and carbuncles. Zentralbl. f. Chir. 51: 2583, Nov. 22, 1924.

25A20: Wein, M.A., L.E. Salutzki & L.M. Königsberg, Own blood treatment in certain skin and venereal affections. Dermat. Wchnschr. 79:1629-1637, December 20, 1924.

25A21: Goljanitski, J.A., Own blood treatment of infected wounds; reply to Wolfsohn. Zentralbl. f. Chir. 52:2344-2347, Oct. 17, 1925.

25A22: Hübner, H., Successful treatment of gonorrheal bartholinitis by deep transfusion of patient's own blood. Zentralbl. f. Gynäk. 49:84-85, Jan. 10, 1925.

25A23: Schmidt, W., Treatment of incipient mastitis with local injections of patient's blood. Zentralbl. f. Gynäk. 49:1893-1895, Aug. 22, 1925; ab. J.A.M.A. 85:1101, Oct. 3, 1925.

25A24: Rausche, C., Treatment of postoperative affections of lungs with intramuscular injections of own blood. Deutsche Ztschr. f. Chir. 193:349-358, 1925 (charts).

25A25: Weicksel, Treatment of pulmonary tuberculosis with autoserum. Deutsche med. Wchnschr. 51:1392-1394, Aug. 21, 1925.

25A26: Vorschütz, J., Treatment with own blood; 208 cases. Arch. f. klin. Chir. 133:509-516, 1924 (in German).

25A27: Rhode, C., Treatment with patient's own blood in internal diseases. München. med. Wchnschr. 72:1107-1109, July 3, 1925.

25E1: Abente Haedo, F., La enfermedad serica; su tratamiento por la autohemoterepia. AN. FAC. DE MED., MONTEVIDEO, 1923-24, ix, 516-532.

25E2: Nourney. Zur Eigenblutbehandlung. FORTSCHR.

D. MED., BERL., 1924, xlii, 177-180.

25E3: Rogers, L.D., AUTOHEMIC THERAPY; ITS SCIENCE AND PHILOSOPHY EXPLAINED. Pan-Therap., Chicago, 1924, lxxii, 1101-1117.

25E4: Levy-Darras. Autohematotherapie. VIE MED., PAR., 1924, v, 2071.

25E5: Tenckhoff, B., Von der Behandlung mit Eigenblut. DEUTSCHE MED. WCHNSCHR., LEIPZ. U BERL., 1924, l, 11748-1752.

25E6: Vorschutz, J., Ueber Eigenbluttherapie. ARCH. F. KLIN. CHIR., BERL., 1924, cxxxiii, 509-516.

25E7: Wein, M.A., Salutzki, L.E., and Konigsberg, L.M., Die Autohämotherapie bei einigen kutanen und venerischen krankheiten. DERMAT. WCHNSCHR., LEIPZ. U. HAMB., 1924, lxxix, 1629-1637.

25E8: Zerbino, V., and Leunda, J.J., Enfermedad de suero y autoseroterapia. AN. FAC. DE MED, MONTEVIDEO, 1923-24, ix, 930-954.

25E9: Ebers, N., Ueber Eigenblutunterspritzungen. MÜNCHEN. MED. WCHNSCHR., 1925, lxxii, 565.

25E10: Tenckhoff. Vergleichsversuch der Wirkung und Wirkungsweise von Eigenblut- und Röntgenbehandlung bakterieller und entzündlicher Affektionen. MÜNCHEN. MED. WCHNSCHR., 1925, lxxii, 581.

25E11: Iaccia, P., Autosieroterapia da vescicante cantaridato. PERIATRIA. NAPOLI, 1925, xxxiii, 89-94.

25E12: Godlewski, H., Procédé d'autohémothérapie par ventouses [cupping]. J. MED. FRANÇ., PAR., 1925, xiv, 119.

25H1: Shamberg, JF and H Brown, "Effects of various agents - ultraviolet light, vaccines, turpentine, neoarsphenamin and autoblood injections - on the enzymes of blood and skin", Archives Int. Med. 35 (May, 1925), 537.

26A1: Graser, E., Autohemotherapy of postoperative bronchitis according to J. Vorschütz. Zentralbl. f. Chir. 52:2514-2518, Nov. 7, 1925 (charts); ab. J.A.M.A. 86:79, Jan. 2, 1926.

26A2: Zerner, Anaphylaxis in autohemotherapy of cancer. Ztschr. f. Krebsforsch. 23:9-11, 1926.

26A3: Mull, W., Autohemotherapy. Zentralbl. f. Chir. 53:463-466, Feb. 20, 1926.

26A4: Reider, W., Autohemotherapy in postoperative pulmonary complications. Zentralbl. f. Chir. 53:205-208, Jan. 23, 1926 (charts); ab. J.A.M.A. 86:919, March 20, 1926.

26A5:  Linhart, W.,
Autohemotherapy in septic
processes. Deutsche Ztschr. F.
Chir. 195:69-72, 1926.

26A6:  Carranza, C.G. & J.
Orgaz, Autohemotherapy in
treatment of asthma. Semana
méd. 2:1527-1531, Dec. 17, 1925;
ab. J.A.M.A. 86:1253, April 17,
1926.

26A7:  Finlayson, A.D. & L. J.
Karnosh, Autoserum treatment of
chronic encephalitis. Ohio
State M.J. 22:309-314, April
1926.

26A8:  Barth, F., Experimental
research on inhibiting action of
mixtures of blood and rivanol on
progressing pyogenic processes.
 Beitr. z. klin. Chir. 135:348-
359, 1925.

26A9:  Rubeska, Local
autohemotherapy of mastitis;
comment on Schmidt's article.
Zentralbl. f. Gynäk. 50:284-286,
Jan. 30, 1926; ab. J.A.M.A.
86:1104, April 3, 1926.

26A10:  Vorschütz, J., Own blood
or own serum? Deutsche med.
Wchnschr. 51:1954, Nov. 20,
1925.

26A11:  Hirsch, L., Survey on
autohemotherapy. Deutsche med.
Wchnschr. 52:551-552, March 26,
1926.

26B1:  Melanin, A. I.,
Autohemotherapy in
uncontrollable vomiting of
pregnancy. Zentralbl. f. Gynäk.

50: 1729-1733, June 26, 1926.

26B2:  Rausche, C.,
Autohemotherapy for acute
hemorrhage from gastric ulcer.
Deutsche med. Wchnschr. 52:1428-
1429, Aug. 20, 1926.

26B3:  Saleras, J. & A. von der
Becke, Autohemotherapy in
gonorrheal epididmitis. Semana
méd. 2:718-723, Sept. 16, 1926.

26B4:  Sorter, A.,
Autohemotherapy of acute
rheumatic polyarthritis. Med.
Klin. 22:725-728, May 7, 1926.

26B5:  Hinze, R.,
Autohemotherapy of pyogenic
processes of face. Zentralbl. f.
Chir. 53:987-989, April 17, 1926
(Illus.)

26B6:  Weicksel, J., Autoserum
treatment of pulmonary
tuberculosis. Ztschr. f.
Tuberk. 45:361-364, 1926.

26B7:  Leesberg, V. C. M.,
autotransfusion. Nederl.
Tijdschr. v. Geneesk 1: 1617-
1619, April 17, 1926 (chart).

26B8:  Erb, K.H., Clinical and
experimental studies on
treatment of local anthrax
infection by blocking with blood
according to Läwen. Beitr. z.
klin. Chir. 137:202-216, 1926;
ab. J.A.M.A. 87:1691, Nov. 13,
1926.

26B9:  Knosp, J., Euphoria after
autohemotherapy. München. med.
Wchnschr. 73:820-822, May 14,
1926.

26B10: Hirsch, L., Influence of autohemotherapy on blood picture. Deutsche med. Wchnschr. 52:1302, July 30, 1926.

26B11: Pette, H., Intraspinal autoserotherapy in sequels of epidemic encephalitis. München. med. Wchnschr. 73:1025-1027, June 18, 1926.

26B12: Descarpentries, M., Preventive injections of hemolyzed autoblood in surgery. Arch. franco-belges de chir. 29:110-114, Feb. 1926.

26B13: Bernard, R., Recurrent exfoliating erythrodermia consecutive to different antisyphilitic remedies; cure by autohemotherapy. Ann. d. mal. vén. 21:692-696, Sept., 1926.

26B14: Rausche, C., Treatment of postoperative gastric hemorrhage with injections of own blood. Deutsche Ztrshr. f. Chir. 198: 108-110, 1926.

26E1: Koenigsfeld, H., Eigenblut oder Eigenserum? DEUTSCHE MED. WCHNSCHR., LEIPZ. U. BERL., 1925, li, 1389-1391.

26E2: Rhode, C., Ueber Eigenblutbehandlung innerer Krankheiten. MÜNCHEN. MED. WCHNSCHR., 1925, lxxii, 1107-1109.

26E3: Riccioli, E., Sull' emosieroterapia ed emoterapia. RIV. DI CLIN. MED., FIRENZE, 1925, xxvi, 496-505.

26E4: Kaum, Ueber Eigenblutbehandlung. ZTSCHR. F. AERZTL. FORTBILD, JENA, 1925, xxii, 655-657.

26E5: Rogge. Beitrag zur Autoserumbehandlung. MÜNCHEN MED. WCHNSCHR., 1925, lxxii, 1555.

26E6: Vorschutz, J., Eigenblut oder Eigenserum? DEUTSCHE MED. WCHNSCHR., LEIPZ. U. BERL., 1925, li, 1954.

26E7: Mull, W., Ueber Eigenblutbehandlung. ZENTRALBL. F. CHIR., LEIPZ., 1926, liii, 463-466.

26E8: Knosp, J., Ueber die euphorisierende Wirkung der Eigenblutinjektionen. MÜNCHEN MED. WCHNSCHR., 1926, lxxiii, 820-822.

26E9: Modinos, P., Il siero da vescicante nella profilassi del morbillo e della grippe. BULL. E ATTI DI R. ACCAD. MED. DI ROMA, 1926, liii, 150-152.

27A1: Goldemberg, L., Autohemotherapy. Semana méd. 2:1025-1029, Oct. 14, 1926.

27A2: Flandin, C., Anti-anaphylactic therapy; contrast with protein therapy. Bull. méd. Paris 40:1393-1395, Dec. 11, 1926.

27A3: Angelucci, A., Autohemotherapy and

iontophoresis. <u>Arch. di ottal..</u> 33:439-463, Oct. 1926.

27A4: Carp, L., Circuminjection of autogenous blood in treatment of carbuncles. <u>Arch. Surg.</u> 14:868-890, April 1927.

27A5: Mouhtar, K. and S. Scandurra, Experimental and clinical observations on autohaemotherapy in surgical conditions. <u>Policlinico (sex. chir.)</u> 33:577-590, Nov. 1926.

27A6: Biebl., M. & F. Barth, Experimental treatment of anthrax. <u>Deutsche Ztschr. f. Chir.</u> 199:226-243, 1926.

27A7: Malinin, A. I., Autohemotherapy for menotoxicosis. <u>Dermat. Wchnschr. (Ergänzungheft Nr. 52a)</u> 83:1881-1883, 1926.

27A8: Arana, M., Autohemotherapy in dermatology. <u>Semana méd.</u> 2:1449, Nov. 25, 1926.

27A9: Schnack, W., Autohemotherapy in prevention and treatment of postoperative lung diseases. <u>Deutsche Ztschr. f. Chir.</u> 199:205-213, 1926.

27A10: Peus, W., Autohemotherapy in pulmonary tuberculosis. <u>München. med. Wchnschr.</u> 74:60, Jan. 14, 1927.

27A11: König, P., Autohemotherapy in treatment of postoperative lung diseases. <u>Deutsche Ztschr. f. Chir.</u> 199:198-204, 1926.

27A12: Vorschütz, J., Autohemotherapy in various conditions. <u>Med. Klin.</u> 23:41-45, Jan. 14, 1927.

27A13: Ludewig, P., Autohemotherapy of influenza. <u>Deutsche med. Wchnschr.</u> 52:2121-2122, Dec. 10, 1926.

27A14: Hinze, R., Autohemotherapy of pyogenic processes in face; case. <u>Zentralbl. f. Chir.</u> 54:200, Jan. 22, 1927.

27B1: Epstein, M.I., Autohemotherapy and collargol treatment of gonorrheal epididymitis. <u>Vrach. Gaz.</u> 31:355-360, March 15, 1927.

27B2: autoserotherapy in chronic eczema, [I. I. Bortolottl] Vrach.dielo 10: 342-346, March 15, 27

27B3: autoserotherapy in internal diseases, [H. Koenigsfeld] Therap.d.Gegenw. 68:104-107, March 27

27B4: autoserotherapy In laryngeal tuberculosis, [A. Luzzatti] Ann.di med.nav. 2:10-15, July-Aug 27

27B5: auto-serotherapy In tuberculous peritonitis, [P. De Michele] Riv.med. 34:101, July 26

27B6: buboes following chancroid treated by autohemotherapy, [F. J. Clusellas] Semana méd. 1:

972-990, April 21, 27

27B7: calcium chloride and auto-serotherapy In treatment of pleurisy, [A.Mincione] Med.prat. 12: 21-29, Jan.31, '27.

27B8: cure of Duhrings disease; case, [G. Liotta] Dermosifilografo 2:118-121, March 27

27B9: effects of reinjection of autogenous blood; modification of stability of suspension by natural and etherized corpuscles [G. Di Macco] Riv.di pat.sper. 2: 29-36, Jan.-Feb. 27

27B10: effects of reinjection of blood in same organism, [L. La Grutta] Riv.di pat.sper. 2:140-149, March-April 27

27B11: experiments of Dr. Caride, [Pagés Maruny] Rev.españ. de med.y cir. 10: 201-204, April 27

27B12: in bubo, [G. Camacho A] Repert.de med.y cir. 18: 299, March 27

27B13: in cancerous diseases, [S. V. Kaufman] Klin.Med, 5: 433-437, 27

27B14: in eczema of nurslings, [G. Roi] Policlinico (sez. prat.) 34: 786, May 30, 27

27B15: in epileptics and insane, [M. Mitlin & E. Posdniakov] Vrach.dielo 10: 502-504, April 15, 27

27B16: in eye diseases, [E. Marri] Arch.di ottal. 34: 241-245, June 27

27B17: in furunculosis, [E. A. Schiriak] Vrach.Gaz. 31: 265-267, Feb. 28, 27

27B18: in gonorrheal epididymitis; 24 cases, [M. Scharman] Wien.klin.Wchnschr. 40: 1384-1387, Nov. 3, 27

27B19: in gynecology, [E. Schwab] Aerztl.Rundschau 37: 85-87, March 25, 27

27B20: in initial stages of poliomyelitis, [Sicard, Haguenau & Wallich] Bull.et mem.Soc.med.d.hop.de Paris 51: 943-946, June 23, 27

27B21: in iritis, [Mallol de la Riva] Med.lbera 2:109, Aug. 6, 27

27B22: in postoperative lung complications, [F. Schwarz] Beitr.z.klin.Chir. 140: 338-342, 27

27B23: in postoperative pneumonia and gonorrheal arthritis. [S. Hoffheinz] Arch.f.klin.Chir. 144: 567-592, 27

27B24: in prurigo, [E. Sotelo Z.] Crón.méd.,Lima 43: 322-329, Nov '26

27B25: in puerperal infection; favorable results in 8 cases,

[Descarpentries] Bull.Soc.d obst.et de gynec. 15: 569-578, Nov. '26

27B26: in sepsis, [W. Linhart] Wien.klin.Wchnschr. 40: 657, May 19, 27

27B27: in surgery [H. Achelis] Deutsche Ztschr.f.Chir. 203-204: 587-601, '27

27B28: in tuberculous ostearthritis and other conditions, [M. Havranek] Rev.med.franç. 8: 329-333, April '27

27B29: in venereal bubo, [R. Smith] Rev.med.cubana 38: 880, Aug.'27

27B30: local; in trachoma. [A Campoy Ibañez] Progresos de la clínica 35:185-206, March '27.

27B31: mechanism of autohemotherapy and its practical application. [O Smirnoff] Vrach. dielo. 10:965-971. July 15, '27.

27B32: mode of action, [A. Lumiere & Mme. Montoloy] Compt. rend.Acad.d.sc. 184 1136-1138, May 9, 27

27B33: practical applications, [a. Finazzi] Cultura med.mod. 6 182-190, April 15, 27

27B34: tabulated data on experimental autoserotherapy, [G. Pergher] Ann.d'ig. 37:349-372, June 27

27B35: treatment of mastitis by autohemotherapy, Bardenhauer's incision and secondary suture, [Harttung] Monatschr.f. Geburtsh. u.gynak. 76 4-7, March 27

27B36: vacuum inoculation with patients own blood in treatment of furunculosis, [F. Kuhn] Munchen.med.Wchnschr. 74 451-453, March 18, 27

27H1:  O'Leary, Arch. Dermat. and Syph.:15:470, April 1927

28A1:  Zuppa, A., Autohemotherapy and ultraviolet rays in herpes recurrens of hands ; 7 cases, Riforma med., 44; 115-117, January 30, '28

28A2:  De Logu, A., Autohemotherapy and autoserotherapy in trachoma, Arch.di ottal. 35: 8-30' Jan. '28

28A3:  Luzzatti, A., Autoserotherapy in case of laryngeal tuberculosis. Ann. di laring., otol. 28:89-95, March '27

28A4:  Cipparrone, E., Eczema in adults cured by automotherapy; 4 cases. Gazz.internationaz.med.-chir. 33:109. March 31, '28

28A5:  Gross, A., Experiments in curative methods of inflammatory diseases with autoserum therapy. Bratisl. lekár. listy 7:492-496. Oct. '27.

28A6:  Reinus, A.M., In angina; case. Ann.d.mal. de 'oreille,

du larynx 46: 1227-1231. Dec.
'27.

28A7: Maimone, D., In eczema; 4 cases Glor.di med.mil. 75:616-620, October 1, '27.

28A8: Kappis, In furunculosis, Therap.d.Gegnew. 69:20-22, Jan '28.

28A9: Cerf, In gastric ulcer; case, Bruxelles-méd. 8:7-9, Nov. 6, '27

28A10: Welsaft, In gonnorrheal bartholinitis, Polska gaz.lek. 7:246-247, April 1, '27

28A11: R. Cohn-Czempin, In gynecological diseases, Zentrabl. f. Gynak. 51:2801, October 29, '27

28A12: in infectious diseases, [N. Morozkin] Vrach.gaz. 31:1643-1647, Nov. 30, 27

28A13: in inflammation of uterine adnexa; 12 cases, [W. Löbner] Zentralbl.f.gynak. 52:437-439, Feb. 18, 28

28A14: in keratoconjunctivitis. [A. De Capite] Pediatria 36:225-236, March 1, 28

28A15: in ovarian and inflammatory hemorrhages, [M Wachtel] Zentralbl.f.Gynak. 52:630-635, March 10, 28

28A16: in skin diseases, [I. Lifschitz] Vrach.Gaz. 31 1359-1361, Sept. 30, 27

28A17: in treatment of fractures, [G. Clemente] Pathologica 20:66-74, Feb. 15, 28

28A18: in typhus, smallpox, syphilis, influenza and various skin diseases, [V. Ivanoff] Russk.Klin. 8:325-340 Sept. 27

28A19: in vernal conjunctivitis; favorable results in 4 cases, [G. Salvati] Gior.di ocul. 8:120-122 Dec 27

28A20: influence of injections of freshly defibrinated blood from patient on defibrination time. [T. Preininger] Wien.klin.Wchnschr. 41:370-374, March 15, 28

28A21: Lawen's local blood injections in treatment of abscesses [O. Wiedhopt] Zentralbl.f.Chir. 54:2818-2821, Nov 5, '27

28A22: methods, [E. Schulmann] Prat.med.trans. 6:460-465, Oct. (A) '27

28A23: of furunculosis in infants. [Z. von Bokay] Jahrb. f. Klnderh. 119: 240-247, March '28

28A24: of recurrent sweat gland inflammations of axilla, [G. Axhausen] Zentralbl.f.Chir. 55:212-214. Jan. 28, '28

28A25: of serum sickness, [J. Morgenstern] Wien.klin.Wchnschr. 41:89-91, Jan. 19, '28

28A26: prophylactic and therapeutic use in postoperative lung complications. [H. Siegenfeld] Wien.med.Wchnschr. 78:381, March 17, 28

28A27: three annulare centrifugal erythemata; bismuth and autohemotherapy: recurrence, [Burnier] Bull.Soc.franç.de dermat.et syph. 35:209-212, March '28

28A28: treatment of pneumonia in infants by glucose injections, and by autohemotherapy, [H. Flesch] Ztsxhr. Kinderh. 44:576-580, '27

228A9: value in spasmodic periodic coryza; 2 cases, [A. Llerena Benito] Arch.de med.,cir.y espec. 28:58-61  Jan. 14, 28

28B1: autohemotherapy, autoserotherapy in tuberculosis, [I.  Menniti] Arch.di biol. 5:21, March-April '28

28B2: autoserotherapy in pleurisy of horse, cases, [Valade]  Rec.de med.vet. 104:336-339, June 28

28B3: clinical and therapeutic study, [J. C. Tassart] Rev. med.latlno-am. 13:1780-1784, June '28

28B4: cure of gonorrheal urinary fistulae; case, [F. Landt] Dermat.Wchnschr. 86:733, June 2 '28

28B5: experimental treatment of alcoholism, [W. Mitkus]  Polska gaz.lek. 7:576-578, Aug 5, 28

28B6: in abscesses of sebaceous glands; [G. Axhausen] Med.  Welt 1:426-428, April 23, '27

28B7: in epidemic encephalitis and in encephalitic influenza [H. Kraus] Munchen.med.Wchnschr. 75:1205, July 13, '28 [Comment by Schmitz, 1458-1459, Aug. 24, '28

28B8: in otorhinolaryngology, [M. Giussani]  Ann.di. laring., otol.  39:  75-83, March '28

28B9: in treatment of herpes zoster, [B. B. Beeson]  Arch. Dermat. & Syph. 18: 573-576, Oct. '28

28B10: injections around abscesses; 5 cases, [Descarpentries]  Bruxeles-méd. 8: 1301-1309, Aug.5, '28

28B11: intravenous injection of sodium salicylate with patient's own blood (Balkowski) in rheumatic fever (Behandlung des akuten Gelenkrheumatismus nach Balkowski), Med. Welt  1: 1313, Oct., '27

28B12: of suppurative dermatitis of extremities in horses; cases, [Lemetayer]  Rev.vét.mil.  12: 157-166, June 30, '28

28B13: treatment of ozena, [C. J. A. van Iterson]  Nederl. Tijdschr.v.Geneesk.  1: 1984, April 21, '28

28B14: value in ocular diseases, [G. Salvati] Gior.di ocul. 9: 17, Feb. '28

29A1: autohemotherapy, [R. Nieto y Vicente] Siglo méd. 82: 401-402, Oct' 27, '28

29A2: aseptic protein shock in nephritis, [G. Kolischer] J.A.M.A. 92: 9~8-970, March 23 '29

29A3: favorable results in trachoma, [h Slutzkin] Klin. Monatebl.f.Augenh. 81: 829-835, Dec. 28' '28

29A4: in asthma, [L. Thuet] Strasbourg-méd. (pt. p 86: 328-339, Sept. 5, '28

29A5: in cancer, [F. Blumenthal] Med. Welt 2: 1819' Dec. 8, '28

29A6: in dermatitis in horses' [Lemetayer] Bull.Acad.vét.de France 1: 404, Dec. '28

29A7: in exudative diathesis, [J. A. Alonso Muñoyerro] Arch.españ.de pediat. 12: 810-81l, Sept. '28

29A8: in herpes zoster, [C. Scudero] Policlinico (sez.prat.) 35: 2550-2557, Dec. 24, '28

29A9: in inguinal bubo' [E. A. Burmeister] Med.Klin. 24: 2011-2012, Dec. 28, '28

29A10: in trachoma, [G. Salvati] Lettura oftal. 5: :,62, Dec. '28

29A11: in treatment of abscess [P. Castagna] Arch.ed atti d. Soc.ital.di chir. (1927) 34:811, '28

29A12: in treatment or acute and chronic infections; case of Iichenoid acanthosis ruber [A. Risi] Studium 18: 479-487' Nov. 20' '28

29A13: of chronic gonorrheal cowperitis, [F. Landt] Dermat. Wchnschr. 87:1842' Dec. 1, '28

29A14: success of integral modified autoserum therapy in inveterate alcoholism; case, [E. Escomel] Crõn. méd., Lima 45: 279-281, Sept. ,28; also, Siglo méd. 83: 217-219, Jan. 12, '29

29A15: value in treatment of warts, [A. Sézary] Bull.Soc. franc.de dermat.et syph. 36: 839' Nov. '28

29A16: value in vernal conjunctivitis; cases' [Cassinuatis] Arch.di ottal. 36: 8-14, Jan. '29

29A17: value of autoserotherapy in serofibrinous pleurisy and peritonitis; cases, [M. Guiffrè] Clin.pediat. 10: 701731, Nov. '28

29A18: value of autoserum irradiated with radium for treatment of cancer' [H. Peters] Ztschr.f.Krebsforsch. 28: 186-190, '28

29B1: autohemotherapy, [L.

Caillon]  Rev.tunishienne
d.sc.méd. 22: 89-95, April '28

29B2: [S. Hoffheinz]  Chirurg
1: 743-749, July 1, '29

29B3: [E. Mühsam]
Ztschr.f.ärztl.Fortbild. 26:
278-281, May 1, '29

29B4: autoserum in chronic
disease, [W. G. Brymer]  M.Rec.
& Ann. 23: 431-433, Nov. '29

29B5: cure of habitual
alcoholism by integral, modified
autoserotherapy; case, [E.
Escomel]  Rev.de méd., Rosario
4: 43-46, Feb. '29

29B6: effect on gaseous
metabolism in nutritional
disturbances, [A. Springsguth]
Ztschr.f.d.ges. exper.Med. 67:
247-252, '29

29B7: in gastric ulcer, [M.
Cerf]  Bruxelles-méd. 9:
827-830, May 19, '29

29B8: in malaria; case, [P.
Sepulcri & E. Vidale]  Riv.di
malariol. 8: 78-80, Jan.-Feb.
'29

29B9: in ocular diseases, [E.
Avalos]  An.Soc.méx.de oftal. y
oto-rino-laring. 7: 208-210,
March-April '29

29B10: in ozena, [A. A.
Aleshkoff]  Vrach.gaz. 33:
2203-2204, Aug. 31, '29

29B11: in surgery, [G. Wolfsohn]
 Therap.d.Gegenw. 70: 399-403,
Sept. '29

29B12: in sympathetic
ophthalmia, [R. & R. J. Guiral]
 Rev. de med.y cir.de la Habana
 34: 337-353, May 31, '29

29B13: in treatment of
exanthematous typhoid fever, [A.
Metzulescu]  Rev.stint.med.  17:
971-997, Nov. '28

29B14: injections of patient's
own blood around boil following
Läwen's method, [K. Erb]
Ztschr.f.ärztl.fortbild.  26:
424-428, July1, '29

29B15: injections with patient's
own blood in treatment of herpes
zoster, [D. Kenedy & E.
Neuwirth]  Dermat. Wchnschr.88:
553-554, April 13, '29

29B16: review of literature, [S.
Hoffheinz]  Ergebn.d.Chir.u.
Orthop.  22: 162-221, '29

29B17: treatment of boils and
carbuncles by circular
injections of patient's own
blood (Läwen), [K. Siätis]
Finska läk.-sällsk.handl.  71:
550-557, July '29

29B18: use of combination of
bismuth, arsphenamine and
patient's blood in treatment of
syphilis resistant to
arsphenamine alone, [Beume]
Dermat. Wchnschr.88: 812, June
8, '29

29B19: various changes of blood
in autohemotherapy in cancer of
uterus and vomiting during
pregnancy, [T. I. Dikoff]

Klin.J.Saratov.Univ. 5: 449-461, April '28

29B20: history, serum fad; looking backward, [J. U. Lloyd] Eclect. M J. 89:521-525, Aug. '29

30A1: autohemotherapy, as therapeutic agent, [E. C. Vivanco] Semana méd. 2: 1256-1265, Oct. 31, ,29

30A2: hemolized autohemotherapy; cases, [Fontoynont] Bull.Soc.path.esot. ~:120-122, ,30

30A3: in chorea, [S. Azmy-Bey & A. El-Agaty] Cong. internat.de méd.trop.et d'hyg., Compt.rend. 2: 727- 729, '29

30A4: in diseases of eyes [J. Jirman] Casop.lék.cesk. 68:1768-1771, Dec. 20, ,29

30A5: in myeloid and In lymphatic leukemia, [W. Bensis Contomercos] Sang 4:49-53, 30

30A6: in ocular diseases, [E. Avalos] An.Soc.mex.de oftal.y oto-rino-laring. 7:361-365, Dec. 29

30A7: in postoperative pulmonary complications [Go-Ko-Rin] Taiwan Igakkai Zasshi, no. 294, p. 58, Sept. '29

30A8: multiforme, bulous erythema, Bazin's hydroa, recurrent for 10 years, cured with autohemotherapy; case, [L. Hufnagel] Bull.Soc.franç.de dermat. et syph. 37:358, March '30

30A9: of chancre bubo' [J. Renner; R. M. Chevalier] Prensa med.argent. 16: 1021-1024 Dec. 30, '29

30A10: of infections [Martin Salazar] Siglo méd. 85: 358-360, April 6, '30

30A11: subconjunctival autohemotherapy in ocular therapeutics in horse; cases, [Marcenac & Lemetayer] Rev.vét.mil. 13:399-408, Dec. 31, '29

30B1: autohemotherapy, autoplastic injections of blood in infected or diseased bone cavities, [E. Leo] Chir.d.org. di movimento 14:703-716, May '30

30B2: arsphenamine-autoserum treatment in syphilogenic diseases of brain and spinal cord, [R. Rotter] Arch.f.Psychiat. 90:824-839, '30

30B3: autosero- and autohemotherapy in internal medicine, [H. Koenigfeld] Med. Welt 4:991, July 12, '30

30B4: autoserotherapy in chronic rheumatism, [P. Le Floch] Presse Méd. 38: 1061-1063, Aug. 6, '30

30B5: autoserotherapy in gonorrheal complications, [T. Egerváry] Orvosi hetil. 74: 693-697, July 19, '30

30B6: autoserotherapy in treatment of skin diseases, particularly psoriasis, [P. Busquet] Gaz.d.hôp. 103: 1085-1090, July 26, '30

30B7: autoserotherapy of sympathetic ophthalmia, [R. & R. J. Guiral] Arch.de oftal. hispano-am. 30: 1-17, Jan. '30

30B8: effect of autohemotherapy and cupping on reticulocyte content of blood, [A. Schapiro] Ztschr.f.d.ges.exper. Med. 71:800-804, '30

30B9: effects of autoproteins in immunity, [G. De Nito] Rassegna di terap.e pat.clin. 2: 193-203, April '30

30B10: favorable results in mental diseases, [A. Hauptmann] Med.Welt 4: 1031-1033, July 19, '30

30B11: general treatment of malignant tumors with special regard to injections of patient's own blood which has been treated with roentgen rays, [S. von Dziembowski] Fortschr.d.Med. 48: 567-571, July 11, '30

30B12: in chronic leukemia, [R. Gusio] Bull.e atti d.r.Accad. med.di Roma 56:179-186, June-July '30

30B13: in chronic malaria; cases, [M. Padoan & M. Frizziero] Riv.di malariol. 9: 135-149, March-April '30

30B14: in convulsive cough, [L. Dàriu] Cluj.med. 11: 405-407, Aug.1, '30

30B15: in several conditions; results in 55 cases, [S. Jouan] Semana méd. 1: 1199-1201, May 8, '30

30B16: in tuberculosis, [I. Jancsó] Orvosi hetil. 74: 750-755, Aug.2, '30

30B17: leukocytic formula in autohemotherapy in surgical infections, [R. Pazzagli] Gior.di med.mil. 78:380-385, July '30

30B18- local autohemotherapy in incipient mastitis, [A. A. Pesaresi] Riv.d'ostet.e ginec.prat. 12: 382, Aug. '30

30B19: macroscopic and microscopic changes in internal organs produced by parenteral administration of autogenous protein, [W. Jelin] Virchows Arch.f.path. Anat. 277: 221-227, '30

30B20: of anthrax; cases, [P. González Montero] Arch. de med., cir.y espec. 32: 597-599, June 7, '30

30B21: of furunculosis, [S. F. Shirokoff] Venerol.i dermat. 7: 36-38, Jan. '30

30B22: results obtained in gonorrheal acute epididymitis from use of ammonium sulphoichthyolate, sodium iodide, autohemotherapy and calcium chloride, [F. Castoldi]

Dermosifilografo 5: 383-400, June '30

30B23: treatment of lobar pneumonia by intrapulmonary injections of patient's whole blood, [K. P. A. Taylor] Clin.Med.&& Surg. 37: 422-426, June '30

30B24: treatment of pneumonia and bronchopneumonia with daily injections of patient's blood, [D. Simici, M. Popescu, A. Lazarescu] Spitalul 50: 260-263, July-Aug. '30

31A1: autohemotherapy, auto-anaphylaxis in course of vesicatory autoserotherapy in tuberculosis; case, [A. R. Nelli] Rinasc.med. 7: 523, Nov.1, '30

31A2- autohemotherapy and autoserotherapy, [f. J. Cramer] Med.Welt 5: 438-440, March 28, '31

31A3- autohemotherapy and autoserotherapy in pulmonary tuberculosis, [V. I. Jancsó] Beitr.z.Klin.d.Tuberk. 76: 549-567. '31

31A4- autoserotherapy; 2 cases, [Schottky] Med.Klin. 26: 1823-1824, De. 5, '30

31A5- continued improvement with injections of patient's own blood mixed with testicular extract, [Filderman] Bull.et Mém.Soc.de méd.de Paris, no. 4. pp. 115-117, Feb.28, '31

31A6- dangers of autohemotherapy without previous exact diagnosis and general physical examination; 4 cases, [S. Jouan] Re.méd.
latino-am. 16: 383-385, De. '30

31A7- effects of Gilbert's autoserotherapy on blood picture in serofibrinous pleurisy; 6 cases, [M. A. Sisti] Diagnosis 10: 237-250, Aug. '30

31A8- erythrodermia from arsphenamine poisoning treated with autohemotherapy but followed by subcutaneous boils and abscesses; case, [J. Gaté, H. Thiers & others] Bull.Soc.franç.de dermat.et syph. (Réunion dermat., Lyon) 38: 400-406, March '31

31A9- fractured neck of femur treated by injection of blood, [E. W. Riches] Brit.M.J. 1:308, Feb. 21, '31

31A10- herpes zoster occurring in course of autohemotherapy; case, [Gougerot & J. Weill] Bull.Soc.franç.de dermat.et syph.38:48, Jan. '31

31A11- in eczema impetiginosum, eczema humida acuta and furunculosis in dogs, [D. J. Kok] Tijdschr.v.diergeneesk. 58: 128-139, Feb.1, '31

31A12- in furunculosis, [A. T. Balmagia] Vrach.gaz. 34: 1586-1588, Nov.15, '30

31A13- in glomerular nephritis, [L. Crosetti] Gior.med.dell'

Alto Adige 3: 12-20, Octo. '30

31A14- in mental diseases, [E. Zara] Riforma med. 47: 330-335, March 2, '31

31A15- in tuberculosis; 114 cases, [V.S. Janesó] Verhandl.d. ungar.ärztl.Gesellsch. 2:230-232, Octo. 30

31A16- injections of patient's own blood, sodium nucleinate and malaria therapy in dementia praecox, [L. Grimaldi] Manicomio 43: 113-138, May-Dec. '29

31A17- late syphilitic disorders (vascular syphilis and neurosyphilis, and late latent cases with persistent positive Wasserman reaction) treated by means of ultraviolet irradiation and of autohemotherapy of irradiated patients, [E. Rajka & E. Radnai] Ztschr.f.d.ges.Neurol. u.Psychiat. 131: 674-705, '31

31A18- spontaneous and provoked leukocytolysis in leukemic patients; autohemotherapy, [M Piazza] Policlinico (sez. med.) 38: 116-138, March '31

31B1: autohemotherapy, autoserotherapy in trachoma, [N. Fehmi] Rev.internat.du trachome 8:68-70, April '31

31B2- autoserotherapy and autohemotherapy in tuberculosis; indications, [I. Jancsó] Beitr.z.Klin.d.Tuberk. 78: 546-558, '31

31B3- autoserotherapy in tuberculosis of eye, [K. Scheider] Orvosi hetil. 75: 821-823, Aug. 8, '31

31B4- biologic evaluation of patient's own blood and serum, [W. Milbradt] Ztschr.f.d.ges.exper.Med. 79: 423-441, '31

31B5- in acute rheumatism of joints, [D. G. Abessalomoff] Klin.med. (nos.11-12) 9: 450-453, '31

31B6- in gonorrhea, [L. Casano Papi] Biol.med. 7:175, July; 227, Aug. '31

31B7- in puerperal fever, [M. J. Litwak] Arch.f.Gynäk, 146: 273-301, '31

31B8- in Rhus toxicodendron dermatitis, [E. Grimes] Arch. Dermat.& Syph. 24: 725-726, Nov. '31

31B9- in undulant fever; case, [G. Bettinardi] Pediatria prat. 8: 268-276, Aug. '31

31B10- in vernal conjunctivitis, [C. Cassimatis] Cong.internat. de méd.trop.et d'hyg., Compt.rend. (1928) 3: 703-711, '31

31B11- indications and technic, [R. Bravo Garcia] Med.ibera 1: 930-934, June 13, '31

31B12- intracutaneous; favorable and unfavorable results, [L.

Alexander]  Med.Klin.  27:
1678-1679, Nov. 13, '31

31B13- mechanism of action;
variations in erythrocyte
sedimentation and protein
content of blood after
autohemotherapy in children, [C.
Sorrentino]  Pediatria  39:
905-914, Sept. 1, '31

31B14- new method of treating
acute articular rheumatism, [M.
Karp]  München.med. Wchnschr.
78: 1913, Nov. 6, '31

31B15- new treatment of
neurosyphilis; association of
actinotherapy and of
autohemotherapy, [C. Brody]
Rev. d'actinol.  7: 334-339,
May-June '31

31B16- of duodenal ulcer, [K.
Hubert]  Wien,med. Wchnschr.
81:744, May 30, '31

31B17- recurrent phlyctenosis of
hands in young persons cured by
autohemotherapy; 2 cases, [J. L.
Carrera]  Prensa méd. argent.
18: 150-151, June30, '31

31B18- ultraviolet irradiation
and autohemotherapy in late
syphilis, [E. Rajka & E. Radnai]
 Arch.Dermat.& Syph.  24:
228-235, Aug. '31; also, Ann.de
dermat. et syph.  2: 956-974,
Sept. '31

31B19- value in mental diseases,
[G. Colucci] Morgagni  73:
1273-1282, July 5, '31

31H1:  Wright, Carroll S.,

"Nonspecific Therapy in
Dermatology, a 5-year Study",
Archives of Dermatology and
Syphilis 23:118-131 (Jan. 1931)

32A1: autohemotherapy, [N.
Burgess]  Brit.J.Dermat.  44:
124-131, March '32

32A2-G. del Vecchio]  Studium
22: 103-107, April 1, '32

32A3-acid-base equilibrium and
skin diseases; influence of
autohemotherapy on alkali
reserve and blood hydrogen ion
concentration, [M. Brozini]
Rinasc. med.  9:  125-127, March
15, '32

32A4-arresting hemorrhage of
female genitals, [M. Oike]
Jap.J.Obst. & Gynec.  14:
461-4623, Oct. '31

32A5-boron compounds in therapy
of epilepsy and their
autohemotherapeutic application,
[G.C. van Walsem]  Psychiat.en
neurol.bl.  35: 466-492,
July-Aug. '31

32A6-calcium chloride and
autoserotherapy  in exudative
pleurisy and serous effusions,
[L. Saighini]  Pensiero med.
20: 671, Oct. 31, '31; 726, Nov.
30, '31

32A7-combined use of
autohemotherapy and endocrine
therapy in various
psychopathies, [R. Biot]
Progrés med., pp.329-333,
Feb.20, '32

32A8-hormonal stimulation by ovaraden (ovarian preparation) and by autohemotherapy, [L. Sternheim]  Med. Welt 6: 164, Jan.30, '32

32A9-in herpes zoster, [S. Cherubino]  Dermosifilografo  6: 708, Dec. '31

32A10-in pulmonary tuberculosis, [K. Szepesi]  Budapesti orvosi ujság 30:  291-293, March 24, '32

32A11-in tuberculosis, [G. Dániel & E. Schiffbeck]  Orvosi hetil.  75: 933-994, Oct. 10, '31

32A12-intraspinal autoserotherapy in poliomyelitic tetraplegia; case, [J. Skoulikides & J. Kostazos] Semaine d.hop. de Paris 7: 613-616, Dec. 15, '31

32A13-intravenous injection of quinine-arsenic preparation and patient's own blood in malaria, [Ritouvanziam & L. V. Xuyen] Monde méd.., Paris  42: 50-55, Jan.15, '32

32A14-new method of treating acute articular rheumatism, [W. Vezér]  München.med. Wchnschr. 78: 2202, Dec. 25, '31  [Comment on Karp's article]

32A15-subconjunctival autohemotherapy in ulcerative keratitis, [Masselin] Bull.Soc.de opht.de Paris, pp.114-119, Feb. '32

32A16-therapy of acute gonorrheal archiepididymitis with intra-orchiepididymal autohemotherapy, [A. Valerio] Folha med. 12: 387, Nov. 25, '31

32A17-therapy of neurodermatitis and eczema by cutaneous distension and local autohemotherapy, [M. Hamburger, P. Mare & A. Waynberger] Bull.méd.., Paris  46: 263-264, April 9, '32

32B1: autohemotherapy, by intradermal autohemolysis, [M. Galioto]  Dermosifilografo  7: 18-24, Jan. '32

32B2-autoserotherapy in tuberculous pleurisy, [D. Schüssler] Wien.med. Wchnschr. 82: 1196-1197, Sept. 17, '32

32B3-efficacious treatment against inveterate alcoholism [J. López Lomba]  Rev. méd. latino-am. 17: 710-714.  Feb. '32

32B4-in acute rheumatic polyarthritis, [F. S. Yurev] Sovet. vrach. gaz., pp.321-324, July 15, '32

32B5-in bronchopneumonia and influenza, [P. I. Glazko & N. I. Gornakov]  Sovet.vrach.gaz., pp.819-821, July 15, '32

32B6-in gastric and duodenal ulcer. [A. O. Villert]  Sovet. klin. 16: 305-312, '31

32B7-in mental diseases, [C. Poli]  Riv.sper.di freniat.  56: 664-679, Sept. 30, '32

32B8-in otitis externa, [G. A. Jarkovskiy] Sovet. vrach. gaz., pp.169-170, Feb.15, '32

32B9-typhoid, [G. Bettinardi] Pediatria 40: 932-943, Sept.1, '32

32B10-iridocyclitis of sympathetic type cured by autohemotherapy; case, [M. Marin Amat. & M. Marín Enciso] Arch.de oftal.hispano.-am. 32: 373-378, July '32

32B11-new method of autoserotherapy in severe asthma and in spasmodic aperiodic coryza. [A. Jacqulein, J. Turiaf, Davous & Réveillaud] Bull.et méd. Soc. méd. d.hop.de Paris 48: 557-567, May 2, '32

32H1: Low, Cranston R., "The Uses of Non-Specific Protein Therapy", Brit. M.J., Sept. 24, 1932, 577-80

33A1 autohemotherapy, after aspiration of abscess, [A. L. Fisanovich] Vrach.delo 15: 637-639, '32

33A2-autoserotherapy of pseudarthrosis, [R. Imbert] Bull. et mém. Soc. nat. de chir. 59: 406-415, March 18, '33

33A3-carbuncle, [I. D. Jones] Sind M.J. 5: 131-132, Dec. '32

33A4-gonococcic rheumatism during puerperium; therapy with antigonococcic vaccine prepared at Pasteur Institute and autohemotherapy, [Auddebert, Ribat & Bec] Bull.Soc. d'obst. et de gynéc. 22: 262-263, Feb. '33

33A5-heliotherapy and autohemotherapy of late syphilitic conditions, [E. Rajka & E. Radnai] Dermat. Wchnschr.95: 1829-1831, Dec. 17, '32

33A6-in herpes zoster, [G. Collosi] Umbria med. 12: 2099-2102, Jan. '32

33A7-in otosclerosis, [L. S. Kavalerchik] Russk.oto=laring. 24: 133-134, '31

33A8-in ozena and atrophic rhinitis, [V. I. Strelova] Russk. oto-laring. 24: 510-519, '31

33A9-in pulmonary tuberculosis, [S. d'Amore] Gazz.d.osp. 54:131-138, Jan. 29, '33

33A10-injection into anterior chamber in tuberculosis of iris; control of results by animal tests, [I. Baer] Klin. Monatsbl.f.Augenh. 90: 485-492, April ' 33

33A11-mechanism of action, [F. Schürer-Waldheim] Deutsche Ztschr.f.Chir. 239: 352-362, '33

33A12-Meller theory on role of tuberculous bacteremia in pathogenesis of sympathetic opththalmia and Schieck method of injecting patient's own blood into anterior chamber in therapy of tuberculous diseases of eye, [W. Riehm] Klin.Monatsbl.f.Augenh. 90: 477-485, April '33

33A13-of erysipelas, [L. Lajos] Zentralbl.f.Gynäk. 57: 586-593, March 11, '33

33A14-of erysipelas, [V. F. Shubert & M. N. Bandin] Klin. med. (nos. 11-12) 10: 368-369, '32

33A15-of puerperal eclampsia, [I. Sztehlo] Gyógyászat 73: 82-83, Feb. 5, '33

33A16-rapid disappearance of profuse eruption of warts after autohemotherapy; discussion of therapeutic value of suggestion, [A. Sézary & P. Auzépy] Bull.Soc. franç. de dermat.et syph. 39: 1625-1626, Dec. '32

33A17-results of injections of own blood into anterior chamber in ocular tuberculosis of anterior part of bulb. [F. Schieck] Klin.Monatsbl.f.Augenh. 90: 1-8, Jan. '33

33A18-tuberculosis of anterior section of eyeball; autohemotherapy by injections into anterior chamber, [Schieck] Ber. ü. d. Versamml. d. deutsch. ophth. Gesellsch. 49: 183-188, '32

33A19-value of injections of hemolyzed blood in deep seated phlegmons; 4 cases, [F. de Macedo Chaves] Med. contemp. 50: 397-398, Dec.25, '32

33A20-vasomotor affections of nose and their relation to bronchial asthma (Flandin method of autoserotherapy), [A.E. Wright] Proc.Roy.Soc.Med. 26: 412-414, Feb. '33; also, J.Laryng.& Otol. 48: 252-256, April '33

33A21 history, forerunners of serum therapy, [M. Neuburger] M: 707-710, De. '32 [Reprint]

33B1 autogenous, autohemotherapy in psychiatry, [Beelitz Med.Welt 7:1330, Sept.16, '33

33B2-autohemotherapy in puerperal fever, [V. Rubeska] Casap.Lek.cesk. 72: 1207, Octo.autohemotherapy 6, '33; 1240, Octo.autohemotherapy 13, '33

33B3-autohemotherapy in zona, [Le Calvé] Prat.méd.franç. 14: 551-557, Aug. autohemotherapy (A-B) '33

33B4-autohemotherapy of erysipelas, [L. Lajos] Orvosi hetil. 77: 755-757, Aug.26, '33

33B5-autoserotherapy in exudative pleurisy and in polyserositis, [B. de Luca & I. Maccherini] Gior.d.med. prat. 15: 392-418, Sept. '33

33B6-autoserotherapy in trachoma and its corneal complications, [R. S. Khursan] Sovet.vestnik oftal. 2: 181-185, '33

33B7-autoserotherapy, using

iodized serum, in therapy of colloidoclastic diathesis, chron. arthritis and hyperthyroidism, [E. Joltrain] Gaz.méd.de France, pp.367-373, May 15, '33

33B8-combined autohemotherapy and vaccinotherapy, [R. Schwarcz & V. López Zabaleta] Rev.méd.del Rosario 22: 728-738, Sept. '32

33B9-fate of own blood injected into various tissues, [K. Maeda] Okayama-Igakkai-zasshi 45: 1681-1682, July '33

33B10-further observations (in skin diseases of allergic origin), [N. Burgess] Brit.J.Dermat. 45: 333-340, Aug.-Sept. '33

33B11-hemostasis of hemophilic hemorrhage with roentgen irradiations of spleen and liver associated with autohemotherapy, [G. B. Costa Starricco] Pediatria 41: 1164-1170, Sept. '33

33B12-in chronic forms of mental diseases, [S. di Mauro] Cervello 12: 263-266, July15, '33

33B13-in grave ulcerative colitis, [R. Bensaude, P. Oury & H. Dany] Arch.d.mal.de L'app.digestif 23: 577-592, June '33

33B14-in mental diseases, [P. Durando] Osp.maggiore 21: 209-213, April '33

33B15-in rheumatic infectious

polyarthritis, [P. I. Glazko] Sovet.vrach.gaz., pp.169-171, March 15-31, '33

33B16-in schizophrenia, [O. Freytag] Psychiat.-neurol. Wchnschr. 35: 322, July1, '33; comment by Magenau 35: 468, Sept.23, '33

33B17-prevention and treatment of serum anaphylaxis by injections of patient's own blood, [C. Rother] Zentralbl.f.Chir. 60: 1336-1338, June 10, '33

33B18-results of ultraviolet therapy and autohemotherapy (Rajka-Radnal method) in syphilis with irreducible Wassermann reaction, [R. Glassner] Bull.Soc.Franç.de dermat.et syph. (Réunion dermat.) 40: 531-532, April '33

33B19-therapy of erythromelalgia by injection of patient's own blood, [T. Kaku] Arch.f.jap.Chir. 10: 916-917, July1, '33

33B20-treatment of acute gonorrheal epididymitis by injection of patient's whole blood, [L. M. Bellin] Illinois M.J. 64: 480-482, Nov. '33

33B21-treatment of anemia with patient's own blood, that has been treated by ultraviolet rays, [C. Fervers] Deutsches Arch.f.klin.Med. 175: 226-240, '33

34A1 autogenous, [M. John] München.med.Wchnschr.

81:177-178, Feb.2, '34

34A2-autohemotherapy in furunculosis, [J. Pou Díaz] Crón. méd., Valencia 37: 931-936, Dec. 15, '33

34A3-autohemotherapy in incoercible vomiting in pregnancy; 2 cases, [L. Henri-Petit] Arch.Méd.-chir.de Province 23: 311-312, Aug.-Sept. '33

34A4-autohemotherapy in malaria, [G. Lio] Riv.san.siciliana 21: 265-268, Feb. 15, '33

34A5-autohemotherapy in otorhinolaryngologic diseases, [J. Garzoni & M. O. Gomes Veiga] Rev.Méd.latino-am. 19: 386-391, Jan. '34

34A6-autohemotherapy in ozena, [Meyrelles do Souto] Rev. de laryng. 54: 1171-1178, Nov. '33

34A7-autohemotherapy in puerperal fever, [V. Rubeska] Casop.lek.cesk. 72: 1260-1263, Oct. 20, '33

34A8-autoserotherapeutic injections into nasal mucosa in asthma and respiratory tract diseases; 9 cases, [A. Jacquelin & G. Bonnet] Presse méd. 42: 249-251, Feb.14, '34

34A9-behavior of homoplastic bone transplants prophylactically treated with blood serum of host; preliminary report, [S. Grisanti] Riv.san.siciliana 22: 3-18, Jan.1, '34

34A10-cure of gonococcic septicemia by autohemotherapy: case, [A. M. Zelasco, N. Bakmas & J. M. Pastoriza] Semana méd. 2: 2025-2027, Dec. 21, '33

34A11-indications for autohemotherapy according to Oliveira Botelho method, [J. G. Gernandes] Gaz.clin. 31: 262-265, Oct. '33

34A12-mechanism of action, [L. C. Waintraub] Bull.Soc.franç.de dermat.et syph. 40: 1798-1802, Dec. '33

34A13-ovarian hemocrinotherapy in scleroderma, [A. Sézary & A. Horowitz] Bull.Soc.franç.de dermat.et syph. 41: 68-71, Jan. '34

34A14-premenstrual liver crises treated by preparation of menstrual blood, [R. Jahiel] Arch.d.mal.de l'app. digestif 23: 1008-1010, Nov. '33

34A15-strengthening defense of syphilitic patients; autohemotherapy, [H. Gougerot & J. Meyer] Bull.gén.de thérap. 184: 337-251, Sept.-Octo. '33

34A16-technic of autogenous blood injection into anterior chamber according to Schieck method, [H. Traumann] Klin.Monatsbl.f.Augenh. 92: 391, March '34

34A17-therapy of gonorrheal epididymitis and arthritis by intravenous injections of hemolyzed autogenous blood, [A.

Ingman] Finska Iäk.-sällsk.handl. 75: 1051-1066, Nov. '33

34A18-therapy of localized pruritus and circumscribed eczema by local injections of novocain (procaine hydrochloride) and patient's own blood, [A. Tzanck, O. Berger & E. Sidi] Bull.Soc.franç.de dermat.et syph. 40: 1728--1734, De. '33

34A19-therapy of tuberculous iridocyclitis by autohemotherapy in anterior chamber of eye, [A. Moreu] Arch.de oftal hispano-am. 33: 699-703, Dec. '33

34A20-treatment of anemias with patient's own blood after it has been irradiated with ultraviolet rays, [C. Fervers] Deutsche med.Wchnschr. 59: 1922-1923, Dec.29, '33

34A21-treatment of pneumonia with patient's own blood defibrinated by ultraviolet rays, [K. Nasvytis] Medicina, Kaunas 14: 649-651, Nov. '33

34A22-vagaries of cancer and deductions therefrom (use of washed autogenous erythrocytes), [H. Gray] Internat.J.Med.& Surg. 46: 578-583, Dec. '33

34A23-history, life of Roux; contributions to development of serotherapy, [A. Bachmann] Bol.Acad.nac.de med.de Buenos Aires (num. extraord.), pp.5-13, '33

34B1-autogenous, autohemotherapy in cerebral hemorrhage; preliminary report, [R. Colella & G. Pizzillo] Rassegna internaz.di clin.e terap. 15: 386-393, April 15, '34; also, Minerva med. 2: 169-173, Aug. 4, '34

34B2-autohemotherapy, [P. E. Morhardt] Presse méd. 42: 1300, Aug.15, '34

34B3-autohemotherapy and gold therapy in tuberculosis, [T. Roux deLaroque] Avenir méd. 31: 205-209, July-Aug. '34

34B4-autohemotherapy in inflammatory gynecologic diseases, [B. Schilling] Gyógyászat 74: 614-616, Octo. 21, '34

34B5-autohemotherapy in schizophrenia. [P. G. Quirós] Arch.de neurobiol. 313: 931-936, July-Dec. '33

34B6-autohemotherapy of acute rheumatism, [A.P. Khokhlov] Klin.med. (no.4) 12: 649-652, '34; abstr., Sovet. vrach. gaz., pp. 544-545, April15, '34

34B7-autohemotherapy of depression, [G. Giehm] Med.Klin. 30: 803-804, June 15, '34

34B8-combined intensive calcium therapy and autohemotherapy in mental diseases, [G. Aschieri] Gior.di pschiat.e di neuropat. 62: 87-94, '34

34B9-exanthematous typhus

successfully treated by autohemotherapy; 16 cases, [A. Babalian] Bull.Soc.path. exot. 37: 235-236, '34

34B10-hemmorhagic rectitis with sanguinary dyscrasia; value of autohemotherapy; case, [L. Morenas] Lyon méd 153: 673-677, June 10, '34

34B11-intraocular autohemotherapy in tuberculosis of anterior portion of eye, [A. Garcia Miranda] Arch.de oftal hispano-am. 34: 349-377, July '34

34B12-local autohemotherapy of arthritis, [U. Rondelli] Minerva med. 1: 704-705, May 19, '34

34B13-prevention of accidents due to reinjection of serums by use of autohemotherapy, [Robert] Bull.Soc.de pédiat.de Paris 32: 435-436, July '34

34B14-serum treatment for opium addicts, [L. S. Huizenga] Chinese M.J. 48: 741-744, Aug. '34

34B15-therapy of ozena with Spiess method (submucous injections of patient's blood), [P. Gritti] Boll.d.mal.d.orecchio, d.gola, d.naso 52: 465-489, Sept. '34

34B16-treatment of pulmonary suppuration with intravenous injections of alcohol in combination with autohemotherapy, [A. S. Salishchev] Klin.med. (no.8) 12: 1158-1162, '34

35A1 autogenous, [Vorschütz] Ztschr.f.ärztl.Fortbild. 31: 703-706, Dec. 15, '34

35A2-autohemotherapy and splenic crinotherapy in elephantiasis of leg; recovery of case, [Filderman] Bull.et.mém.Soc.de méd.de Paris 138: 566-567, Nov.24, '34

35A3-autohemotherapy as new method in asthma, [P. Levin] Rev.Asoc.méd.argent. 48: 1494-1498, Dec.'34

35A4-autohemotherapy in anemia using blood irradiated with ultraviolet solar rays, [B. Boggian & F. Canova] Riv.di idroclimat.,talassol.e terap.fis. 46: 31-39, Jan. '35

35A5: autohemotherapy in bronchial asthma, [K. Maddox & R. Back] M.J.Australia 1: 277-278, March 2, '35

35A6: autohemotherapy in cerebral apoplexy, [N. Ronco] Terapia 24: 335-337, Nov. 34

35A7: autohemotherapy in trachomatous pannus and corneal ulcers, [A. P. Zakharov] Sovet.vestnik oftal. 5: 437

35A8: autohemotherapy in various diseases of children (recurrent vomiting, chorea minor and nocturnal enuresis), [C. Cardinali] Pedlatria prat. 12:1-4, Jan. 35

35A9: autohemotherapy;

indications and its use as vehicle for medicaments, [E. Achitouv] Presse med. 42: 2016-2017, Dec. 15 '34

35A10: autohemotherapy of puerperal mastitis, [L. Sinn] München.med.Wchnschr, 82: 133-134, Jan. 24, 35

35A11: autohemotherapy of verruca; results in 11 cases, [A. Sezary & A Horowitz] Bull.Soc.franç.de dermat.et syph. 42: 308-312, Feb. 35

35A12: further study on autohemotherapy, with special reference to its use in some forms of otorhinolaryngology, [A. della Vedova, Jr.] Gazz.d.osp [56]:403-406, April 14, 35

35A13: injection of autogenous blood into anterior chamber in tuberculous iritis, [H. Serr] Ber.u.d.Versamml.d. deutsch.ophth.Gesellsch. 50:41-48, 34

35A14: intramuscular autohemotherapy, new treatment for cerebral hemorrhage; 7 cases; preliminary report, [R Colella & G Pizzillo] Ztschr.f.d.ges.Neurol.u. Psychiat. 152: 337-344, '35: also, Med.argent. 14:1-5, Jan. 35; also, Riv.di pat.nerv. 45:116-127, Jan.-Feb. 35, also, Forze san. 4: 212-219, Feb. 10, 36; also, Wien.med.Wchnschr. 85: 341-344, March 23 '35; also, Presse med. 43: 574-576, April 10, '35

35A15: introduction of autogenous blood into anterior chamber according to Schieck method In tuberculosis iridocyclitis, [M. L. Krasnov] Sovet.vestnik oftal. 5: 522-527, 34

35A16: leukocytic formula in trachoma before, during and after autohemotherapy, [G. Bossalino] Boll.d'ocul. 14: 225-235 Feb. '35

35A17: mechanism of action of autohemotherapy in cerebral hemorrhage, study of isohemolytic and iso-agglutination and hemagglutination phenomena In blood; 16 cases, [G. Rabboni & S. F. Gurrieri] Policlinico (sez, med.) 42: 163-168, March '36

35A18: procedure for arsenical autohemotherapy (exohemophylaxis) with highly diluted injections in syphilis [L. C. Waintraub] Ann.d.mal.ven. 30: 265-270, April '36

35A19: technic and mechanism of injections of autogenous blood into anterior chamber according to Schieck method in tuberculous iridocyclitis, [W. Kyrieleis] Ztschr.f.Augenh. 85:16-23, Dec. 34

35A20: therapy of psoriasis by injection of patients own blood which has been treated by ultraviolet rays. [M. Murayama] J.Orient.Med. (Abstr. Sect.) 22:40, March'35.

35A21: treatment of erythema nodosum with injections of patient's own blood. [J. Heimbeck], Norsk mag. f. lægevidensk. 96:390-394, April '35

35A22: ultraviolet irradiation and autohemotherapy of syphilis. [K. Pogany] Orvosi hetil. 79:214-215, Feb. 23, '35.

35A23: use of patient's own serum in combating opium addiction, [L. S. Huizenga & P. H. Jukao Ku], Geneesk. tijdschr. v. Nederl. Indië 75:22-23, Jan. 8, '35.

35A24: value of autohemotherapy in arterial hypertension, [V. M. Buscaino & V. Longo] Rassegna Internaz.di clin.e terap. 16: 124-127, Feb. 15, 36

35B1: autogenous, action of autohemotherapy on nitrogen fractions of blood, [C. Negri & G. Terzi] Gior.di clin. med. 16: 739-752, June 30, 35

35B2: action of autohemotherapy on plasmatic and globular cholesteremia, [C. Negri] Gior.di clin.med. 16: 725-738, June 30, 35

35B3: action of hemotherapy on calcemia and on chlorides in blood and urine, [C. Negri & C. Chiodarelli] Gior.di clin. med. 16: 858-869, July 20, 35

35B4: action of hemotherapy on diastases in blood and urine, [C. Negri & G. Tattoni] Gior. di clin.med. 16: 870-880, July 20, 35

35B5: application of intra-ocular autohemotherapy according to Schieck in heredosyphilitic parenchymatous keratitis, [I. Brecher], Klin. Monatsbl.f.Augenh. 95: 83-87, July 35

35B6: arterial pressure after autohemotherapy, [L. Gipperich] Ateneo parmense 7:173-176 May-June 35

35B7: ascites treated by autohemotherapy; case [B. L. Kamra] Indian M.Gaz. 70: 626, Nov. '35.

35B8: attempts at therapy of ozena with autohemotherapy; clinical study [E. Tavani] Ann.di laring.,otol. 35:1-22, '35

35B9: autohemotherapy in arterial hypertension [G. Pizzillo] Riforma med. 51:1505-1508 Oct. 5 '35

35B10: autohemotherapy in certain forms of allergic supprations [O. Coquelet] J.de chir.et Ann.Soc.belge de chir. 34-32: 203-208 April 35

35B11: Autohemotherapy in epilepsy [V. A. Lukashev] Klin. med. 13: 600-601 April 35

35B12: autohemotherapy of anterior chamber in tuberculous iridocyclitis [P. Mata] Arch.de oftal.hispano-am. 35: 270-273 May 35

35B13: autohemotherapy of cerebral hemorrhages, cases, [R. Colella & G. Pizzillo] Arch.lnternat.de neurol. 54: 145-152 March 35; also J.Nerv.& Ment.Dis. 82: 652-659, Dec. '35

35B14: autohemotherapy of pneumonia: 10 years of experience. [G. Tillmann] München.med.Wchnschr. 82:1604-1607      Oct. 4, 35

35B15: autoserotherapy with blister serum in therapy of toxicomania [R. E. Carratali] Rev.Asoc.med.argent. 49: 641-645 May 35; also Rev.de criminol. psiquiat.y med.leg. 22: 362-366 May-June 35

35B16: effect of autohemotherapy on blood picture [L. Gipperich] Gior.di clin.med. 16: 952-961 Aug. 10 '35

35B17: injection of tuberculous patients with their own blood, preliminary communication [O. Amrein] J.State Med 43: 426-429 July 35

35B18: injections into nasal mucosa in bronchial asthma; 11 cases [D. Moruzzi] Policlinico (sez. prat.) 42: 905-911 May 13 35

35B19: local autohemotherapy in trachoma, [J. Balza & R. Romano Yalour] Arch.de oftal.de Buenos Aires 10: 502-504 July 35

35B20: morphine addiction; treatment by autogenous serum; Modenos phlyctenar method; preliminary report [T. D. Lee] Northwest Med. 34: 313 Aug. 35

35B21: new treatment for chronic ulcers of leg and foot (injection of autogenous blood in varicose and syphilitic ulcers) [C. H. Verovitz] Ohio State M.J. 31: 850-854 Nov. 35

35B22: therapy of chronic encephalitis (parkinsonism) by intraspinal injection of patient's own blood [V. Seletskiy, D. M. Mitnitskiy & A. A. Fridman] Vrach. delo 18: 61-62 35

35B23: value of autohemotherapy in juvenile asthma [K. Maddox & R. F. Back] Arch Dis.Childhood 10: 381-388 Oct. 35

36A1: autogenous autohemotherapy [J. de Oliveira Botelho] Gaz.clin. 33: 296-297 Nov. 35

36A2: application of intra-ocular autohemotherapy according to Schieck in heredosyphilitic parenchymatous keratitis [A. Linksz] Klin.Monatsbl.f.Augenh. 96: 233-234 Feb. 36 [Comment on Brecher's article]

36A3: autohemotherapy in hypertrophic gingivitis [A. Zona] Stomatol. 34:117-126 Feb. 36

36A4: autohemotherapy in schizophrenia [S. Cagilero] Studium 26: 73-76 April 1, '36

36A5: behavior of leukocyte count and formula in pulmonary tuberculosis treated by autoserotherapy [G. Tumino] Riv.di pat.e clin.d.tuberc. 10:164-170 March 31 36

36A:6 effect of local injection of blood on healing of fractures; experimental studies [T. Mitsutake] Nagasaki Igakkwai Zassi 14: 390 March 25 36

36A7: Immediate and late results of autohemotherapy In apoplexy [F. Lloret Gil] Siglo med. 96: 560-562, Nov. 16 35

36A8: prophylactic autohemotherapy for reduction of postoperative pulmonary complications, [G. Karpati] Zentralbl.f.Gynak. 60: 516-523 Feb. 29 36

36A9: statistical results of treatment of various dermatoses with patient's own blood which has been subjected to ultraviolet irradiation [M. Murayama] J.Orient Med. (Abstr. Sect.) 23:104 Dec. 35

36A10: symptoms of pulmonary suppuration and its therapy with methenamine combined with autohemotherapy [V. S. Tredlov] Sovet.vrach.gaz. pp. 1735-1744, Nov. 30, 35

36A11: therapy of chronic toxi-infectious diseases of neuraxis by autohemotherapy associated with provoked aseptic meningitis (autohemoneuraxotherapy) [G. Boschi] Rev.neurol. 64: 951-955, Dec. 35

36A12: therapy of headache due to hypertension by autohemotherapy [Blas Moia] Rev.argent.de cardiol. 2: 239-245, Sept.-Oct. 35

36A13: variations in amino-acid curve in blood after protein colloid and autohemotherapy, [G. de Nito & G. Calore] Pathologica 28. 76-80 Feb. 15 36

36B1: Autogenous autohemotherapy in cerebral hemorrhage; 3 cases [A. Salamero Castillón] Clin.y lab. 23: 479-487, June 36

36B2: autohemotherapy in cranial hemorrhages; recovery of case [Benigno de Araujo & L. Rapouso] Rev.med de Pernambuco 6: 336-338 Sept. 36

36B3: autohemotherapy of children's diseases [G. Kellhammer] Monatschr.f.Klnderh. 65: 385-406 36

36B4: autohemotherapy of sleeplessness [H. Haenel] Psychiat.-neurol.Wchnschr.38: 429-430 Aug. 22 36

36B5: autotherapy by de Oliveira Botelho method [T. Miraglia] Gaz.clin. 34: 230-232 Aug. 36

36B6: behavior of granulofilamentous substance of erythrocytes during autohemotherapy [S. Acquaviva] Studium 26: 97-101 May 1 36

36B7: hemocrinotherapy of bacterial particularly

staphylococcic inflammations [L. & M. Filderman] Rev. franç.d'endocrinol. 14: 235-245 June 36

36B8: intracutaneous injection of patient's blood In vitiligo vulgaris [N. Nishikawa] Okayama-Igakkai-Zasshi 48: 2196-2197 Sept. 36

36B9: serum treatment of narcotic addiction, [D. M. Black] Canad.M.A.J. 35: 177-179, Aug. '36

36B10: specific pressor effects of autohemotherapy according to hour of administration; therapeutic value, [G. B. Cacciapuoti & G. Reale] Gazz.internaz.méd.-chir. 46: 345-350, June 30, '36

36B11: treatment of acute gonorrheal epididymitis and acute gonorrheal arthritis by means of injection of autogenous blood; influence of treatment on rapidity of red cell sedimentation of patients [T. Sakurai] Bull.Nav. M.A.Japan (Abstr. Sect.) 25: 38-39, July 15, '36

37A1: autogenous, [C. Fischer] Med.Welt 10:1659-1661. Nov. 14, '36

37A2: autohemotherapy and its uses, [M. Moroni] Gazz.d. osp. 58: 393-395, April 25, '37

37A3: autohemotherapy and procaine hydrochloride in therapy of lesions of crucial and lateral ligaments of knee joint, [F. Mandl] Wien.klin.Wchnschr. 50: 625-626, May 14, '37

37A4: autohemotherapy by subconjunctival injections in therapy of trachoma; 2 cases, [E. Sel-a Martinez] Rev. internat.du trachome 14: 19-22, Jan. '37

37A5: autohemotherapy; experimental study. [T. Aoki] Mitt. a.d.med.Akad.zu Kioto 19: 1859-1861, '37

37A6: autohemotherapy in certain diseases of lungs and pleura, [G. A. Lvovich] Sovet.vrach.zhur. 41: 357360, March 15, '37

37A7: autohemotherapy in epilepsy, [G. I. Mirzoyan] Klin. med. 14: 1546-1547, '36

37A8: autohemotherapy in primary arterial hypertension in menopause, [F. Graziano] Riv.san.siciliana 25: 143-153, Feb. 1, '37

37A9: autohemotherapy of depression and melancholia, [T. von Lehoczky] Psychiat.-neurol.Wchnschr. 39: 180-183, April 24, '37

37A10: autoserotherapy for drug addiction, [M. Vivian] Lancet 1: 1221-1223, May 22, '37

37A11: autoserum treatment for opium addicts observation on 1,000 cases, [A. W. Woo] Chinese M.J. 51: 8.0-90, Jan. '37

37A12: bacteriologic studies on polyarthritis; attempts at specific (enterococcic) autovaccinotherapy and autoserotherapy' [N. Svartz] Acta med.Scandinav. supp. 78. pp. 327-338. '36

37A13: behavior of Pagano-Hering, reflex (carotid sinus cardiovascular reflex) after autohemotherapy, especially in arteriosclerosis, [A. Geremia] Gior.med.d.Alto Adige, 3: 473-488, Aug.'36

37A14: biologic autosatotherapy (autohemotherapy), [A. Y. Rubinov] Vrach.delo 19: 1113-1116, '36

37A15: desensitizing action of autogenous serum irradiated with ultraviolet rays; experimental study, [M. Murayama] J.Orient.Med. (Abstr. Sect.) 26: 56-57. April '37

37A16: direct irradiation of autogenous blood with ultraviolet rays (Havlicek method) as potential method of therapy in tuberculoses, [O. H. Bueher] Beitr.z.Klin.d. Tuberk. 89: 377-384, '37

37A17: effect and mode of action of autohemotherapy in agranulocytosis, [T. Sakurai] Klin.Wchnschr.. 16: 564-565, April 17, '37

37A18: habitual luxation of shoulder and rupture of crucial ligaments of knee; therapy by injections of patient's own blood, [F. Mandl]

Zentralbl.f.Chir. 64: 1030-1033, May 1, '37

37A19: Havlicek method of treating pulmonary tuberculosis with autogenous blood irradiated with ultraviolet rays, [K. Glombitza] Deutsches Tuberk.-Bl. 11: 65-69, March '37

37A20: influence of autohemotherapy on resorption of blood infected under bulbar conjuntiva, into anterior chamber and into vitreous humor: experimental study, [A. Bellavia] Riv.san.sicilianna 25: 333-337, April 1, '37

37A21: therapy of abscess of axillary sweat glands by injection of patient's own blood, [O. Adam] Zentralbl.f. Chir. 64: 26-31, Jan. 2, '37

37A22: therapy of craniocerebral trauma by dehydrating forced drainage of cerebrospinal fluid and autohemotherapy, [Gomez Durán] Cir.ortop.y traumatol., Madrid 1: 1351 5~, '36

37A23: therapy of solitary nonparasitic cyst of femur (intracystic autohemotherapy by simple puncture); 2 cases, [M. Chaton] 'Mém.Acad.de chir. 63: 473-485 April 14, '37

37A24: total otitic zona of Sicard or complete syndrome of Souques' geniculate ganglion rapid recovery of case after autohemotherapy, [E. Cornet] Bull.Soc.méd.chir.de l'Indochine 14: 1273-1274, Nov. '16

37A25: treatment of carbuncle by autohemotherapy, [P. Rit] Calcutta M.J. 32: 31-82, Feb. '37

37A26: use of autohemotherapy G. Lyon] Bull.méd., Paris 51: 113-120, Feb. 20, '37

37A27: history, priority of Antonio Cesaris Demel in conception of serotherapy (Priorita di pensiero di Antonio Cesaris Demel nella concezione della sieroterapia), Biochim. e terap. sper. 24: 109-113, March 31' 37

37B1: autogenous, autohemotherapy combined with serotherapy in pneumonia; case in infant' [A. Diaz Padróni] Bol.Soc.cubana de pediat. 9:161-174, April , 37

37B2: autohemotherapy in depression and melancholia, [T. Lehoczky] Gyógyásezat 77: 344-347, May 30-June 6' , 37

37B3: autohemotherapy in dermatology especially in psoriasis and herpes zoster) , [J. W. Jones & M. S. Alden] South.M.J. 30: 735-737, July '37

37B4: autohemotherapy in hyphemia, [A. Licheri] Rassegna ital.d'ottal. 6: 62-71, Jan.-Feb. , 37

37B5 -autohemotherapy in paralysis of ocular muscles: 2 cases [R. Campos] Riforma med. 53:1439-1442 Oct. 9, '37

37B6 -autohemotherapy in pleurisy [G. A. Lvovich] Probl. tuberk., no. 6 pp. 73-75, '37.

37B7 -autohemotherapy in Tonsillitis, [K. Thurn] München. Med. Wchnschr. 84: 1139, July 16, '37

37B8 -authemotherapy of corneal ulcers, [A. B. Kolenko] Vestnik oftal. 10: 820-840, '37

37B9 -autohemotherapy of trachomatous pannus, [B. P. Lerner] Vesnik oftal. 10: 841-843, '37

37B10 -autoserotherapy in gonorrheal arthritis; experimental and clinical observations; preliminary report, [A. Goldey] Urol.& Cutan.Rev. 41: 556-558, Aug. '37

37B11 -autoserotherapy of drug addiction, [E. Bello] Rev.méd peruana 9: 340-344, July '37

37B12 -different types of rheumatism and their treatment with sulfur, sunlight, vitamins and autohemotherapy. [J. Le Calvé] Presse Med. 45: 1409-1410, Oct. 6, 37

37B13 -endonasal autoserotherapy in spasmodic rhinitis, [V. A. Carando & J. Robbio Campos] Semana méd. 2: 604-606, Sept 9, 37

37B14 -etiopathogenesis and therapy of menorrhagia and metrorrhagia in puberty; value or autohemotherapy, [F. Putzu

Doneddu] Ann.di ostet.e ginec. 59: 787-823, July 31, 37

37B15 -failure of attempted prophylaxis of postoperative embolism by autohemotherapy [H. Fobe] Bull.Soc. d'obst.et de gynec. 26: 368-370, April '37

37B16 -Havlicek method of injecting autogenous blood irradiated with ultraviolet rays in therapy of seropositive latent lues resisting all treatment, [M. von Hecht-Eleda & G. Riehl, Jr.] Arch.f.Dermat.u.Syph. 176: 8-15, '37

37B17 -new applications of autohemotherapy in genital disturbances in women, [P. Abrami, J. Dalsace & R. Wallich] Presse méd. 45: 713-715, May 12, '37

37B18 -production of aseptic meningitis and administration of autohemotherapy in small doses in case of sclerosis in plaques and case of amyotrophic lateral sclerosis, [C. Roncati] Policlinico sez. prat.) 44: 1832-1837 Sept. 27, '37

37B19 -seasonal asthma cured by autohemotherapy; 2 cases, [F. Dazé & P. Dumas] J.de l'Hôtel-Dieu de Montréal 6: 145-152, May-June 37

37B20 -staphylococcic septicemia; natural process and its therapeutic use (autohemotherapy); 2 cases with recovery of 4 and 5 years duration, [A. Raiga] Bull.et mém.Soc.d.chirurgiens de Paris

29:102-113, Feb. 5, '37

37B21 -subconjunctival autohemotherapy in trachomatous pannus, cases [Delord] Bull.Soc.d'opht.de Paris 49: 372-375. July 37

37B22 -therapy of chronic toxi-infectious diseases of neuraxis by autohemotherapy associated with provoked aseptic meningitis (autohemoneuraxotherapy); application to case of amyotrophic lateral sclerosis, [E. de Aguiar Whitaker] Rev.assoc.paulista de med. 10: 80-90, Feb. '37.

37B23 -therapy of postoperative pulmonary complications with injections of autogenous blood, [J. Philipowicz] Zentralbl.f.Chir. 64: 1698-1699, July 17, '37

37B24 -treatment with auto-blood for so-called auto-intoxication, [N. Sata] Orient.J.Dis.Infants 21: 31-32, March '37

37B25 -ultraviolet irradiation and autohemotherapy in syphilis; treatment of persistent serologic positive and latent syphilis, [H. L. Baer] Pennsylvania M.J. 40: 943-948 Aug., '37

37B26 -use of autohemotherapy in treatment of psoriasis and herpes zoster; preliminary report. [E. E. Barksdale] Virginia M.Monthly 64: 378-381, Oct. 37

38A1 -autogenous, autohemotherapy in mental diseases; advantages or use of hemolysed blood in distilled water; cases, [P. Tenconi] Note e riv.di psichiat. 66: 449-470, Oct.-Dec., '37

38A2 -autohemotherapy and heteroprotein therapy in dichloroethyl sulfide intoxication in dogs; experimental study, [R Andreoni] Profilassi 11 1-3, Jan-Feb '38

38A3 -autohemotherapy by subconjunctival route in complications of trachoma; results in 9 cases, [E. Selfa Martinez] Rev.Internat.du trachome 16:87-92, April '38

38A4 -autohemotherapy in arterial hypertension, [D.Boccia, M.Bonafina & D.Ugazio] Rev.sud-am.de endocrinol. 21:107-117, Feb. 15, '38

38A5 -autohemotherapy in arterial hypertension, [P E Perret] Schweiz. med. Wchnschr.68:285-288, March 12, '38

38A6 -autohemotherapy in pulmonary tuberculosis, [E. B. Freilich and G. C. Coe] Illinois M. J. 73:154-157, Feb. '38

38A7 -autohemotherapy of lobar pneumonia, [K. T. V. Simon] Jahrb. f. Kinderh. 150:157-181, '37

38A8 -autohemotherapy of pneumonia, [Tillmann] Deutsche med. Wchnschr. 64:1687-169, Jan. 28, '38

38A9 -autohemotherapy of stenocardia and peripheral vascular spasms, [H. O. Wachsmuth] Deutsche med. Wchnschr. 63:1795-1798, Nov.26, '37

38A10 -autoserum treatment of opium addiction, [W.B. Weng] Malayan J. J. 12:157-158, Nov. '37

38A11 -behavior of blood dextrose after autohemotherapy, [A. Germia & C. Dalmata Mian] Gior.di clin. med.19:114-120, Feb. 10, '38.

38A12 -comparison of results obtained by dicephalospinal therapy (production of aseptic meningitis followed by autohemotherapy and autocerebrospinal fluid therapy) in 40 cases of sclerosis in plaques [G.Tanfani] Minerva med. 1:225-229, March 3, 38

38A13 -experience with Havlicek method of injections of autogenous blood irradiated with ultraviolet rays,[S Litzner] München med Wchnschr 86:280-281, Feb 25, 38

38A14 -hemocrinotherapy of epilepsy, [L.Abad Colomer] Crón méd., Valencia 41:255-280, Nov-Dec 37

38A15 -hypotensive action of autohemotherapy in hypertension and cerebral hemorrhage; review of literature and personal

contribution,[V. Longo]
Clin.med.ital.68:825-866, Dec.
'37

38A16 -intravenous
autohemotherapy with hemolyzed
blood; technic and leukopoietic
response; Preliminary report
[S.R. Dean & H.C. Solomon] J Lab
& Clin Med. 23:775-786, May 38

38A17 -local autoserotherapy in
trachoma; cases [H. Jourdan] Ann
d'ocul 175:254-258, March 38

38A18 -new nonspecific therapy
for stubborn chronic ascending
infection in female by
reinjection of patient's own
blood after it has been
irradiated with ultraviolet rays
(Havlicek method) [V Föderl]
Wien klin.Wchnschr.51:528-532,
May 13, 38

38A19 -technic and results [R
Stahl] Ztschr.f.ärztl.Fortbild
35:93-98 Feb 15 38

38B1: autogenous,
autohemotherapy and therapeutic
meningitis in sclerosis in
plaques; 2 cases, [O Bonazzi]
Gazz. d. osp. 59:643-650, June
19, 38

38B2 -autohemotherapy; case of
purpura rheumatica with new
method of treatment [L.Saxon]
Illinois MJ 74:191-193. Aug. '38

38B3 -autohemotherapy in
dystrophy and in pretuberculous
conditions of infants, [M
Rignani] Gior di clin med
19:664-671, July 20, '38

38B4 -autohemotherapy of
acanthosis rubra lichenoides;
case,[A Risi] Dermat Wchnschr
107:1142-1147 Sept 24, '38

38B5 -autohemotherapy of
apoplectic ictus, case [Amic]
Lyon med [162] 88-92 July 24, 38

38B6 -autohemotherapy of
tropical ulcer, cases, [A
Menghetti] Ann di med nav e
colon 44:328-336 July-Aug., '38

38B7 -autoserotherapy of
nonpurulent pleural effusions [S
A Savitz & N Blumberg] M Rec
148:406-408, Dec 7, '38

38B8 -autoserotherapy with
blister serum in toxicomania;
experimental study, [R.E.
Carratala] Rev. de psiquiat. y
criminol. 2:725-732, Nov.-Dec.,
'37; also An. Fac. de cien.
med.de La Plata 3:127-135, '38;
also Rev. med. latino-am
23:1042-1048, June '38

38B9 -experimental study on
healing of wound influenced by
own blood injection. [K.Tei] J.
Chosen M. A. (Abstr. Sect )
28:45, July 20, '38

38B10 -influence of autoprotein
therapy (autogenous blood) and
of heteroprotein therapy on
induced aminoacidemia curve;
study in gonorrhea patients, [A
Baccaredda]
Boll.d.Soc.med.-chir.,Pavia
52:421-453, '38

38B11 -menstrual hepatic crises
cured by menstrual
autohemotherapy; case, [E May,

Mme Logeals & R Tiffeneau] Bull et mem Soc med d hop de Paris 54:835-839, May 23, '38

38B12 -quinine combined with autohemotherapy in treatment of malaria, [A.A. Guseyn-Zade] Klin. med., 16 425-426, '38

38B13 -results with injections of autogenous blood irradiated with ultraviolet rays, [Grossekettler & Lühdemann] Deutsche med Wchnschr 64 897-898, June 17, 38

38B14 -use of autogenous irradiated blood and laparophos, Havlicek lamp, in gynecology and obstetrics [Burgkhardt] Arch f Gynak 166:535-536, '38

39A1: autogenous, association of histadine and hemotherapy in treatment of gastric and duodenal ulcers [Séta] Rev med du centre-ouest 10:248-253 Dec '38

39A2 -ambulatory autohemotherapy in hypertension [A della Vedove] Rev med de Rosario 29:111-142 Feb '39

39A3 -autohemotherapy; new method of treating hyperemesis gravidarum [L Sax☺on & J. E. Stoll] Illinois MJ 75:352-355, April '39

39A4 -hemocrinotherapy in angiospasm of extremities [L.Filderman] Rev.de path comparee 38:1390-1395, Dec '38

39A5 -hemotherapy in apoplexy

[L.I.Larina] Sovet.vrach zhur 42:763-768, Nov 30, '38

39A6 -hemotherapy in pulmonary tuberculosis [R Pfaffenberg] Ztschr.f.ärztl Fortbild 35:551-552, Oct 1 '38

39A7 -injection of blood into anterior chamber in certain diseases of eyes [L B Zats & N I Medvedev] Vestnik oftal (No.1) 14:61-65, '39

39A8 -intracerebral autohemotherapy of mental diseases [E Mariotti & M.Sciutti] Riv. sper.di./freniat. 61:870-876, Dec. 31, '37

39A9 -intramuscular injection of irradiated blood as new method of treating posthemorrhagic anemia [P Patat] Ginecologia 5:29-35, Jan '39

39A10 -severe hemoptosis treated exclusively with autohemotherapy; 10 cases [C P Tonegaru] Rev san mil Bucuresti 37:1019-1028, Dec 38

39A11 -treatment of chronic pemphigus by serum taken from bullae [S W Smith] Brit J Dermat 51:213-214, May '39

39B1: autogenous artificial antisyphilitic dermo-immunization and its importance in transforming therapy and prophylaxis; new conception of actino-autohemotherapy and actino-chemotherapy of syphilis; favorable effect of cutaneous lesions [E Radnai] Ann d mal ven

34:325-342, June '39

39B2: autohemotherapy in disturbances of menopause [M Repetti] Ann di osted e gnec 61:603-628, Man 31 '39

39B3: autohemotherapy in peptic ulcer [O E Amchislavskaya] Vrach delo 21:385-390, '39

39B4: autohemotherapy in treatment of tuberculosis of anterior half of eyeball [D M Rolett] Bull Russ Med Soc New York, pp 91-95, Sept '39

39B5: effect of injections of fresh and hemolyzed blood on erythropoiesis [J Schernhardt] Folia haemat 62:93-96, '39

39B6: hemocrinotherapy (combined hemotherapy and endocrinotherapy) [L Filderman] Bull.et mem Soc de med de Paris 142: 662-669, Nov 4, '38; abstr,Harefuah 16:ii May 39

39B7: Irradiated blood in therapy of chronic recidivating stomatitis aphthosa [A.Arai & T Maruoka] Otorhino-laryng 12:845, Oct '39

39B8: local autohemotherapy in hidrosadenitis [S.Popesco & N Hodos] Rev de chir Bucuresti 42:433-435, May-June '39

39B9: use of autohemotherapy reinforced with artificial fever in treatment of rheumatic disease [W K Ishmael] J Oklahoma M A 32:337-343, Sept '39

40A1: autogenous,autohemotherapy in glaucoma [V.Delfin] J. Philippine Islands M.A.19 683-695, Nov '39

40A2: autohemotherapy [R Koschade] Deutsche med Wchnchr 66:178-179, Feb 16, '40

40A3: autohemotherapy in treatment of arterial hypertension and disorders of menopause [G.Alexianu Buttu & E.Lichtig] Bull et mem Soc roumaine d'endocrinol 6:67-71, Feb-March '40

40A4: autohemotherapy of bronchial asthma in children [G Tamasi] Budapeste orvosi ujság 37:933-935, Dec 7, '39

40A5: hemocrinotherapy (combined hemotherapy and endocrine therapy) [L Filderman] Clinique Paris 35:6-9, Jan. '40

40A6: hemotherapy with blood irradiated with ultraviolet rays [E Sehrt] Med Welt 13:1554-1558, Doc 9, '39

40A7: hypotensive action of autohemotherapy [U Miglioccio] Athena 9:56, Feb 40

40A8: Indications for and technic of whole-blood injections [C Hardwick] Practitioner 144:79-82, Jan 40

40A9: Injection of blood in therapy of progressive vacial furunculosis and inflammation of axillary sweat glands, [M.Mennenga] Deutche Ztschr. f. Chir. 253:62-75, '39

40A10: late results of autohemotherapy of subjective symptoms of chronic arterial hypertension [B Moia] Rev med latino-am 25:10-15, Oct '39

40A11: therapy of acute supprative circumscribed mastitis with proteolytic antiferments (autohemotherapy) [D Maragliano] Accad. med Genova 54:593-596

40A12: treatment (autohemotherapy) of carbuncle in outpatient department, [C.R. Dutt] Indian M. Gaz. 75:75-76, Feb. '40.

40B1: autogenous, autohemotherapy combined with artificial fever; further observations on rheumatic disease [W.K. Ishmael] Arch. Phys. Therapy 21:335-339, June '40

40B2: autohemotherapy, blood cholesterol and erythrocyte sedimentation in pulmonary tuberculosis, [A.A. Raimondi,M. Albertal & F. M. Gonzalez] Arch. argent. de fisiol. 16:276-283, July-Sept. '40

40B3: autohemotherapy in so-called intestinal or cryptogenic fever as a means of releasing latent allergy; clinical study [C. Grassi Bertazzi] Minerva med.2:16, July 7,'40

40B4: autohemotherapy of carbuncles and furuncles of face, [Y.I.Koen] Sovet.med. (no.8) 4:31-32, '40

40B5: autohemotherapy of typhoid, [V. Boico & G. Ravalico] Minerva med. 2:155-159, Aug. 11, '40

40B6: endocrine clinical diagnosis and its application to hemocrinotherapy, [M.Filderman] Bull.et.mem.Soc.de med. de Paris 141:845-851, Dec. 24, '37

40B7: indications and technic, [W. Ruge] Ztschr.f.arztl.Fortbild. 37:237-239, April 15, '40

40B8: irradiated blood in gynecology, [F. Burgkhardt] Zentralbl.f.Gynak. 64:845-848, May 18, '40

40B9: irradiated blood in therapy of anemia and leukemia, [V.Rao] Rinasc.med. 17:187-188, April 15, '40

40B10: local autohemotherapy of chronic diseases of joints, [M.E.Volskiy] Sovet.med. (no.3) 4:31-32, '40

40B11: treatment of asthma in children with injection of autogenous blood [G. Tamasi] Kinderarztl.Praxis 11:248-251, Aug., '40

40H1: Becker, William S. and Maximillan E. Obermayer, Modern Dermatology and Syphology, J.B.Lippincott Co., Phila. (1940), discusses autohemotherapy for herpes zoster (p. 480), and recommends it for psoriasis, chronic urticaria, and in Wassermann - fast or relapsing early syphilis" (p. 32)

41A1: autogenous, autohemotherapy in craniocerebral trauma; 4 cases. [A.Tarabini Castellani] Policlinico (sez.prat.) 47:2141-2143, Dec. 16, '40

41A2: autohemotherapy as reactivating agent in syphilis; importance in ocular syphilis; preliminary report [O. Perez Siliceo] Bol.d.Hosp.oftal.de Ntra.Sra.de la Luz 1:165-168, Jan-Feb., '41

41A3: autohemotherapy in postoperative iritis after cataract extraction, [V. Popoviciu & O. Lungu] Romania med.19:58-59, March 1, '41

41A4: combined autohemotherapy and sulfanilamide therapy in infectious arthritis, [F. Paunescu] Romania med 19:45, Feb. 15, '41

41A5: diacephalospinal therapy of diseases of nervous system by production of aseptic meningitis and by autohemoneuraxotherapy, [D. Paulian and M. Chiliman] Arch de neurol.4:159-171, '40

41A6: herpes simplex; case of unusually extensive, recurrent type, apparently cured after autoserotherapy, [C.C. Thomas] Arch Dermat & Syph. 43:817-821, May '41

41A7: intermittent claudication treated by Caride Massini

autohemotherapy; 10 cases, [H. Basabe] Rev. med. latino-am. 26:505-514, Feb. '41

41A8: microautohemotherapy in whooping cough; preliminary report, [W. Lages] Brasil-med. 55:35-36, Jan. 18, '41

41A9: reinjection of patient's own blood irradiated with ultraviolet light using new model of Kromayer lamp as source of radiation, [R. Bottler and J. Lehmann] Strahlentherapie 68:460-472, '40

41A10: therapy of uterine hemorrhages in ascending gonorrhea by means of hemolyzed autogenous blood, [F.M. Monosova and E.L. Rossiyanskaya] Sovet.med. (no.20) 4:12-13, '40

41A11: year's campaign against trachoma, with special reference to therapy with salicylazosulfanilamide mixed with autogenous blood [L. Dor] J.de med.de Lyon 21:377-379, Dec. 5, '40

41B1: autogenous, autohemotherapy in cases of fixed serologic reactions (Hinton) with negative results, [I. Kopp and H. C. Solomon] Am. J. Syph., Gonor. and Ven. Dis. 25:591-594, Sept. '41

41B2: autohemotherapy as new treatment of eclampsia, with report of cases [C. Galve Raso] Medicina, Madrid 9:156-161, Aug., '41

41B3: autohemotherapy in

croupous pneumonia, [A.F. Grozev] Vrach.delo (no.3) 23:191-196, '41

41B4: autohemotherapy; indications and technic, [H.G.B. Reinhard] Ztschr.f.arztl.Fortbild. 38:69-72, Feb. 1, '41

41B5: autoserotherapy with blister serum in toxicomania; experimental study [R. Carratala] Jorn.neuropsiquiat.panam., actas (1939) 2:781-791, '41

41B6: experiences with autogenous blood in urticaria and asthma. [K. and H. Kondo] Okayama-Igkkai-Zasshi 53:886-887, April '41

41B7: intradermal autohemotherapy of pain [V.F. Pataro] Dia med. 13:575, June 30, '41

41B8: intraglandular autohemotherapy in fourth venereal disease, with report of cases [G.Amato] Gaz.clin.39:127-133, April '41

41B9: local application of patient's blood in cutaneous leishmaniasis [M.V. Bobrov] Vrach.delo (nos. 11-12) 22:785-788, '40

41B10: local autohemotherapy in ulcers of cornea, [N.O. Blyumenfeld] Vestnik oftal. 18:373-377, '41

41B11: malarial disease uncovered by autohemo-fever therapy after 35 years, [T.P.Prout & C. A. Losada] J.M. Soc. New Jersey 38:647-648, Dec. '41

41B12: perifocal autoserotherapy of ulcers and wounds [P. Valentie de Oliveira] Publ.med.Sao Paulo 12:13-17, June-July '41

41B13: treatment of chorea minor with intraspinal injections of patient's own serum, [H. Broekema] Maandschr.v.kindergeneesk. 9:477-487, Sept. '40

41C1 Hall, A.Z., The use and limitations of auto-hemic therapy. NAT. ECLECT. M. ASS. Q., 1940-41, 32: No. 3, 42-4 [619.1]

42A1: Magerl, J.F., Influence of ultraviolet radiation on immunobiologic activity of blood. Ztschr. f. Immunitätsforsch. u. Exper. Therap. 99:378-385.

42A2: Lapp., A.D., Asthma treated with patient's blood serum, Brit.M.J. 1:552, May 2, 1942.

42A3: Arias, P., Autohemotherapy (Caride Massini) in epilepsy, Semana Méd. 2:1113-1115, Nov. 6, 1941.

42A4: Rietti, E., Autohemotherapy in dysmenorrhea, Semana Méd. 2:593-4, Sept. 4, 1941.

42A5:   de Mienicki, M., Effect of autoserum administered by intradermal route on psoriasis patients. Ann. de Dermat. et Syph. 10:1054-1063, 1939-1940.

42B1:   Marks, M.M., Lymphopathia venereum, autoserum as specific antigen, South.M.J. 35:1092-1097, Dec. 1942.

42B2:   Moreno, B.O., Therapy of inflammatory forms of chronic rheumatism, with special reference to autohemolysotherapy; preliminary report. Bol. d. Inst. Clin. Quir. 18:435-437, July, 1942.

43A1:   Alvaro, M.E., Attempted autohemotherapy in genuine arterial hypertension. Hospital, Rio de Janiero 22:599-604, Oct. '42.

43A2:   Forster, E., Therapy of infections and allergic diseases with autogenous blood treated with short wave irradiation. Deutsche med. Wchnschr. 68:86, Jan. 23, 1942.

43A3:   Naide, M., Treatment of leg ulcers with blood and concentrated plasma (lyovac). Am. J. M. Sc. 205:489-493, April 1943.

43B1:   Ruiz Moyano Flores, J., Autohemotherapy in malaria and its interpretation in light of new pathogenic knowledge. Semana Méd. Españ. 6:70, Jan. 16, 1942.

43B2:   Kondo, K. & H., Cure of urticaria and bronchial asthma by intramuscular autohemic injection. Far East. Sc. Bull. 1:41, Sept. 1941 [abstract].

43B3:   Barbosa, R. F., Intracutaneous autoserotherapy in essential hypertension; preliminary report. Med. Cir. Pharm., pp. 197-199, April 1943.

43B4:   Prudente, A., Regeneration technic in plastic surgery, using blood as "nutritive bed"; illustrative case of wound of buttock. Arq. de cir, clín. e exper. 6:272-280, Aptil-June 1943.

43B5:   Bobrov, M.V., Treatment of cutaneous leishmaniasis with blood dressings. Trop. Dis. Bull. 40:441, June 1943 [abstract]

44A1:   Kreyes, H., Application and technic of autogenous blood dressings in leg ulcers resistant to therapy. Ztschr. f. ärztl. Fortbild. 39:360-362, Aug. 15, 1942.

44A2:   Desai, D.B., Autohemotherapy, Antiseptic 40:608-10, Nov. 1943.

44A3:   Jofre de Villegas, F., Autohemotherapy in cerebral hemorrhage. Semana Méd. Españ. 6:49, July 10, 1943.

44A4:   Raettig, H., Convalescent serum in combination with autohemotherapy. Bull. War Med. 4:473, April, 1944 [Abstract]

44A5:   Zuñiga P., S.T.,

Intracisternal injection of arsphenamine treated serum in therapy of neurosyphilis. Med. y cir., Bogotá 8:204-214, Feb. 1944.

44A6: Rabinovitz, E., Treatment of typhoid fever by autohemotherapy. Harefuah 26:87, March 1, 1944.

44B1: Duék, H., Autohemotherapy in gravidic vomiting. An. brasil. de ginec. 17:197-203, March 1944.

44B2: Vieira de Rocha, R., Nicolas-Favre disease, with special reference to new technic of therapy; use of autohemotherapy and salicylazosulfanilamide (sulfonamide). Med.cir.pharm., pp. 167-176, March 1944.

44B3: Raettig, H., Treatment of typhus fever by convalescent serum in combination with autohemotherapy. Trop. Dis. Bull. 41:275-276, April 1944 [abstract]

44B4: Consales, P.A., and W. T. O'Connell, Use of blood in treatment of duodenal fistula. New England J. Med. 231:582-4, Oct. 26, 1944.

45A1: Massini, P. Caride, Cerebral hemorrhage: Caride Massini autotherapy. Semana méd. 1:269-273, Feb. 4, 1942.

45B1: Boccia, D., M. Bonafina & D., Ugazio, Autohemotherapy in arterial hypertension. Prensa Méd, La Paz 4:130; 140, July-August, 1944.

45B2: Mohanty, J.K., Local autohemotherapy in carbuncle; analysis of 27 cases. Antiseptic 42:384-390, July 1945.

45D1: Stevanin, M., Autoemolisoterapia in alcune dermopatie. DERMOSIFILOGRAPHO, 1944, 19 (May-June) 67-76. [1103 n]

45D2: Sammartino, E.S., Sistema universal para la practica de la hemoterapia flebo e hipodermoclisis. SEM. MED., B. AIR., 1945, 52: pt 2 (Sept. 13), 407-425. [1129 o]

46A1: Erkun, S., Autohemotherapy in hemorrhagic cystitis. Türk tip cem.mec. 11:394-5, 1945.

46A2: Orbach, E.J., Use of blood-kaolin-penicillin paste in treatment of varicose and torpid leg ulcers. Am. J. Surg. 71:253-255, Feb. 1946.

46B1: Cardoso, L. E., Increasing surgical field in intra-abdominal surgery by intraperitoneal injection of patient's blood. Brasil méd.-cir. 8:1-6, Feb. 1946.

46B2: Pezzarossa, G., Presumed power of autohemotherapy to turn syphilitic seroreactions negative; recent syphilis (primary and secondary period), Ateneo parmense 16:159-167, 1945.

46B3:   de Reyes Pugnaire, M., Stenosing rectitis; attempted therapy by perirectal autohemotherapy; cases. Med. colon., Madrid 8:38-50, July 1, 1946.

46B4:   Bessone, L., Therapy of psoriasis by means of intracutaneous autoserotherapy according to de Mienicki. Dermosifilografo 17:463-49\80, August 1942,

46B5:   Kook, N., Treatment of recurrent shoulder dislocation with autohemo-injections. Acta med. orient. 5:277-279, August 1946.

46D1:   Reyes Pugnaire, M. de., Rectitis estenosantes; ensayos de su tratamiento por la autohemoterapia perirrectal. MED. COLON, MADRID, 1946, 8: No. 1. (Jul. 1), 38-50. [468 l]

47A1:   Vivian, M., Autoserotherapy for treatment of drug addiction. M. Press 217:338-341, April 23, 1947.

47A2:   Schiassi, B., Critical study of hemocrinotherapy of various inflammations. Policlinico (sez. prat.) 49:1377, Oct. 5, 1942; 1421, Oct. 12, 1943.

47A3:   Ross, B., and P.J. Richeson, Intensive autohemotherapy of acne. U.S.Nav.M.Bull. 47:154-155, Jan.-Feb., 1947.

47A4:   Fradà and S. Onorato, Relation between autohemotherapy

and blood groups. Boll. Soc. Ital. biol. sper. 22:36-37, Jan.-Feb. 1946.

47B1:   Saasa and Daire, Asthma of anaphylactic origin cured by progressive intradermal autoserotherapy; case in child 4 years old. Algérie méd., pp. 495-6, June-July, 1947.

47B2:   Lazoravits, L., Combined therapy of circulatory disorders of heart with autogenous blood and circulatory hormone (cardiokinetic muscle extract). Orvosok lapja 3:195-197, Feb. 16, 1947.

47B3:   Brocq, P. & T. Stephanopoli, Metabolic role of erythrocytes in reparation and upkeep of cellular tissues; new data on hemotherapy. Bull. Acad. nat. méd. 131:408-410, June 10-17, 1947.

47C1:   Ryss, S. & Stroikowa, X., La transfusion de l'homosang dans la théraupeutique de la maladie ulcéreuse de l'estomac et du duodénum. ARCH. MAL. APP. DIGEST, 1945, 34: (Oct.-Dec.), 307-322. [61 a]

47D1:   Wallis, R., Application of auto-hemotherapy in gynecological cases. 671-3, M. MOUNT SINAI HOSP., N. YORK, 1947, 14: No. 3 (Sept. - Oct.) [1256 s]

47D2:   Stern, H.J., Autohaemo-therapy in hordeolosis., 766-9, BRIT. J. OPHTH., 1947, 31: No. 12 (Dec.) [1618 s]

48A1:  Hussenstein, J., Autohemotherapy and penicillin in phlebitis.  Semaine d. hôp. Paris 23:2861-2864, Dec. 21, 1947.

48A2:  Orator, V., combination of sulfonamide or penicillin with stimulant therapy; injection of penicillin mixed with patient's own blood.  Wien. med. Wchnschr. 98:20-22, Jan. 10, 1948.

48B1:  Battaglini, S., Intracutaneous autoserum therapy of psoriasis (de Mienicki). Dermosifilografo 23:89-93, March-April, 1948.

48B2:  de Reyes Pugnaire, M., Therapy of inflammatory rectal stenosis; perirectal autohemotherapy and reaction of presacral sympathetic (superior hypogastric plexus).  Rev.españ. cir., traumatol.y ortop. 7:54-67, July-August 1947.

48B3:  Hasche-Klünder, R., Traumatic muscular tuberculosis following autoserotherapy. Deutsche med. Wchnschr. 73:371-372, Sept. 3, 1948.

48C1:  Tolone, S., La regolazione autoemoterapica della resistenza capillare; meccanismo d'azione del-autoemoterapia. [546 h]

49A1:  Meyer, F., Autoserotherapy of furunculosis; 2 cases.  Deutsche med. Wchnschr. 74:546, April 29, 1949.

49A2:  Greval, S.D.S., Serologic technic.  Indian M. Gaz. 83:549-551, Dec. 1948.

49A3:  Sperber, P.A., Whale oil, trichophytin and autoserotherapy in treatment of epidermophytosis.  Ann. Allergy 7:91-102, Jan.-Feb., 1949.

49B1:  Poth, D.O., Autohemotherapy of herpes zoster; results in 154 cases. Arch. Dermat. & Syph. 69:636-638, Oct. 1949.

49B2:  Dostrovsky, A., & A. Ticho, Case of ocular leprosy treated with autoserum from cantharides blisters.  Internat. J. Leprosy 17:434-47, Jan.-June, 1949.

49D1:  Weissenbach, R.J., L'autohémothérapie intradermique. HOPITAL, 1949, 37: No. 576 (July), 147. [568 h]

49D2:  Poth, D.O., Autohemotherapy of herpes zoster; results in 154 cases. 636-8.  ARCH. DERM. SYPH., CHIC., 1949, 60: No. 4 (Oct.) [989 b]

49H1:  Saxon, Leo, "Treatment of herpes zoster with special reference to autohemotherapy", J. Am. Inst. Homeop. Oct. 1949, 213.

49H2:  Mease, "Modified Autohemic Therapy", J.Florida M.A.,, SSSVI July 1949, 22-25.

50A1:  Urso, F., Effect of

spleen on absorption time of blood injected into muscles; experimental study. Pathologica 41:77-84, March-April, 1949.

50A2: Giese, R., Shortening of bleeding time and coagulation time following operations and injections of autogenous blood. Zentralbl. Chir. 74:565-569, 1949.

50A3: Agneta, J.O., and A.A. Cordero, Therapy of various dermatoses in female by means of autogenous premenstrual serum. Prensa méd.argent. 37:83-88, Jan. 13, 1950.

50B1: Desmonts, T., N. Rière & G. Sournies, Acute purpura in course of undulant fever; intramedullary autohemotherapy for arrest of hemorrhage; case. Sang. 21:552-553, 1950.

50B2: Goldschmied, A., Simple modification of tissue therapy (subcutaneous injections of patient's own blood), with special consideration of peptic ulcer. Polski tygodnik lek. 5:967-973, 1950.

50B3: Friederich, H.C., and H. Ruther, Therapy of cutaneous ulcers with autogenous blood dressings. Neue med. Welt. 1:1405-1407, October 28, 1950.

50C1: Desomonts, T., Riére N., Sournies, G., Acute purpura in the course of brucellosis, intramedullary autohemotherapy, arrest of hemorrhage, SANG 21:6 (1950), p. 552-3. [21341]

50C2: Rojas, J.C., Histaminic autohemotherapy, PRENSA MÉDICA ARGENTINA 37: 26, 30 June 1950, p. 1461-5. [31314]

51A1: Nase, H., Prevention of serum sickness following tetanus prophylaxis by injecting patient's own blood together with antiserum, Zentralbl. Chir. 76:284-288, 1951

51A2: Stender, A., Transorbital leukotomy and a new variant; intrafrontal injection of autogenous blood, Nervenarzt 21:514-517, Dec. 1950

51B1: Baniewicz, N., Injection of patient's own serum into cisterna magna and spinal canal in therapy of virus diseases of nervous system, Polski Tygodnik Lek. 6:342-346, 1951

51C1: Botar, G., allergic eye disease and autohemotherapy - pericardial fluid in myxedema], ORVOSI HETILAP 91:29 (16 July 1950), p. 923-4. [59827]

51C2: Haferkamp, H., Effect of autohemotherapy on the blood and the blood picture, HIPPOKRATES 21: 15-16 (31 Aug 1950), p. 475-8 [3641]

51C3: Nase, H., Autohemoprophylaxis of serum sickness/prevention of shock following inoculation against tetanus, ZENTRALBLATT FUR CHIRURGIE, LEIPZIG. 76:4 (1951), p. 284-5. [61279]

51C4: Frühauf, H., Autohemotherapy with ultraviolet

rays irradiation, MEDIZINISCHE KLINIK 45:46 (17 Nov. 1950), p. 1469-72. [37218]

51C5: Meco, O., "Autoemopiretoterapia associate; rapporto preliminare della casistica e preliminari considerazioni." [Associated autohemo-pyretotherapy - autohemotherapy and fever therapy of psychoses, RIVISTA DI PATOLOGIA NERVOSA E MENTALE, 71:2 (1950) p. 303-13. [17761]

51C6: Meco, O., Effect of autohemopyretherapy (autohemotherapy and fever therapy) on the autonomic nervous system/neurovegetative components of various diseases], RIVISTA DI PATOLOGIA NERVOSA E MENTALE, 71:2 (1950) p. 333-342. [17763]

51C7: Sauer, G.C., and Simm, F., "Evidence of adreno-cortical stimulation by autohemotherapy." JOURNAL OF INVESTIGATIVE DERMATOLOGY, 16:3 (March 1951), p. 177-192. [56822]

51C8: Auto-serotransfusion into the cisterna magna and the spinal canal in viral diseases of the nervous system, POLSKI TYGODNIK LEKARSKI 6:11 (12 March 1951), p. 342-6. [97739]

51C9: Gába, V., Skácel, J., Sabata, J., Treatment of eye diseases with refrigerated autogenous blood. II CESKOSLOVENSKI OFTHALMOLOGIE. PRAHA. 7:4 (1951), p. 271-286. [92799]

51C10: Dvorák, M., Autoserotherapy in supprative skin diseases/furunculosis, LÉKARSKÉ LISTY 5:24 (15 Dec. 1950), p. 735-7. [36474]

51C11: Reddick, R. H., "Autohemotherapy in chronic mental disorders; a preliminary report.", JOURNAL OF THE AMERICAN INSTITUTE OF HOMEOPATHY 43:10 (Dec. 1950), p. 263-9. [34410]

52A1: Ksenofontova, M.A., Intramuscular injection of autohemolyzed blood in therapy of peptic ulcer, Klin. Med. (2) 30:69-70, 52 [R]

52A2: Jucovsky, J., Sulfonated autoserum therapy of leprosy, Rev. Brasil. Leprol. 19:166-192, Sept. 1951 [P]

52B1: Bondurant, C.P., Use of attenuated or inactivated blood serum in management of pemphigus vulgaris; case, A.M.A. Arch. Dermat. & Syph. 66:394-6, Sept. 1952

52C1: Flandin, C., "L'auto-serotherapie desensibilisatrice." [Desensitizing autoserotherapy], VIE MEDICALE. (Paris) 32:8 (August 1951) p. 53-4. [7170]

52C2: Haferkamp, H., Non-specific alternative therapy with special reference to autohemotherapy; homeopathy, HIPPOKRATES (Stuttgart) 23:2 (31 Jan. 1952) p. 29-33. [37513]

52C3: Novotny, J., Kubelka, V.,

Local autoserotherapy with antibiotics in operative dentistry, CESKOSLOVENSKA STOMATOLOGIE (Praha) 51:10 (Oct. 1951), p. 395-401. [36070]

52C4: Jucovsky, J., Sulfone autoserotherapy in leprosy, REVISTA BRASILEIRA DE LEPROLOGIA (Sao Paulo) 19:3 (Sept. 1951) p. 166-192. [22702]

53A1: Przemeck, H., Ultraviolet irradiation of circulating blood and results of its intravenous or intramuscular reinjection, Strahlentherapie 88:522-526, 1952 [G]

53B1: Strakisch, W., Autogenous blood in therapy of ovarian migraine; preliminary report, Zentralbl. Gynäk. 75:961-063, 1953 [G]

53B2: Chamorro, J., Autohemotherapy of malaria, Rev. Clín. Españ. 49:121-123, April 30, 1953 [S]

53B3: Gualdi, G., Autoplasm in corneal wounds; experimental study, Rass. Ital. Ottal. 22:393-400, July-Aug. 1953 [I]

53B4: Gualdi, G., Autoplasm in therapy of conjunctival wounds; experimental study, Rass. Ital. Ottal. 22:176-183, March-April 1953 [I]

53B5: Friederich, H.C., G. Riedel & H. Ruther, Clinical use of corpuscular blood constituents in local therapy of crural ulcers, Medizinische, pp. 776-778, June 6, 1953 [G]

53B6: Sperling, E., Intrafrontal injection of patient's own blood as variant of leukotomy; results of after-examination, Arch. Psychiat. 190:377-388, 1953 [G]

53B7: Heimark, J.J. & R.L. Parsons, Spinal injection of blood to lower blood pressure in essential hypertensive patients; 2 cases, Minnesota Med. 36:738-739, July 1953

53C1: Mercier, R., Autohemotherapy and antibiotic therapy (especially in tuberculosis), CONCOURS MEDICAL. (Paris) 74:35 (30 August 1952), p. 2867-70. [12886]

53C2: Bertazzi, C.G., The results of treatment with triphenyl, sulfoidol and autohemotherapy in two cases of a chronic fever of unknown nature, ACTA MEDICA ITALICA DI MALATTIE INFETTIVE E PARASSITARIE. (Napoli), 7:9 (Sept. 1952), p. 225-8. [41071]

53C3: Peters, H., Therapeutic venous and muscular stimulation as supportive treatment in carcinosis; pyrogenated serotherapy and autohemotherapy, PRAKTISCHE ARZT (Wien) 6:63 (15 August 1952), p. 447-8. [51647]

53D1: Komorowska, A., Autochemotherapy in allergic diseases of the skin, PRZEGLAD DERMATOLOGII I WENEROLOGII (Warszawa) 2:4 (Oct.-Dec. 1952), p. 607-616. [17846]

53D2: Chamorro, J., Treatment

of malaria by autohemotherapy, REVISTA CLINICA ESPAÑOLA (Madrid) 49:2 (30 April 1953) p. 121-3. [45591]

53D3: Strakosch, W., Migraine treatment with own blood, HIPPOKRATES (Stuttgart) 24:9 (15 May 1953), p. 277-9. [39585]

53D4: Heimark, J.J., and R.L. Parsons, "Spinal injection of blood to lower blood pressure in essential hypertensive patients; report of two cases.", MINNESOTA MEDICINE (St. Paul) 36:7 (July 1953), p. 738-9. [42860]

54A1: Binda, B., Infiltrations of novocain (procaine hydrochloride) in anal pruritus; surgical therapy of essential anal pruritus, Minerva Anestesiol. 20:104-106, March 1954 [I]

54B1: Mease, J.A.Jr., Blood extract therapy in intractable arthritic, Med. Times 82:750-752, Oct. 1954.

54C1: Horanyi, J., Ganglion of hand, therapy with prothrombin and autohemother., ORVOSI HETILAP (Budapest) 94::32 (9 Aug. 1953), p. 887-8. [8872]

54C2: Geller, F.C., The treatment of initial puerperal mastitis and general pyogenic/micrococcal infections, THERAPIE DER GEGENWART (Berlin), 92:11 (Nov. 1953), p. 412-4. [56328]

54C3: Strakosch, W., Autohemotherapy of ovarian

migraine; preliminary report, ZENTRALBLATT FÜR GYNÄKOLOGIE (Leipzig) 75:25 (1953), p. 961-3. [24784]

54C4: Filichev, T.E., Treatment of pyoderma with staphylococcal antiphagin mixed with patient's blood, VESTNIK VENEROLOGII I DERMATOLOGII (Moskva) 3 (May-June 1953), p. 13-14. [11356]

54C5: Lages, W., Treatment of whooping cough by associated microautohemotherapy, JORNAL DE PEDIATRIA (Rio de Janeiro) 18:8 (August 1953), p. 343-54. [29573]

54D1: Jochmus, H., Treatment of arterial hypertension by the reinjection of hemolysed blood, HIPPOKRATES (Stuttgart) 25:7 (15 April 1954), p. 215-8. [37020]

54D2: Marshall, K.G., "Sanguinary sketches." - hemotherapy history, McGILL MEDICAL JOURNAL (Montreal) 23:2 (April 1954), p. 59-72. [15889]

54D3: Felder, H., Autohemotherapy with sodium citrate injections in therapy of hay fever; preliminary report, MEDIZINISCHE KLINIK (Berlin) 49:18 (30 April 1954), p. 748-9. [27644]

54D4: Zábelková, Z., Role of autohemotherapy in effectiveness of penicillin in pyoderma, BRATISLAVSKÉ LEKARSKE LISTY 33:9 (1953), p. 809-811. [3235]

54D5: Kubelka, V., Perner, K.,

Local autoserotherapy with antibiotics in dermatology, BRATISLAVSK; LEKHRSKE LISTY 33:9 (1953), p. 807-8. [3234]

55A1:  Reddick, R.H., Autohemotherapy in psychiatry, Maryland M. J. 4:22-31, Jan. 1955

55A2:  Frandsen, V.A. & T. Samsoe-Jensen, Effect of Autohemotherapy, Acta Allergol. 8:26-30, 1955

55B1:  Cantoni, L., E. Cassi & G. Suppa, Autohemoantibodies; formation by autohemosensitization experimentally by means of autohemotherapy, Boll. Ist. Sieroterap. Milanese 34:273-283, May-June 1955 [I]

55C1:  Prusak, L., Treatment of diseases of the nervous system with patients hemolyzed blood with special reference to multiple sclerosis; preliminary communication, POLSKI TYGODNIK LEKARSKI (Warszawa) 9:46 (15 Nov. 1954), p. 1471-5. [48905]

55C2:  Reddick, R.H., "Autohemotherapy in psychiatry.", MARYLAND STATE MEDICAL JOURNAL (Baltimore), p. 22-31. [47013]

55C3:  Schwendy, J., Intracutaneous autohemotherapy of bronchial asthma, DEUTSCHE GESUNDHEITWESEN (Berlin) 9:18 (6 May 1954), p. 562-5. [2650]

55D1:  Herberger, W., The treatment of annoying axillary sweat (hyperhidrosis) with autohemotherapy in local injections, HIPPOKRATES (Stuttgart) 26:11 (15 June 1955), p. 341-3. [53650]

55D2:  Enkelmann, A., Clinical studies on autohemotherapy with irradiation, intravenous administration; comparison with other methods of fever therapy. HIPPOKRATES (Stuttgart) 26:9 (15 May 1955), p. 280-5. [53633]

55D3:  Ozegowski, P., Therapy of bronchial asthma with hemolyzed blood of the patient, POLSKI TYGOD LEK 10:17 (25 April 1955), p. 555-6. [46104]

56B1:  Lipton, R.A., Paradoxic reaction following administration of laked, incubated autogenous blood, Ann. Allergy 14:370-373, Sept.-Oct. 1956

56C1:  Cantoni, L., Cassi, E., and Suppa, G., Research on auto-antibodies.  II. Formation of auto-antibodies by experimentally induced auto-sensitization by autohemotherapy, BOLLETTINO DELL'ISTITUTO SIEROTERAPICO MILANESE 34:5-6 (May-June, 1955), p. 273-83. [1869]

56C2:  Shaposhnikov, M.S., Treatment of stenocardia/angina pectoris, intracutaneous autohemotherapy in head zone. SOVETSKAIA MEDITSINA (Moskva) 19:11 (Nov. 1955), p. 72-3. [43293]

56D1:  Gruger, A., Therapeutic use of patient's hemolysed

blood, in aqueous solution. HIPPOKRATES (Stuttgart) 27:10 (31 May 1956), p. 316-22. [39875]

56D2:  Orlov, T.K., Shevchuk, K.S., and Sen'ko, V.M.  Use of penicillin with autohemotherapy, in abscess. AKUSHERSTVO I GINEKOLOGIIA (Moskva) 32:1 (Jan.-Feb. 1956), p. 69-70. [21689]

56D3:  Otto, E., Treatment of spontaneous pneumothorax with autohemotherapy, intrapleural administration.  HIPPOKRATES (Stuttgart) 27:7 (15 April 1956), p. 215-8.  [39849]

56D4:  Porras, T., and Porras, J., New contributions in autohemotherapy locus dolenti in septic processes/furunculosis, SEMANA MEDICA (Buenos Aires) 108:6 (9 Feb. 1956), p. 200-3. [6937]

56D5:  Prusak, L.,m Laskowska, D., Charal, N., Wierzbicka, I., Radomska, M., and Zimny, S., Further observations on application of hemolyzed autogenous blood in certain diseases of the nervous system, POLSKI TYGODNIK LEKARSKI (Warszawa) 11:9 (27 Feb. 1956), p. 395-8. [58232]

57C1:  Heller, S., Therapy of allergic states, MEDICINA INTERNA (Bucuresti), 7:4 (Oct.-Dec., 1955), p. 151-2. [46236]

57C2:  Strakosch, W., Autohemotherapy in gynecology, indications and technic, ZENTRALBLATT FÜR CHIRURGIE (Leipzig) 78:45 (10 Nov. 1956), p. 1783-6. [48809]

57C3:  Ansfield, F.J., and J. L. Rens, "Autohemotherapy; an effective treatment for herpes zoster." WISCONSIN MEDICAL JOURNAL (Madison) 55:12 (Dec. 1956), p. 1319-1320. [27579]

57C4:  Riskin, M., Venous allergy; recurrent phlebitis and desensitization, ANGÉIOLOGIE ET ANNALES DE LA SOCIÉTÉ FRANCAISE D'ANGÉIOLOGIE ET E'HISTOPATHOLOGIE (Paris) 8:3 (May-June 1956), p. 1-4. [1046]

57D1:  Ghins, J., Interpretation of relative adrenal insufficiency in asthma; variations of eosinophilia in asthma caused by certain disorders; autohemotherapy, SCALPEL (Bruxelles) 110:9 (2 March 1957, p. 195-206. [30824]

57D2:  Otto, E., Treatment of traumatic and spontaneous pneumothorax, MÜNCHENER MEDIZINISCHE WOCHENSCHRIFT 99:13 (29 March, 1967), p. 436-7. [28867]

57D3:  Theurer, K., Immunotherapy of chronic rheumatism; counter-sensitization by activated autoserum, ÄRXTLICHE FORSCHUNG (MÜnchen) 11:5 (10 May 1957), p. I/259-263. [33313]

58C1:  Válová, M., Rejchrt, B., Treatment of caustic injuries of the eye with subconjunctival injections of patient's own blood with penicillin, CESKOSLOVENSKI OFTHALMOLOGIE (Praha) 13:5 (Sept. 1957), p. 383-7.   [32845]

58C2:   Sereni, F., and M. Nonato, The efficacy of autovaccinotherapy in asthmatic syndromes in children, CLINICA PEDIATRICA (Bologna) 39:8 (August 1957), p. 624-634. [22919]

58D1:   Prusak, L., Treatment of multiple sclerosis using hemolyzed blood of the patient, NEUROLOGIA, NEUROCHIRURGIA I PSYCHIATRIA POLSKA (Warszawa) 8:2 (March-April 1958), p. 173-6.   [59138]

59D1:   Polonskii, K.V., Treatment of bronchial asthma with hemolyzed autoblood, subcutaneous admin., SOVETSKAIA MEDITSINA (Moskva) 23:1 (Jan. 1959), p. 124-5.   [20863]

59D2:   Sviridov, N.A., Autohemopenicillinotherapy in purulent inflammation of the skin and subcutaneous tissue/furuncles and carbuncles, KHIRURGIIA (Moskva) 35:4 (April 1959), p. 103-4.   [29415]

60F1:   Bolzani, L., & M. Isotti, Delirium tremens and autohemo-therapy.  Riv. Sper. Freniat. 13:1372-82, 31 Dec. 1959  (It)

60H1:   Schiff, Bencel L., "Autohemotherapy in the treatment of post-herpetic pain", Rhode Island Med.J. 43 (Feb. 1960), 104.

61F1:   Bikfalvia, A., & Ecke, H., Treatment of chronic osteomyelitis with autogenous blood-antibiotic plombage. Bruns. Beitr. Klin. Chir. 201:190-207, 1960 (Ger)

61F2:   Oettingen, E.N. von, Treatment of inhalation allergies by the local administration of the patient's dried serum.  Med. Klin. 55:1649-50, 9 Sept., 1960 (Ger)

62F1:   Monti, P.C., Lysozome therapy and autohemotherapy in oto-rhinolaryngology. Sem. Med. (B. Air.) 119:1038-42, 25 Sept. 1961 (Hun)

63F1:   Bacskulin, J., Subconjunctival auto-blood injections in fresh and old burns. Klin. Mbl. Augenheilk. 142:728-33, 1963 (Ger)

63F2:   Calcagnino Ricceri, J., Original treatment of eczema. Intradermal autohemotherapeutic procedure. Outline of its technic: method and clinical criterion regulating its use. Results. Conclusions. Sem. Med. (B. Air.) 121:330-4, 26 July 1962 (Sp)

64F1:   Bikfalvi, A., etal., Autogenous blood-antibiotic plombage therapy of chronic osteomyelitis. Results of a 4-year treatment series. Mschr. Unfallheilk. 66:257-61, July 1963 (Ger)

64F2:   Bauer, E., On micromed-autohemotherapeutic injections and their significance in the treatment of degenerative rheumatic states. z. rheumaforsch 22:398-401, Oct. 1963 (Ger)

65F1:  Bacskulin J, & Bacskulin E, Further experiences with subconjunctival autohemotherapy in fresh and old corrosions. Amer. J. Ophthal. 59:674-80, Apr. 1965

65F2:  Bacskulin, J., Further experiences with subconjunctival autogenous blood injections in burns. Ber. Deutsch. Ophth. Ges. 65:528-31, 1964 (Ger)

65F3:  Bacskulin, J., Treatment of eye injuries with the subconjunctival injection of the patients' own blood and with microwaves. Rehabilitation (Bonn) 17:88-9, Dec. 1964 (Ger)

65F4:  Litricin, O., etal., Use of subconjunctival autohemotherapy in chemical eye diseases, Srpski. Arh. Celok. Lek., 92:173-9, Feb. 1964 (Ser)

66F1:  Gassler, H., Treatment of chemical eye burns with Passow's operation and Tolazoline, with reference to subconjunctival auto-blood injection. Klin. Mbl. Augenheilk. 147:79-86, Sept. 65 (Ger)

66F2:  Barin, V.A., Combined treatment of eye burns using autoserum-penicillin-novocaine. Oftal. Zh. 20:172-4, 1965 (Rus)

66F3:  Alezzandrini, A.A., etal., Autohemotherapy in the treatment of ocular burns caused by alkalies. Arch. Oftal. B.

Air. 40:397-400, Dec. 1965 (Sp)

66P1:  Findings on therapy )autovaccine therapy and antibiotic therapy in rheumatic fever of tonsillar, post-tonsillectomy origin.  Di Lauro E.  Bol Mal Orecch 84:1-9, Jan-Feb 66  (It)

66P2:  Autovaccines for the treatment of cancer.  Snegotska O.  Folia Clin Int (Barc) 15:303-8, Jun 65 (Sp)

68F1:  Baumann, E., On the practice-related modification of the filling of the bone defects using the patient's own blood with Gelastypt and on the problem of its tolerance. DDZ 22:313-5, 22 June 1968 (Ger)

68F2:  Sallai, S., etal., Experience with autologous blood therapy in burns. Klin. Mbl. Augenheilk 150:879-86, 1967 (Ger)

68F3:  Sóvágó, J., etal., Experiences with simultaneous administration of tetanus serum and autogenous blood. z. Aerztl. Fortbild. (Jena) 61:588-90, 1 June 1967 (Ger)

69F1:  Colucci, G., Local autohemotherapy in idiopathic vulvar irritation. Friuli Med. 22:571-80, May-June 1067 (Ita)

70F1:  Colucci, G., etal., Therapy of essential pruritus valvae and kraurosis vulvae with local autohemotherapy. Ann. Ostet. Ginec. 91:601-13, Sept. 1969 (Ita)

70F2: Bacanu, C.G., etal., Results of administration of a total cellular-microbial disintegrated autovaccine in a case of chronic marginal parodontopathy. Stomatologia (Bucar) 16:469-70, Sept.Oct. 1969 (Rum)

71F1: Amoile, S.P., etal., Cryotherapy and autogenous serum therapy. Arch. Ophthamol. 86:113-4, July 1971

72F1: DiGiovanni, A.J., Epidural injection of autologous blood for postlumbar-puncture headache. II. Additional clinical experiences and laboratory investigation. Anesth. Analg. (Cleve) 51:226-32, Mar.-Apr. 1972

72F2: Marcove, R.C., etal., A clinical trial of autogenous vaccine in osteogenic sarcoma in patients under the age of twenty-five. Surg. Forum 22:434-5, 1971

72F3: Schwarz, P., Modification of Theurer's autohemotherapy. Treatment with antibody fragments (immunologic enhancement). z. Allgemeinmed. 47:1576-9, 31 October 1971 (Ger)

73F1: Dolezalová, V., etal., Subconjunctival injection of autogenous blood in the eye after thermical and chemical burns. Cesk. Oftalmol. 29:207-12, May 1973 (Eng. Abstr.) (Cze.)

74F1: Reuter, S.R., etal., Control of abdominal bleeding with autogenous embolized material. Radiologe 14:86-91, Feb. 1974

75F1: Artamonov, V.P., Case report of successful treatment of an acute keratoconus by introduction of autologous blood into the anterior chamber. Vesta Oftalmol. 5:76-7, Sept.-Oct. 1974 (Rus)

80F1: Shapiro, V.I., Experience in treating acne vulgaris and conglobata with penicillin in autologous blood in combination with staphylococcal antiphagin. Vesta Dermatol. Venerol. 7:52-4, July 1979 (Engl. Abstr.) (Rus)

81F1: Orculas, E., Use of a collyrium with autoserum in trophic corneal diseases. Rev. Chir. [Oftalmol.] 24(4):289-91, Oct.-Dec. 1980 (Eng. Abstr.) (Rus)

81F2: Xue, Q.C., Autohemotherapy in the treatment of chemical and thermal burns of the eye (author's transl.). Chung Hua Yen Ko Tsa Chih 15(3):195-7, 1979 (Chi)

83F - - ["SEROTHERAPY see IMMUNIZATION, PASSIVE (300+ articles)]

88H1: Shakman, S.H., "Cuyugan's Malaria Treatment; Aid vs AIDS?", AAAS Pacific Division Proceedings Vol. 7:42 (1988)

ABSTRACT OF PRESENTATION (6-20-88): Cuyugan's Malaria Treatment - Aid vs. AIDS?
[Shakman SH, Proc.Pac.Div. AAAS

7, 1988, 42]

In 1941 Filipino Dr. Eutiquiano Cuyugan treated approx. 40 malaria patients as follows: Blood (10 cc) was drawn from the arm, put in a culture dish for 2-3 mins. (swirled a bit to keep coagulation even), & injected into the same patient's buttock muscle. After 8-10 hours the site of injection became red. After 1 day chills would cease but fever remained. Over 2-3 days, fever would diminish and then disappear. By the 4th day patients could generally resume normal activity. A dose of about 3cc was not effective for a 10-year-old but a subsequent dose of about 5cc was. Cuyugan's son Roberto performed the procedure on others and self and believes it safe, suggesting possible use against AIDS.* Cuyugan's (anti-protozoa) method may be viewed as a synthesis of Sir Almroth Wright's studies**: (a) "auto-inoculation"{350-1} of blood undergoing (b) coagulation [as may be related to blood's "antibacterial power"{301}] into (c) the tissues where "bacteriotropic substances are manufactured"{353} [incl. (d) "opsonins"{83}]; comprising (e) "vaccine-therapy" with preferred "vaccines prepared from the original patient"{375}. Antibody known to opsonize bacteria (e.g. IgG & IgM)*** may also relate to viruses: IgG may neutralize (polio) virus in bloodstream***; and a deficient IgM response is associated with AIDS ****.

*Interviews with R. Cuyugan, San Francisco, USA, Jan.,1988.
**WRIGHT, A.E., Studies on Immunization (1909). ***CLARK, W.R., Experimental Foundations of Modern Immuniz. (1986), 416.
****FAUCI, A.S., Science 239 (5 Feb. 1988), 620.

APPENDIX D:   AUTO-VACCINE BIBLIOGRAPHY

Key: All listings indicate year, source, and sequential item (e.g., 10N2 is from 1910, source "N", second article.)

Autovaccinotherapy:

J,K = QUARTERLY CUM. INDEX MED. Vaccinetherapy 1916-1956

L,M = CURRENT LIST "Vaccinotherapy"  1941-1959

N = INDEX MEDICUS "Vaccinotherapy", 1903-1927

P = CUMULATED INDEX MEDICUS "Vaccine Therapy", 1960-1982

03N1:  Wright, A.E., On therapeutic inoculations of bacterial vaccines; and their practical exploitation in the treatment of disease.  BRIT. M. J., LONDON, 1903, 1069-1074.

07N1:  Ohlmacher, A.P., A series of medical and surgical affections treated by artificial autoinoculation, according to Wright's theory of opsonins.  J. AM. M. ASS., Chicago, 1907, xlviii, 571-577. [Discussion], 639-641.

07N2:  Ohlmacher, A.P., A series of medical and surgical affections treated by artificial autoinoculation, according to Wright's theory of opsonins. ILLINOIS MED. J., Springfield, 1907, xi, 343-350.

07N3:  Wright, Sir A.E., The opsonic theory. PEDIATRICS, N.Y., 1907, xix, 6-21.

09N1:  Berghausen, O., Some experiences with autogenous bacterial vaccines.  LANCET-CLINIC, Cincin. 1909, ci, 55-61.

10N1:  Wolfer, L., Vaccine auto inoculation.  ARCH. F. KINDERH., Stuttg., 1909, liii, 122-133.

10N2:  Dodds, W.T.S., Technic of making concomitant autogenous vaccines from sputum. INDIANAPOLIS M. J., 1910, xiii, 3-5.

10N3:  Forrester, C.R.G., Auto-vaccine in traumatic infections.  ILLINOIS M. J., Springfield, 1910, xvii, 733-735.

11N1:  Wood, F.M., Autogenous vaccines; a new method for their preparation and use by the surgeon (a resume of four years' experience with vaccine therapy).  RAILWAY SURG. J., Chicago, 1910-11, xvii, 148-153.

11N2:  Callison, J.G., Streptococcus mucosus septicemia clinically resembling typhoid; blood culture; treated with an autogenous vaccine.  POST-GRADUATE, N.Y., 1911, xxvi, 553.

11N3:  Herschman, F., Practical value of autogenous vaccines in modern medicine; description of method; illustrative cases. INDIANAPOLIS M.J., 1911, xiv, 413-416.

11N4: Craig, H.A., The principles and application of autogenous bacterial vaccines in the treatment of diseases. MED. REC., N.Y., 1911, lxxx, 1015-1021.

12N1: Sellwood, J.J., Autogenous vaccines. MED. SENTINEL, Portland, Oreg., 1912, xx, 135-139.

12N2: Scott, T.B. and Scott, G.B. A record of the treatment of bacterial infections by autogenous vaccines. LANCET , LOND. 1912, ii, 879.

12N3: Craig, H.A., Observations on 395 cases treated with autogenous bacterial vaccines. J. VACCINE THERAPY, Lond., 1912, i, 318-327.

13N1: Vrijburg, A. Opsonogeen (vaccine) en auto-therapie. TIJDSCHR. V. VEEARTSENIJK., Utrecht, 1913, xl, 137-147.

13N2: Mazzitelli, P. La thérapeutique par les autovaccins (méthode de Wright). RÉPERT DE MÉD. INTERTNAT., Par., 1913, iii, fasc. 27, 16-18.

14N1: Hanson, H. Observations on preparation and administration of autogenous vaccines. SOUTH. M. J., Nashville, 1914, vii, 154-159.

14N2: Gould, C.W. Autogenous versus stock vaccines. J. MED. ASS. GEORGIA, Augusta, 1913-14, iii, 364-366.

14N3: Stone, W.B. Autogenous vaccines in colon bacillus infections. ALBANY M. ANN., 1914, xxxv, 135-140.

15N1: Allen, J.D. The preparation and use of autogenous vaccine. KENTUCKY M.J., Bowling Green, 1915, xiii, 27-32.

15N2: Tutt, J.F.D., Three cases treated by autogenous vaccines. VET. M., LONDON, 1915, lxxi, 224.

15N3: Pierce, C.H., The practical value of autogenous vaccine therapy, with cases. JOURNAL-LANCET, Minneap., 1915, n.s., xxxv, 414-419.

16J1: Wohl, autosensitized vaccines in, MED. REC. 89: 770, April 29, '16

16J2: Wohl, autoserobacterins in, AM. J. M. SC. 152: 262, Aug. '16

16N1: Hekman, J., Over de behandeling van verschillende ziekten met autovaccins. NEDERL. TIJDSCHR. V. GENEESK., Amst., 1916, i, 2161-2171.

17J1: Bunce, A. H., Autogenous vaccine, summary of views and experiences of some of foremost physicians in United States on use of, J. M. A. GEORGIA 6: 241, April '17.

17N1:  Bunce, A.H., Observations on the use of autogenous vaccine; a summary of the views and experiences of some of the foremost physicians in the United States. J. MED. ASS. GEORGIA, Augusta, 1916-7, vi, 241-246.

17N2:  Meader, Isabel M., Autogenous vaccines. WOMAN'S M.J., 1917, xxvii, 131-134.

18J1:  Womer, W.A., Autogenous vaccine, 100 cases treated with, PENN. M. J. 22, 137, Dec. '18.

18J2:  Bazy, L. and L. Cuvillier, Sensitized autovaccine, PRESSE MÉD. 26:219, April 25 '18; ab. JAMA 70: 1898, June 15, '18

18J3:  Cecil, R.L., Sensitized vaccine in prophylaxis and treatment of infections, Am. J. M. Sc. 155: 781, June 1918

18N1:  Valée, A. & Potvin, R., Traitement de la furonculose et de l'acne par les auto-vaccins antistaphylococciques.  BULL. MÉD. DE QUÉBEC, 1917-8, xix, 135-143.

19J1:  Tehon, L.R., Autogenous, formulas for use in standardizing autogenous vaccines, JAMA 73: 1063, Oct. 4, 1919

19N1:  Womer, W.A., One hundred cases treated with autogenous vaccines.  PENN. M. J., Athens, 1918-19, xxii, 137-140.

19N2:  Tehon, L.R., Formulas for use in standardizing autogenous vaccines.  J.AM.M.ASS., Chicago, 1919, lxxiii, 1063.

20N1:  Rizzi, S., Gli autovaccini nelle forme bronco-polmonari.  POLICLIN., ROMA, 1919, sez. prat., xxvi, 1089.

20N2:  Tehon, L.R., Formulas for use in standardizing autogenous vaccines.  AM. J. PHARM., PHILA., 1919, xci, 807.

20N3:  De Blasi, D., Autovaccinazione in malattie da virus filtrabili.  ANN. D'IG., ROMA, 1919, xxix, 717-726.

20N4:  Wright, Almroth E., etal., VACCINETHERAPY: ITS ADMINISTRATION, VALUE, AND LIMITATIONS.  London, 1919, Longmans, Green & Co., 216p.

20N5:  Miller, E.C.L., The theory and practice of autogenous vaccines.  VIRGINIA M. MONTH., Richmond, 1920-21, xivii, 213-215.

21J1:  Jenkins, C.E., Autogenous, a misuse of autogenous vaccines, [C.E. Jenkins] PRACTITIONER 107: 123, Aug. 1921

21J2:  H. K. Mulford Company, report from, Serobacterins (sensitized bacterial vaccines), CHINA M. J. 35: 131, March 1921

21J3: Jaquelin, B. and A., Autovaccine therapy in 2 cases of staphylococcemia, PARIS MÉD 11:169, Aug. 27, 1921; ab. JAMA 77:
1289, Oct. 15, 1921

21N1: Vallet & Villa, "Vaccinothérapie par les auto-vaccins préparés selon une méthode nouvelle." MONTPÉL. MÉD. xliii (1921), 161-163.

21N2: Dore, J., "Contribution a l'étude de l'autovaccinothérapie. Étude expérimentale sur la production des anticorps. TOULOUSE, 1921, C. Dirion, 155p., 8&

21N3: Vallet, G., "Vaccinothérapie par les autovaccins auto-sensibilisés." COMPT. REND. SOC. DE BIOL., Par., lxxxiv (1921), 5-7.

21N4: Vallet, G., "Pyothérapie et ptysmathérapie; méthodes d'autovaccination curative. COMPT. REND. SOC. DE BIOL., Par., lxxxiv (1921), 710.

21N5: Vallet, G. "Vaccinothérapie par les auto-vaccine préparés selon une méthode nouvelle. MONTPÉL MÉD. xliii (1921), 179-184.

22J1: Jaureguil, F., Autovaccines in therapeutics, SEMANA MÉD. 2: 530-531, Oct. 20, 1921; ab. JAMA 78:621, Feb. 25, 1922

22J2: Parisot, J. & P. Simonin, Autovaccines in vaccine therapy, REV. DE MÉD. 39:392-423, July 1922; ab. JAMA 79:1804, Nov. 18, 1922

22N1: Jenkins, C.E., "A misuse of autogenous vaccines." PRACTITIONER, LOND. cvii (1921), 123-125.

22N2: Parisot, J., and P. Simonin, "Réactions locales a l'inoculation d'autovaccins; étude pathogénique. COMPT. REND. SOC. DE BIOL., Par., 1922, lxxxvi, 400-402.

23J1: Pauron, Autogenous, recent literature on autovaccines, ARCH. DE. MÉD. ET PHARM. MIL. 78: 157-174, Feb. 1923

23N1: Parisot, J., and Simonin, P., Étude sur la vaccinothérapie par les auto-vaccins. REV. DE MÉD, PAR., 1922, xvii, 8.

23N2: Pauron, "La vaccinothérapie par les autovaccins". ARCH. DE MÉD. ET PHARM. MIL., PAR., 1923, lxxviii, 157-173.

24J1: Zezschwitz, P.V., Treatment with autovaccine, MUENCHEN MED. WCHNSCHR. 71:237, Feb. 22, 1924

24J2: Buzello, A., Autogenous vaccines in surgery, MED KLINIK 20:1218-1221, Aug. 31, 1924 (chart)

24J3: Tietz, L., Experiences with autogenous vaccines,

DEUTSCHE MED. WCHNSCHR. 50:432, April 4, 1924

24J4:  Clark, J.H., Use of autogenous vaccines in pulmonary diseases with special reference to Cohen-Heist method, J. LAB. & CLIN. MED. 10: 243-248, Dec. 1924

24N1:  Grimberg, A., "Les autovaccins."  J. DE MÉD DE PAR., 1922, xli, 740-742.

24N2:  Maurin, E., "La législation des autovaccins." RÉPERT. DE PHARM., PAR., 1924, 3. s., xxxvi, 65-67.

24N3:  Candido, G., "Le cure auto ed eterovacciniche e la loro efficacia."  RIFORMA MED., NAPOLI, 1924, xl. 293-295.

25J1:  Gaehlinger, H., Autogenous vaccines in treatment of colon bacillus infection of intestines, PARIS MED. 1:428-431, May 9, 1925.

25J2:  autovaccine treatment in cerebrospinal meningitis, [G. Etienne, Francfort and Dombray] Bull. et mém. Soc. méd. d. hop. de Par. 49:316-320, Feb. 27, 1925 (charts); ab. JAMA 84:1306, April 25, 1925

25J3:  Ryti, E. & F. Saltzman, Autovaccine treatment of septicemia, particularly streptococcus septicemia, [E. Ryti & F. Saltzman] FINSKA LÄK.-SÄLLSK. HANDL. 67:303-326, April 1925 (charts); ab. JAMA 85:80, July 4, 1925.

25J4:  Breitkopf, E., Autovaccines in surgery, BEITR. Z. KLIN. CHIR. 134:458-9, 1925

25J5:  Breitkopf, E., Experiences with autogenous vaccines in surgery, BEITR. Z. KLIN. CHIR. 134:145-152,1925

25J6:  Kauntze, W.H., Infection with coliform bacilli as cause of rheumatoid arthritis and chronic rheumatism; its diagnosis and its treatment by autogenous vaccines.  J. HYGIENE 23: 389-420,

April 1925

25J7:  Merle, L., Meningococcus septicemia; partial improvement from serum treatment; recovery from autovaccine, BULL. ET MÉD. D. HOP DE PAR. 49:1004-1005, June 26, 1925.

25J8:  Becker, A., Mixed infection in pulmonary tuberculosis and experiments in treatment with autogenous mixed vaccine, [A. Becker] ZTSCHR. F. TUBERK. 42: 118-136, 1925; ab. JAMA 84: 1791, June 5, 1925.

25J9:  Orsós, E.J., Simple preparation of autovaccines, MUENCHEN MED. WCHNSCHR. 72: 1823-1826, Oct. 23, 1925

25J10:  Went, S., Specific treatment of chronic catarrh of colon. DEUTSCHE MED. WCHNSCHR. 51: 1695-1697, Oct. 9, 1925; ab. JAMA 85: 1679, Nov. 21, 1925

25J11: Borgbjaerg, Vaccine therapy of supprative colitis, UGSK. F. LAEGER 87: 909-912,

Oct. 15, 1925

25J12: Heymann, A., Vaccine treatment of gonorrhea, [A. Heymann] ZTSCHR. F. UROLOG. 19:355-358, 1925

25J13: Dick, J.S., Vaccines in chronic and recurring catarrh of respiratory tract, PRACTITIONER 115:416-419, Dec. 1925

25J14: Monziols, R., Weinberg's tilotherapy in chronic enteritis, COMPT. REND. SOC. DE BIOL. 93:521-523, July 24, 1925; ab. JAMA 85:1337, Oct. 24, 1925

25J15: Fuss, E.M., Action of autogenous vaccines on blood picture, ZTSCHR. F. KLIN. MED. 101:467-472, 1925

25J16: V. René, Hexamethylenamin in preparation of vaccines, CAS. LEK. CESK. 64:755-756, May 9, 1925; ab. JAMA 85:236, July 18, 1925

25N1: Bessemans, A., "La pratique de l'autovaccinothérapie." ANN. DE L'INST. CHIR. DE BRUX., 1924, xxv, 121-131.

26J1: Stahl, R. & H. Nagell, Autogenous, treatment of septic conditions, especially endocarditis lenta, with vaccinated human serum and autovaccine, KLIN. WCHNSCHR. 4, 2392-2395, Dec. 10, 1925 (chart); ab. JAMA 86:384, Jan. 30, 1926

26J2: Hagens, G., Case of chronic bronchitis with asthmatic attacks treated with autogenous mixed vaccine, UGESK. F. LAEGER 87:1195-1196, Dec. 31, 1925; ab. JAMA 86:992, March 27, 1926

26J3: Ciesaynski, K., Case of paranephritis in infant, aged 16 months, cured by autovaccine, ARCH. DE MÉD. D. ENF. 28:762-767, Dec. 1925; ab. JAMA 86:912, March 20, 1926

26J4: Joronha, A.J., Preliminary note on 2 cases of asthma treated with an autogenous vaccine prepared from a gram-negative bacillus isolated from sputum during attack, INDIAN M. GAZ. 411:75, Feb. 1926

26K1: v. Adler-Racz, Autogenous, autovaccine therapy in urology, ZTSCHR. F. UROL. 20: 336-346, 1926; ab. JAMA 87:375, July 31, 1926

26K2: Went, S., Bacteriology and specific treatment of infections of urinary passages, ZTSCHR. F. UROL. 20:4010-415, 1926

26K3: Schil, L., Chronic metritis caused by intestinal bacteria, PARIS MÉD. 2:85-87, July 24, 1926; ab. JAMA 87:1074, Sept. 25, 1926

26K4: Halbe, A., Effect of injections of autovaccines on

leukocyte number and on leukocyte picture in bronchial asthma. COMPT. REND. SOC. DE BIOL. 94:1045-1046, April 23, 1926

26K5: Halbe, A., Local immunity, COMPT. REND. SOC. DE BIOL. 94:1043-1044, April 23, 1926

26K6: v. Berde, K., Orsós' autovaccine, MUENCHEN MED. WCHNSCHR. 73: 1031-1032, June 18, 1926

26K7: Barfurth, W., Treatment of inflammatory processes and infections by products of inflammation. DEUTSCHE MED. WCHNSCHR. 52:996-997, June 11, 1926; ab. JAMA 87:452, Aug. 7, 1926

26K8: Courtois-Suffit & G. Garnier, Two cases of cerebrospinal meningitis treated by autovaccine after failure of serotherapy, BULL. ET MÉM SOC. MÉD. D. HOP. DE PARIS 60:1185-1193,

July 2, 1926 (charts)

26K9: Velasco Blanco, L., Use of autogenous vaccine in treatment of infections of childhood, ARCH. PEDIAT. 43:697-706, Nov.

1926

26K10: Hemeleers, Vaccine therapy applied in affections of ear, ARCH. MÉD. BELGES 79:241-245, June 1926; ab. JAMA 87:708, Aug.

8, 1926

26K11: Hilgermann, Valuation of specific vaccine treatment in infectious diseases, MUENCHEN MED. WCHNSCHR. 73:898-902, May 28, 1926

26K12: Bakscht, G., Autohemotherapy in hemorrhagic metropathies, uterus, ZENTRALBLK. F. GYNAEK. 50: 1390-1393, May 22, 1926; ab. JAMA 87: 211, July 17, 1926

26N1: Breitkof, E., "Erfahrungen mit der Autovakzinetherapie in der Chirurgie." BEITR. Z. KLIN. CHIR., BERL. U. WIEN. 1925, cxxxiv, 145-152.

26N2: Orsós, E.J., Ueber eine neur, einfache Herstellungsmethode von Autovakzinen. MÜNCHEN MED. WCHNSCHR., 1925, lxxii, 1823-1826.

26N3: von Berde, K., "Meine Erfahrungen ueber die Autovakzine von Orsós. MÜNCHEN MED. WCHNSCHR., 1926, lxciii, 1031.

26N4: Blanco, L.V., "The use of autogenous vaccine in the treatment of some infections of childhood." ARCH. PEDIAT., N.Y., 1926, xliii, 697-706.

27J1: autogenous vaccines in infections of respiratory tract, [L. Utz and A.M. Fitzgerald] M.M. Australia 1:15-20, Jan. 1, '27; also Eye, Ear, Nose and Throat Monthly 6:24-27, Feb. '27

27J2: autogenous vaccines in

treatment of chronic nasal catarrh in horses, ]C. Davenport]   Vet.J. 83:78-83, Feb. '27

27J3: chronic case treated with autovaccines of Bacillus coli; permanent recovery,[J.Rubinstein] Arch.f.Verdauungskr. 39:117-123, Oct. '26

27J4: good results in gonorrhea, [R. Darget and A. Boileau] Bull.Soc.Franç.d'urol. 6:33-46, Jan. 17, '27

27J5: in asthma, [Haibe] J.de med de Paris 45:1075-1080, Dec. 27, '26

27J6: in furunculosis; cure of 5 cases, [G. Lodato] Arch. Ital.di.sc.med.colon. 8:35-37, Jan. '27

27J7: in gonorrhea, [P.G. Castellino] Gior.ital.di dermat.e sifil. 67:1606-1617, Dec. '26

27J8: in leprosy, 'G.Lanteri] Gior. ital.di dermat.e.sifil. 67:1573-1576, Dec. '26

27J9: injection of patient's own pus, [K. Lutz] Deutsche med. Wchnschr. 52:1818-1819, Oct. 22, '26

27J10: septicemia cured by autovaccine; case [B.Botta] Gior. di batteriol.e immunol. 1:412-421, Aug. '26

27J11: treatment of

inflammations with pus of patient, [A. Levinson] München med. Wchnschr. 74:241, Feb. 11, '27

27K1: autogenous, acrodermatitis cured by auto-vaccination; case [H.Oltramare, J.Golay and A. Staropinsky] Ann. de dermat. et syph. 8:193-200, April '27

27K2: arthritis and chronic urethritis cured by use of gonorrheal pus, [G. Lodato] Arch. ital.di sc. med. colon. 8:77-80, Feb. '27

27K3: autopyotherapy in cold abscesses [E.Makai] Zentralbl. f. Chir. 54:2452-2455, Sept. 24,'27

27K4: autopyotherapy; remarks on Makai's article, [M.Havranek] Zentralbl.f.Chir. 54:1683-1685, July 2, '27

27K5: by mouth in treatment of typhlocolitis, [Gaehlinger] Paris med. 2:37-41, July 9, '27

27K6: colon bacillus autovaccines in cystopyelitis of pregnancy, [G.Ajello Rabboni] Terapia 17:269-271, Aug. '27

27K7: dosage, [G.Petragnani] Policlinico (sez.prat.) 34:1279-1281, Sept. 5, '27

27K8: effect of polyvalent atypical coli autovaccine on peripheral blood picture and on place of injection, [K.von Knorr and L. Nemeth] Wien.klin.Wchnschr. 40:554,

April 28, '27

27K9: experiments with autovaccines in treatment of leprosy, [G. Lanteri] Boll.Soc.ital.di biol.sper. 2:162, Feb. '27

27K10: Friedlander bacillus as causative agent of tonsillar abscess, and preparation of autovaccines from capsular bacteria, [B. Busson] Monatschr.f.Ohrenh. 61:325-328, April '27

27K11: in acne keratosa, [G.Lanteri] Arch.ital.di dermat.,sif. 2:274-280, Feb. '27

27K12: in chronic colitis and eterocolitis, [J. Leontieff] Vrach.Gaz. 32:829-833, June 30, '27

27K13: in colitis, [K. von Knorr] Wien.klin.Wchnschr. 40:935-937, July 21, '27

27K14: in cutaneous spirotrichosis; mode of action of vaccine, [A. Sezary, E. Combe and F. Benoist] Bull.et mem.Soc.med.d.hop.de Paris 51:619-622, May 19, '27

27K15: in infections of urinary passages, [A.V. Adler-Racz] Urol. and Cutan.Rev. 31:489-494, Aug.'27

27K16: in influenzal pneumonia, [V.D. Vischegorodtzeva] Varch.dielo 10:329-334, March 15, '27

27K17: in various infections, [M.Friesleben] Med.Klin.23:1257-1258, Aug. 19,'27

27K18: nasal infection in children; analysis of 85 cases treated by autogenous vaccine, [L. Mackey] Brit.M.J. 1:1004, June 4, '27

27K19: principles of treatment with inflammatory products (autopyotherapy), [E.Makai] Deutsche med. Wchnschr. 53:570-572, April 1, '27

27K20: pyo-and autopyo-vaccination in pyogenic infections of animals, [E.Bemelmans] Tijdschr.v.diergeneesk. 54:610, July 1, '27

27K21: quick process of preparing yatren autovaccines at patient's bedside; 10 cases, [E.Negru and S. Staniloiu] Cluj.med. 8:324-328, Aug. '27

27K22: streptococcic septicemia cured by auto-vaccine; case, [G. Etienne and M. Verain] Rev.med.de l'est. 55:301-306, June '27

27K23: theoretical bases and fields of application, [O.Kirchner] Ztschr.f.arztl.Fortbild. 24:489-494, Aug. 1, '27

27K24: treatment of skin diseases with auto-enterovaccines, [P.G.Castellino] Riforma med. 43:300-302, March 28, '27

28J1: aseptic pyotherapy in treatment of wounds, [M.Belin] comp.rend.Soc.de biol. 97:1581-1582, Dec. 16'27

28J2: autopyotherapy of empyema of infants, [H.Flesch] Monatschr.f.Kinderh. 37:149-152, '27

28J3: autoserum treatment of furunculosis and certain other purulent infections of skin, [A.Zenin] Klin.Med. 5:892-895, Sept. '27

28J4: autovaccinotherapy and sympathectomy ion suppurated unhealerminated successfully; treatment with autogenous vaccine, [C.H.McIlraith, W. Turner & J.A. B. Hicks] Lancet 2:68-60, July 14, '28

28K2: favorable results of cutaneous autovaccines (Ponndorf_ in various infections, [A. Daiber] Med.Kor.-Bl.f.Wurttemberg 98:333-335, June 16, '28

28K3: for treatment of phtisical patients, [S. Mallanah] Indian M. Rec. 48:260, Sept. '28

28K4: in gonorrhea, [V.Manca-Pastorino] Gior.ital.di dermat. e sifil. 69:582-590, June '28

28K5: in gonorrheal arthritis; cases, [P.Fabry] Liege med. 21:439-448, April 1, '28

28K6: in ozena, P Carco] Bol.d.Soc.ital.di biol.sper. 3:595, May '28; also

Boll.d.mal.d.orecchio,d.gola e d.naso 46:73-82, July '28

28K7: in pulmonary form of distemper in dogs, [S.Mglej] Berl.tierarztl.Wchnschr. 44:557-560, Aug. 24, '28

28K8: in pyelocystitis of childhood, [A. Lubrano and A Nastasi] Pediatria 36:756-765, July 15, '28

28K9: inflammation of kidney, renal pelvis and bladder due to staphylococcus cured by autovaccine, [L. Velasco Blanco] Arch.latino-am.de med. 4:108-110, Oct. 1, '28

28K10: local skin reactions in selection of antigens for autogenous vaccines, [S.Dorst and W.B. Wherry] Ohio State M.J. 24:539-543, July '28

28K11: local treatment of puerperal infection with Besredka's autogenous bouillon vaccine, [G. Aschermann and L. Rosenblum] Monatschr.f.Geburtsch.u.Gynak. 79:293-301, July '28

28K12: of chronic articular rheumatism, [P. Rudback] Acta med. Scandinav. (supp. no. 26) pp. 140-146, '28

28K13: of gynecologic infections, [G.J.Pfalz] Deutsche med. Wchnschr.54:1121-1125, July 6, '28

28K14: of ulcerative colitis, [E. Bucka] Arch.f.Verdauungskr.

42:561-568, April '28

28K15: protein-vaccine-pus therapy in puerperal infection, [G. Ajello] Rev.sud-am.de endocrinol. 11:393-401, June '28

28K16: rapid technic for autovaccine therapy in pneumonia; clinical results [J. Gate and H. Gardere] Compt. rend. Soc. de biol. 99:817-819, Sept. 18, '28

28K17: treatment of intestinal parasites in epilepsy with autogenous vaccines of Entameba histolytica; preliminary report, [R. A. Ashbaugh]  Illinois M.J. 54: 129-134, Aug. '28

29J1: autogenous, cure of case of otitis media with autovaccine combined with yatren, [W. Cuntz] forschr. d.Therap. 4: 694, Nov. 10, '28

29J2: cerebrospinal meningitis; treatment by spinal lavage and autovaccine therapy; case, [I. Constandache & M. Francke] Bull.et mém. Soc. méd.d.hop.de Bucarest  10: 353-357, Dec. '28

29J3: in gonorrheal arthritis, [Audebert & Planques]  Bull. Soc. d'obst.et de gynéc.  18: 176-178, Feb. '29

29J4: in unusual severe pseudomembranous streptococcic conjunctivitis; case, [C. Marlotti]  Boll.d'ocul.  7: 1118-1139, Nov. '28

29J5: local autovaccinotherapy in pediatric practice, [F.

Cantani]  Pediaria  36: 1100-1106, Oct.15, '28

29J6: of enterocolitis in children; cases, [Ayuso y o'Horibe] Gac.méd. de México 59: 689-697, Dec. '28; also, Crón méd.-quir.de la Habana 55:73-81, Feb. '29

29J7: of persistent nasal catarrh in horses, [A. A. Pryer] Vet.J. 85: 113-117, March '29

29J8: preparation of autovaccines in deep tubes for pulmonary gangrene and other respiratory diseases; injections by artificial tracheal fistulae or by transthoracic route, [G.Rosenthal] Bull.et mem.Soc.de med.de Paris, no.10, pp. 300-303, May 26, '28; also J. de med. de Paris 48:141, Feb. 14, '29

29J9: simple method of filling autovaccine ampules, [T. Kertész]  München.med. Wchnschr. 75: 1721, Oct. 5, '28

29J10: treatment of chronic arthritis with streptococcic vaccines, [P. M. Keating]  Texas State J.Med.  24: 691-693, Feb. '29

29J11: vaccine and allied therapy, [H. M. Banks & I. Anderson]  J.Indiana M.A.  22: 192-194, May' 29

29K1: autogenous, in case of septicemia from middle ear disease, [Roediger] Verinsbl.d.pfälz.Aerzte  41: 80-83, March 15, '29

29K2: behavior of bacteriolytic, opsonic and bacteriotropic indices and of skin tests in therapeutic autovaccination in urinary diseases, [C. Chiaudano] Gior.di bacteriol.e immunol. 3: 868-874, Sept. '29

29K3: general furunculosis due to Sarcina tetragena, treated by autovaccine and antivirus, [B. Galli-Valerio & M. Bornand] Schweiz.med. Wchnschr. 59: 730, July 13, '29

29K4: in closed, suppurative processes (osteomyelitis), [S. I. Spassokukotzky & I. I. Mikhalevsky] Vestnik khir. (nos. 48-49) 16-17: 155-167, '29

29K5: in empyema in children; cases, [A. Sementini] Terapia 19: 141-149, May '29

29K6: in gonorrhea, [Tedeschi] Gazz.internaz.med.-chir.37:360, June 15, '29

29K7: in gonorrhea in pregnant; 3 cases, [J. Audebert & J. B Giscard] Rev.franç de. gynéc.et d'obst. 24: 145-147, March '29

29K8: in pyelitis, [M. Nikhamkina] Vrach.dielo 12: 338-342, March 15, '29

29K9: in pyelonephritis of pregnancy; delivery of child with mortal melena as result of pyloric ulcer, [Bonnet & Imbert] Bull.Soc.d'obst.et de gynéc. 18: 369, May '29

29K10: local autovaccinotherapy in carbuncular pustule, [A. Battista] Riforma med. 45: 527-531, April 20, '29

29K11: of implanted mouse carcinoma (M. 63), [T. Lumsden] Lancet 2: 814-816, Oct. 19, '29

30J1: autogenous, in cerebrospinal meningitis, [G. I. Tchuevskaya] Klin.j.saratov.Univ. 6: 37-40, June '28

30J2: in cerebrospinal meningitis with Diplococcus crassus, [G. Candido] Riforma med. 45: 1190-1191, Aug 1.31, '29

30J3: in gonorrhea of puerperium, [Audebert & J. B. Giscard] Bull.Soc.d'obst. et de gynéc. 18: 652-655, Nov. '29; also, J.de. méd. de Paris 48: 1029, Nov. 28, '29

30J4: in gynecologic infections; cases, [A. Albaneses] Riv. ital.di ginecol. 9: 569-580, June '29

30J5: in intestinal infections of infants, [D. Price] Irish J.M.Sc., pp. 59-63, Feb. '30

30J6: in meningococcus meningitis, [E. Appelbaum] Arch. Pediat. 47: 61-63, Jan. '30

30J7: in ulcerative epitheliomas of uterine cervix, [F. Speciale] Policlinico (sez. prat.) 36:

1425-1427, Oct. 7, '29

30J8: in pyuria in early childhood, [A. Romeo Lozano] Arch.españ.de pediat.  13: 641-657, Nov. '29

30J9: preparation and use of autogenous vaccines, {R. A. Keilty] J.A.M.A.  94: 95-100, Jan. 11, '30

30J10: treatment of gonorrhea in pregnancy by Giscard's autovaccine; case, [Audebert & E. Estienny]  Bull. Soc.d'obst. et de gynéc.  18: 678, Nov. '29

30K1: autogenous, in grave colitis, [H. Surmoont & R. Buttiaux]  Presse méd.  38: 956-959, July 16, '30

30K2: acute articular rheumatism; recovery with specific autovaccine, [P. Ivanissevich]  Semana méd.  2: 731-736, Sept. 4, '30

30K3: bacterial hypersensitivity of intestinal tract; treatment with autogenous vaccine and sodium ricinoleate, [S. E. Dorst & R. S. Morris]  Am.J.M.Sc. 180: 650-656, Nov. '30

30K4: danger of possible reinoculation of disease, [J. Lembeye]  Presa méd. argent. 17: 417-419, Aug.10, '30

30K5: enterococcic septicemia with manifestations in throat, mouth and skin cured with autovaccine therapy; case, [S. Barbera] Arch.ital.di otol. 41: 324-31, July '30

30K6: for infections of urinary tract in infants; 13 cases, [L. velasco Bianco]  Rev.de especialid.  5: 194-202, April'30; also, Arch.am.de med. 6: 47-60, April 1, '30

30K7: for pulmonary abscess from Staphylococcus aureus in nursling; case, [P. Lereboullet, M. Lelong & F. Benoist]  Bull.et mém. Soc.méd.d.hop.de Paris (54): 1284-1289, July 21, '30

30K8: local immunization with polyvalent autovaccine of capsulated diplobacillus in ozena, [W. Jelin] Ztschr.f.Laryng., Rhin.  19: 434-437, July '30

30K9: of gonorrhea, [Memmesheimer & Dieckmann] Arch.f.Dermat.u.Syph.  160: 252-256, '30

31J1: autogenous, conditions for success, [H. Surmont & R. Buttiaux]  Echo méd.du nord 34: 539-596, Dec.13, '30

31J2: endotracheal injections in chronic pneumonia; case, [F. Giordano] Gazz.internaz.med.-chir.  39: 160-164, March 15, '31

31J3: in case of puerperal septicaemia, [C. C. B. Gilmour] Malayan M.J. 6: 23-24, March 1, '31

31J4: in sepsis of urinary tract in children, [L. Auricchio] Pediatria  39: 457-456, May 1, '31

31J5: in ulcerative colitis, [G. K. Lavsky] Russk.Klin. 13: 323-328, '30

31J6: phagedenic ulcer of penis; isolation of staphylococcus pathogenic for animals; autovaccination; case, [P. Chevallier, Lévy-Bruhl & R. Moricard] Bull.Soc.franç de dermat.et syph. 38: 448-455, March '31

31K1: autogenous, autopyo-urovaccine in gonorrhea and its complications, [L. I. Litwak & I. S. Schister] Dermat.Wchnschr. 93: 1735-1739, Nov. 7, '31

31K2: autopyovaccine in therapy of putrid lung suppurations, [L. Bernard & Pellissier] Bull.et mém.Soc.méd.d.hop. de Paris 47: 1696-1702, Nov.23, '31

31K3: simple and practical autovaccine therapy in gonorrhea, [C. Tedeshi] Cong. internat. de méd. trop. et d'hyg., Compt. rend. (1928) 3: 941-943, '31

31K4: treatment of psoriasis with vaccine from scales, [A. Toma] Annde dermat. et syph. 2: 1110-1113, Oct. '31

32J1: autogenous, in asthmatic syndromes, [E. Frola] Riforma med. 48: 46-50, Jan. 9, '32

32J2: disseminated sclerosis, clinical and serological observations during experimental vaccine treatment, [J. Purves-Stewart & F. D. M. Hocking] Lancet 1: 605-609, March 19, '32

32J3: in chronic colitis and enterocolitis, [V. A. Beliaeva] Klin.med. (no.16) 9: 717-719, '32

32J4: in primary gonorrheal meningitis treated by auto-lystaevaccine; case. [P. E. Weil, Duchon & Bertrand] Bull.et mém.Soc. méd.d.hop.de Paris 47: 1799-1803, Dec. 7, '31

32J5: streptococcic autovaccines in infectious endocarditis, [C. Dimitracoff] Bull.méd., Paris 46: 6-9, Jan.2, '32

32J6: ulcerative colitis due to chronic infection with Flexner-Y bacillus; case with cure by autogenous vaccine, [T. T. Mackie] J.A.M.A. 98: 1706-1710, May 14, '32

32J7: value, [P.Levey] Nebraska M.J. 17:75-76, Feb. '32

32K1: autogenous, practical contribution to bacteriology and treatment of otitis, [L. C. D. Hermitte] Tr.Roy. Soc. Trop. Med & Hyg. 26: 189-194, Aug. '32

32K2: Myelitis caused by Staphylococci aureus; recovery after autovaccine therapy; 2 cases, [N. Flessinger, H. R. Olivier & A. Arnaudet] Rev.de méd., Paris 49: 487-499, Oct. '32

32K3: osteomyelitis of cranial vault secondary to acute sinusitis; early operation and injections of autovaccine; recovery, [E. M. Nattino & N. Caubarrere]  An.de oto-rino-laring.d. Uruguay  2: 20-35, '32

32K4: treatment of puerperal septicemia caused by hemolytic streptococci with large doses of serum and autovaccine; anatomicopathologic study of 19 cases, [J. C. Estol & C. M. Dominguez]  An.Fac.de med., Montevideo  17: 201-280, March-April '32

32K5: treatment of putrid pulmonary suppurations by autopyovaccine prepared by animal passage of sputum of patients, [L. Bernard & Pellissier]  J.de méd. de Paris  52: 503-505, June 23, '32

33J1: autogenous, allergy in staphylococcic infections treated with autovaccines, [P. Costantini]  Boll.d.Ist. sieroterap. milanese  11: 691-702, Oct. '32

33J2: important role of colon bacilli in pathology of digestive tract in man and animals; efficacy of autovaccine therapy, [T. V. Simitch, S. Moatchanine & S. Mrchevitch] Paris méd 2: 389-392, Nov. 12, '32

33J3: in prevention of complications in conservative surgical treatment of infected reno-ureteral lithiasis, [E.

Jeanbrau]  Ztschr.f.urol.Chir. 36: 188-190, '33

33J4: pathogen-selective cultures in relations to vaccine therapy, [F. Boerner & M. Solis-Cohen]  Am.J. Clin. Path. 3: 125-131, March '33

33J5: results of therapy with vaccine prepared from hemoculture in various types of rheumatic fever. [P.Ivanissevich] Semana med. 1:575-579, Feb. 16, '33

33J6: value in osteomyelitis of cranial bones, [P. Carco] Oto-rino-laring.ital. 2:547-558, Dec. '32

33K1: autogenous, in actinomycosis, [E.Payr] Muenchen med. Wchnschr. 80:1001-1003, June 30, '33

33K2: intravenous vaccine (streptococcic) therapy in chronic arthritis, [W.B. Rawls, B.J. Gruskin and A. Ressa] An. Int. Med. 7:566-581, Nov. '33

33K3: of acute coryza, [L.Hoyle] Brit.M.J. 1:996-997, June 10, '33

33K4: of chronic sinus infections and nasal allergy, [W.C.Cox] Mil.Surgeon 73:121-128, Sept., '33

33K5: of metastatic pneumococcic supprations, [du Bourguet and Crosnier] Soc.de.med.mil.franç., Bull.mens. 27:96-98, March '33

33K6: purulent pleurisy caused by Pfeiffer's bacilli in infant; autovaccine therapy; case, [L.Velasco Blanco and C.P. Montagna] Arch.am.de med. 9:140-146, '33

33K7: transitory bacteremia due to Streptococcus viridans; autovaccinotherapy; 2 cases, [T.de Sanctis Monaldi] Riforma med. 49:1127-1133, July 29, '33

33K8: urticaria of 17 years' duration; case treated successfully (by colon bacillus vaccine), [J.L.Emmett and A.H.Logan] JAMA 101:1966, Dec. 16, '33

34J1: autogenous, clinical significance of B. coli hemolyticus (use of autogenous vaccines), [W.L.Niles and J.C. Torrey] Am.J.M.Sc. 287:30-36, Jan. '34

34J2: cure of unilateral parotitis following rhino-stomatogenic infection; case, [H. Zumsteeg] Med.Welt 7:1819-1822, Dec. 23, '33

34J3: desensitization in colitis, [H.G. Mogena] Arch.de med., cir.y especialid. 37:361-363, April 7, '34

34J4: in rheumatoid arthritis; clinical study and critique, [c.L.Short, L. Dienes and W. Bauer] Am.J.M.Sc. 187:615-623, May, '34

34J5: in trachoma, [A. Cusumano] Rassenga ital.d'ottal. 2:725-735, Sept.-Oct. '33

34J6: in trachoma, [Perez Llorca] Rev.cubana de oto-neuro-oftal. 2:262-265, Sept.-Oct. '33

34J7: in ulcerative blepharitis, [K.V.Snegirev] Sovet.vestnik oftal. 4:208-209, '34

34J8: of purulent pleurisy caused by influenza bacillus; case in infant, [L.Velasco Blanco and C.P. Montagna] Arch.argent.de pediat. 4:875-881, Dec., '33

34J9: otitic meningitis caused by Streptococci; surgical and autovaccine therapy, [P. Hernandez Gonzalo and M. Chediak] Rev.med.cubana 44:1458-1466, Dec. '33

34J10: phagedenic ulcer of penis successfully treated by subcutaneous injections of staphylococcic autovaccine, [P.Chevallier, M. Levy-Bruhl, A.Fiehrer and B.Hahn] Bull.Soc.franc.de dermat.et syph. 40:1748-1751, Dec. '33

34J11: selective vaccine in treatment of bronchial asthma; preliminary report, [H.M. Banks and T.J. Beasley] J.Indiana M.A. 27:151-156, April, '34

34K1: autogenous, [R.Freund] Schweiz.med.Wchnschr. 64:921-923, Oct.6, '34

34K2: according to Citella in ozena; comparison of results with those of arsphenamine and diphtheria vaccines, [G.Russo

Frattasi] Riforma med. 50:1192-1198, Aug.4, '34

34K3: autolysate therapy for verruca vulgaris, [F.E.Cormia] Arch.Dermat. and Syph. 30, P.44-48, July, '34

34K4: combined with dietetic therapy of chronic colitis, [L.B.Berlin, B.S.Levin, P.L. Isaev and O.O. Shmidt] Klin.med. (no.6) 12:910-914, '34

34K5: desensitizing therapy in colitis, [H.G.Mogena] Arch. argent. de enferm.d.ap.digest.y de la nutricion 9:245-252, Feb.-March, '32

34K6: in chronic sinus infections and nasal allergy; further studies, [W.C.Cox] Mil.Surgeon 75:317-324, Nov. '34

34K7: massive autovaccine in acute blenorrhagic urethritis, [E.Tarantelli] Gior.ital.di dermat.e sif. 75: 1283-1292, June '34

34K8: milk vaccine therapy in surgical treatment of peritonitis, [J.G.Anderson] Am.J.Surg. 25:521-524, Sept. '34

34K9: of chronic secretion from enucleation cavity, [Hudelo and Bruneau] Bull.Soc.d'opht.de Paris, pp.94-114, March '34

34K10: of embolic glomerulonephritis; role of focal infection in production of nephritis, [G.Battistini] Minerva med. 1:801-810, June 9, 1934

34K11: preliminary autovaccination in surgery of patients with urinary infections, [Bonnet] Progres med., pp.753-754, May 5, '34

34K12: Streptococcus viridans vaccine in endocarditis lenta; 3 cases, [C.Dimitracoff] Arch.d.mal.du coeur 27:246-260, April, '34

34K13: therapy of cardio-articular rheumatism; author's method of tonsillectomy immediately followed by autovaccination, [R. Cirera Volta] Rev.med.de Barcelona 22:100-109, Aug., '34

35J1: autogenous, general immunization in blepharitis and eczema of eyelids, [A.A.Yakovleva] Sovet.vestnik oftal. 5:234-238, '34

35J2: autobacteriotherapy; attempt at replacing vaccine therapy by method better suited to use in colonial medicine, [S.Golovine] Presse med. 43:579-581, April 10, '35

35J3: in pyelonephritis in pregnancy; 28 cases, [P.Trillat] Gynec.et obst. 30:497-516, Dec. '34

35J4: in septicemia caused by Proteus vulgaris; cure of case, [A.Deshons] Montpelier med. 6:201-206, Oct. 15, '34

35J5: rapid recovery of case of erythrodermia desquamativa (Lenier-Moussous' disease) after peroral administration of infinitesimal doses of enterococcic vaccine [G.Blechmann and Mme. P.J. Menard] Nourrisson 23:89-98, March '35

35J6: simple rapid method of preparation of auto-antivirus for use in therapy of infected cancers of uterine cervix, [A.Rouslacroix] Compt.rend.Soc.de biol. 117:17-18, '34

35J7: successes and failures in staphylococcic supprations, [T. Messerschmidt] Fortschr.d.Therap. 11:156-159, March '35

35J8: value of auto-uro-vaccine therapy in acute hemorrhagic nephritis, {R. Tiberi] Diagnosi 14:183-196, June '34

35K1: autogenous, eczema cured by vaccine made from strain of bacillus furnished by gingival hemoculture; case, [R. Vincent and Resnik] Rev.de stomatol.37:420-421, June, '35

35K2: auto-antivirus therapy in chronic supprative dacryocystitis, [c. Suhateanu, Dinulescu, Albescu and Paraipan] Rev. san. mil., Bucuresti 34:471-474, Oct., '35

35K3: autovaccine and antivirus therapy of chronic colitis, [D.Gutierrez Arrese, D. Lopez Blanco and J.M. Lastra] Arch.f.Verdauungskr. 58:167-180, Oct., '35

35K4: for diphtheria carriers, [A.C. Buthrie] Brit.M.J. 2:341, Aug.24, '35

35K5: general immunization in dacryocystitis, [A.A. Yakovleva] Sovet.vestnik oftal. 6:392-394, '35

35K6: local intradermal therapy in chronic purulent otitis media, [U.Secondi] Ann.di laring.,otol. 34:59-75, '34

35K7: meningococcemia in boy; recovery of case after therapy with septicemine (iodine preparation) and autovaccine, [Rocaz and Fiot] J.de med. de Bordeaux 112:299-300, April 20, '35

35K8: of protracted pneumonias, [N.A. Kurshakov] Vrach.delo 18:217-220, '35

35K9: Streptococcus vaccines, [M.J. Breuer] Nebraska M.J. 20:398-399, Oct., '35

35K10: subacute malignant pemphigus with extensive bullae (Brocq's form) due to gram-positive Diplococci; local therapy associated with autogenous vaccine therapy, [G.Guardali] Arch. ital. di dermat., sif. 11:437-445, Sept., '35

35K11: technical and clinical aspects, [R. Freund] Fortschr. d. Therap. 11:391-397, July, '35

35K12: therapy of disseminated furunculosis with autogenous and

heterogenous vaccines,
[J.M.Lewin] Dermat. Ztschr.
71:85-88, April '35

35K13: value of autogenous
vaccine prophylaxis and therapy
in streptococcic otitis media;
experimental study, [S. Vitale]
Gior.di med. mil. 83:749-770,
aug., '35

36J1: autogenous, of asthma,
[H.M. Rozendaal and C.K. Maytum]
Proc. Staff Meet., Mayo Clin.
11:90-91, Feb. 5, '36

36J2: in pediatrics, [C.J.
Bloom] New Orleans M. and J.J.
88:738-746, June, '36

36J3: intravenous therapy in
sepsis due to Staphylococcus
aureus; 3 cases, [V. de Antoni]
Policlinico (sez. prat.) 43:763-
777, April 27, '36

36J4: of rheumatism; preliminary
report, [J.M.Pardo, E. Conde
Gargoll and A. van Baumberghen]
An. de med. int. 4:1191-1196,
Dec., '35

36J5: prognostic value of
variation in Arneth count in
cases of treated asthma, [L.E.
Napier and Dharmendra] Indian M.
Gaz. 71:139-143, March '36

36J6: purulent pleurisy caused
by Pfeiffer's bacillus; case in
child cured by autovaccine
therapy, [G.Negro] Soc.
internaz. di microbiol., Boll.
d. sez. ital. 8:9-12, Jan., '36

36J7: study of effects of
injections upon skin

sensitivity, [M. D. Touart, W.S.
Thomas and W.L. Tucker] J. Lab.
and Clin. Med. 21:365-375, Jan.,
'36

36K1: autogenous, [Oliveira
Botelho] Gaz.clin. 34:218-220,
July, '36

36K2: bacillary (Friedländer
type} vaccines in asthma;
assessment of results, [E.T.
Conybeare and F.A. Knott] Guy's
Hosp. Rep. 86:420-430, Oct., '36

36K3: continuous subarachnoid
drainage for influenzal
meningitis by means of ureteral
catheter and vaccine, [H.A.
Stribley] J.Iowa M. Soc. 26:300-
303, June '36

36K4: importance and variations
of bactericidal power of whole
blood in localized and
generalized surgical infections;
action of vaccine therapy, [F.
Bordonaro] Arch. Ist. biochim.
ital. 8:71-98, March '36

36K5: in acute tympanic
suppration with incipient
mastoiditis; 18 cases, [G.B.
Fornari] Riforma med. 52:676-
682, May 16, '36

35K6: in allergic bacterial
dermatoses; preliminary report,
[T.N. Graham and E.R. Traub]
Arch.Dermat. and Syph. 34:484-
489, Sept. '36

36K7: late results in massive
therapy of ozena, [P.F. Pieri]
Oto-rino-laring. ital. 6:304-
318, Aug., '36

36K8: of purulent otitis media, [Westphal and G. Willführ] Muenchen. med. Wchnschr. 83:1344-1345, Aug. 14, '36

36K9: of staphylococcic abscess on edge of eyelid, [Z. Jablonska] Klin. Monatsbl. f. Augenh. 97:362-370, Sept., '36

36K10: of staphylomycoses, [H. Gross and E. König] Fortschr. d. Therap. 12:610-612, Oct., '36

36K11: polyvalent group autovaccine in local immunization against scarlet fever, [T.K. Maslovskiy] Sovet. vrach. zhur., pp. 1389-1391, Sept., 30, '36

36K12: results of fecal autovaccine therapy of chronic bacterial colitis and in intestinal amebiasis during an amebic phase; technical and clinical study; 18 cases, [L. Pontoni] Policlinico (sez. med.) 43:502-522, Oct., '36

36K13: Schönlein's disease cured by therapeutic serum sickness induced by Streptococcus viridans vaccine; case, [L. Cotti and G. Rettanni] Gior. di clin. med. 17:767-783, Aug. 30, '36

37J1: autogenous, bacteriologic studies on polyarthritis; attempts at specific (enterococcic) autovaccinotherapy, {N. Svartz] Acta med. Scandinav., supp. 78, pp. 327-338, '36

37J2: secondary infections

during pulmonary tuberculosis and autovaccine therapy, [M. Jaquerod] Rev. de la tuberc. 3:185-191, Feb., '37

37K1: autogenous, author's method of autovaccine and autoprotein therapy of favus, [G. Balice] Riv. di chir. 3:341-347, June '37

37K2: effect of blood transfusion, autovaccination and silver salts on immunity in supprative processes, [A.G. Zebrin] Novy khir. arkhiv 38:285-289, '37; also Khirurgiya, no. 3, pp. 20-23, '37

37K3: in hay fever, [W.c. Behen] J. Michigan M. Soc. 36:852-853, Nov., '37

37K4: of urinary infection in infants; 30 cases, [L. Velasco Blanco] Arch. am. de med. 13:85-98, '37

37K5: results, [J. W. Wolff] Nederl. tijdschr. v. geneesk. 81:5106-5114, Oct. 23, '37

37K6: therapeutic value of so-called "parasitic vaccines" in pyoderma and gonorrheal complications, [H. Reiss and T. Piatek] Deramat. Wchnschr. 105:948-956, July 24, '37; also Polska gas. lek. 16:591-593, July 25, '37

38J1: autogenous, in asthma; preliminary report, [W. C. Sacks] Univ. Hosp. Bull., Ann Arbor 4:11, Feb. '38

38J2: cerebrospinal otitic meningococcic meningitis; surgical and autogenous vaccine therapy followed by recovery of patient [L. Maryssael] Bruxelles-méd. 18:803-807, April 17, '38

38J3: in postoperative period of appendectomy, [A. Bernardes de Oliveira] Ann. paulisst. de med. e cir. 35:225-248, March '38

38J4: in purulent diseases of lungs, [L. M. Yanovskaya] Klin. med. 16:2450250, '38

38J5: oral administration in Lenier-Moussous' disease; case, [G. Blechmann and P. Peyron] Progrès méd., pp. 597-598, April 23, '38

38J6: preparation of autogenous pyovaccine and its utilization in therapy of supprative infectious diseases, [I. Orsós] Dermat. Wchnschr. 106:438-445, April 16, '38

38J7: prontosil (sulfanilamide derivative) and autovaccine in conservative therapy of osteomyelitis, [Kasarcoglu] Türk tib cem. mec. 4:48-52, '38

38J8: seronegative typhoid with multiple relapses cured by autovaccination; case, [P. Depetris and G. Elkeles] Semana Méd. 2:1396-1399, Dec., 16, '37

38J9: therapy of pemphigus by active immunization with contents of pemphigus bullae; further experiment, [A.E.H.

Binger] Wien. klin. Wchnschr. 51:237-238, Feb. 25, '38

38J10: treatment of osteomyelitis, using B.I.P.P. (pertolatum preparation) and autogenous vaccine, [M.T. Myers] J.M.A.Georgia 26:565-569, Dec. '37

38K1: autogenous, in cerebral circulatory diseases, k[P. Kormos] Orvosi hetil. 82:764-766, July 30, '38

38K2: in pyelitis, [Reinaldo Márquez and A. Curbelo] Vida nueva 42:307-316, Oct. 15, '38

38K3: in trichomoniasis in female, [J. Adeodato Filho and A. Dourado] Rev. de gynec. e d'obst. 1:680-691, June '38

38K4: leukocyte oxydase and peroxydase reaction in shock due to therapy, [C. Zelaschi] Clin. med. ital. 69:301-323, May-June, '38

38K5: production of autovaccine in vivo by electrocoagulation of tonsils, [A.P. Seltzer] M. Rec. 148:65-67, July 20, '38

38K6: rapid production of vaccine for treatment of pneumonia with notes on its use, [F. P. G. de Smidt] Brit. M. J. 2:1140-1142, Dec. 3, '38

39J1: autogenous, as therapeutic measure for pyelocystitis in children, [K. Tohjimbara, K. Hirata and T. Morita] Taiwan Igakkai Zasshi 37:1810, Nov., '38

39J2: autoserovaccine therapy of septicemias and gonorrheal arthritis, [A. Grimberg] J. de méd de Paris 59:47-48, Jan. 19, '39; also Bull. et mém. Soc. de méd. de Paris 142:81-85, Jan. 29, '38

39J3: in chronic and focal infections, [M. Solis-Cohen] Internat. Clin. 2:214-233, June '39

39J4: psoriasis cured by intestinal autovaccine, prepared with colibacilli; case, [S. Prat] Gaz. d. hôp. 112:331-332, March 8, '39

39J5: specific vaccine treatment of otomycosis; preparation of vaccine, [G. M. Mood] Am. J. Trop. Med. 18:703-714, Nov. '38

39J6: streptococcus vaccines in treatment of allergic conditions, with special reference to their use in bronchial asthma; cases, [R. S. Yivisaker] Minnesota Med. 22:6-12, Jan. '39

39J7: tonsillectomy and autovaccine in therapy of polyarthritis, [Laval] Ztschr. f. Hals-, Nasen- u. Ohrenh. 44:381-383, '38

39K1: autogenous, septicemia due to Friedländer's pneumobacillus; case cured by autovaccine, [J. Rouffart-Marin] Bruxelles-méd. 19:1145-1146, July 16, '39

39K2: associated with specific serotherapy of pneumococcic meningitis; case, [F. Schiappoli] Riforma med. 55:1439-1446, Sept. 30, '39

39K3: asthma in children treated with autogenous (bronchoscopic) vaccine, [J. Crump] Am. J. Dis. Child. 58:768-777, Oc. '39

39K4: of typhoid, [M. Braunsas] Medicina, Kaunas 20:736-749, Sept. '39

40J1: autogenous, rapid dual-purpose media for autovaccines, [K.P.A. Taylor and F. Mason] South. Med. and Surg. 102: 53-55, Feb., '40

40J2: chronic supprative diseases of adnexa due to Friedländer's pneumobacillus, successfully cured with autovaccine, [A. Fingerland, M. Hub and J. Marsálek] Casop. Lék. cesk. 78:1145-1147, Oct. 20, '39

40K1: autogenous, appendectomy and appendicular autovaccines in complicated appendicitis, [F. Teixeira da Silva] Rev. méd. brasil. 5:213-226, Aug. '39

40K2: acute periarticular rheumatism treated successfully by autogenous staphylococcal vaccine of intestinal origin, [A.G. Shera] Brit. M. J. 2:629, Nov. 9, '40

40K3: associated toxoid-autovaccine therapy of infections in children, [R. Scapaticci] Boll. Soc. ital. biol. sper. 15:432-433, April, '40

40K4: auto-antivirus in chronic purulent otitis, [S. Nemirovsky] Rev. méd. de Rosario 30:619-648, June '40

40K5: autopyovaccination in gonorrhea, [J. Krecek] Dermat. Wchnschr. 110:482-485, June 8, '40

40K6: bacteriology of bile; autovaccine therapy of hepatovesicular diseases, [N. Romano, S. Rey and A. Rottgardt] Rev. Asoc. méd. argent. 54:361-368, May 15, '40

41J1: autogenous, probable Staphylococcus albus origin of herpes zoster and polyarthritis; case with recovery after autovaccine therapy, [V. A. N. d'Angelo] Rev. argent. de reumatol. 5:235-238, Dec. '40

41J2: therapy of whooping cough by means of lysed autovaccine of bronchial exudate, [P. Salmerón Mora] Rev. clín. españ. 2:167-169, Feb. 1, '41

41J3: transformation of typical paratyphoid B bacilli into mucous form during autovaccine therapy of carrier, [P. vor dem Exche] Ztschr. f. Immunitätsforsch. u. exper. Therap. 98:75-89, April 22, '40

41K1: autogenous, nonfilament-filament ratio changes following administration to persons with low-grade chronic illness, [M. H. Stiles] J. Lab. and Clin. Med. 26:1453-1460, June '41

41K2: application of autofiltrate in fistulous forms of osteoarthritic tuberculosis in children, [E. L. Vishnyakova] Probl. tuberk., no. 3, pp. 80-81, '41

41K3: chemical inactivation of vaccines, [J. N. Frazer] Am. J. M. Technol. 7:233-235, Sept. '41

41K4: post-traumatic streptococcic meningitis with recovery after treatment with sulfanilaminde alone and combined with autovaccine respectively; 2 cases, [K. Bronø] Ugesk. f. læger 103:648-650, May 15, '41

42J1: autogenous, advantages of chemically inactivated vaccines, [J. N. Frazer] Am. J. M. Technol. 8:89-94, May '42

42J2: in puerperal and pelvic infections, [C. A. Garber] J. Am. Inst. Homeop. 35:119, March, '42

42J3: specific therapy in sinusitis, [M. Solis-Cohen] Arch. Otolaryng. 35:623-630, April, '42

42J4: utilization of pus (autopyovaccine) in treatment of pyogenic disorders, [I. J. Arnsson] New York State J. Med. 42:770-772, April 15, '42

43J1: autogenous, intestinal autointoxication as cause of severe chronic blepharocon-junctivitis; vaccine therapy, [L. Szerdahelyi] Gastro-enterologia 67:147-151, '42

43K1: autogenous, appendectomy and appendicular autovaccines, [F. Teixeira da Silva] Rev. flum. de med. 7:179-193, July '42

43M1: Fairbanks Barbarosa, J., Vaccinotherapy and serotherapy in otorhinolaryngology, REV. BRASIL. OTORINOLAR., 1943, 11: 215-243. [1013 d]

43M2: Lopes Ferreira, Autogenous vaccine in association with serum and sulfonamide, GAC. MED. MEXICO, 1943, 73:41-3 [1076 cd]

44J1: autogenous, importance of coproculture in therapy of enteric infections, [g. Arias] Bol. Soc. cubana de pediat. 15:1134-1140, Dec. '43

44J2: medicinal aerosols; therapy of asthma with aerosols of pneumodilating substances and autovaccines [L Dautrebande, E. Philippot, R. Charlier, and E. Dumoulin] Presse méd. 50:566-567, Sept. 12, '42

44K1: preparation of bacterial vaccines; autovaccines, [J. F. Bedini] Rev. san. mil., Buenos Aires 43:348-354, March, '44

45J1: autogenous, biliary autovaccines, [P.A. Sainz] Inform. méd. 8:111-122, July, '44

45J2: recent trends in bronchologic use of chemotherapeutic and biotherapeutic agents (including sulfonamides, penicillin and autogenous vaccine), [G. Tucker and J. P. Atkins] Ann. Otol., Rhin. and Laryng. 53:777-786, Dec. '44

45K1: autogenous, specific autovaccine in therapy of severe ulcerative colitis, [A. Hämmerli] Gastroenterologia 68:36-41, '43

46J1: autogenous, salmonellosis due to Salmonella london: intracutaneous vaccine therapy; case, [A. Curbelo y Hernández and J. R. Alfonso] Rev. cubana pediat. 18:161-165, March '46

47J1: autogenous, problem of rheumatic carditis; decline of one doctrine and origination of better theory; 34 new cases of carditis clinically cured following autovaccine therapy, [F. Gonzalez Suarez] Gac. méd. españ. 20:483-488, Dec., '46

47J2: treatment of contagious impetigo contagiosa and furunculosis by autovaccines injected by intracutaneous route, [F. van Deinse] Presse méd. 54:750-751, Nov. 9, '46

47K1: autogenous, in female genital trichomoniasis, [J. Adeodato, Jr.] Obst. y ginec. latino-am. 5:31-39, Jan.-Feb. '47

47K2: in ulcerative colitis, [Z. Maratka and V. Wagner] Casop. lék. cesk. 86:133-139, Feb. 7, '47

47K3: treatment of postgonorrheal infections with massive injections, [T. V. Williamson] Urol. and Cutan. Rev. 51:224-226, April '47

48J1: autogenous, in cervical actinomycosis; case, [P. J. Kooreman] Nederl. tijdschr. v. geneesk. 85:1896-1898, May 3, '41

48J2: therapy of inoperable gastric cancer with autovaccinations with patient's gastric juice, [C. Finkelstein] Gastroenterologia 73:45-55, '48

48J3: treatment of chronic ulcerative colitis with staphylococcus autovaccine; preliminary report, [W. A. Heazlett] Gastroenterolgy 10:634-642, April '48

48K1: autogenous, extensive roentgen ulcer cured by autovaccine combined with antireticular cytotoxic serum of Bogomolets, [M. Dvorácek and V. Kubelka] Casop. lék. cesk. 87:644-648, May 28, '48

48K2: treatment of non-specific ulcerative colitis; correlated bacteriologic and immunologic studies, [Z. Maratka and V. Wagner] Gastroenterology 11:34-49, July, '48

48M1:  Merten, A., Healing of a surgical wound after mastoidectomy, through autovaccine. MSCHR. OHRENH., 1948, 82, No. 4 (April, 1948), 180-2.  [134 m]

49J1: autogenous, local autovaccine therapy of nasopharyngeal infections, [A.R. Prévot] Semaine d. hôp. Paris 25:160-162, Jan. 14, '49

49K1: autogenous, autovaccine, polysaccharide therapy of scleroma; 2 cases, [L. Cioglia and E. Pirodda] Oto-rino-laring.ital. 18:1-11, '49

49K2: treatment of intrinsic bronchial asthma with autogenous vaccine, [A.C. Grorud] Ann. Allergy 7:540-549, July-Aug. '49

49L1:  Van Der Ghinst, M., Remarks on the treatment of grave furunculosis; value of radiotherapy and of vaccination. BRUXELLES MÉD, 1949, 29: No. 14 (Apr. 3, 1949), 730-3. [1124 s]

50J1: autogenous, autovaccine therapy of acute and subacute diffuse glomerulonephritis in first and second stage and in advanced stage, [G. Izar] Bull. schweiz. Akad. med. Wissensch. )supp. 1) 6:152-160, '50

50K1: autogenous, in cases of furunculosis resistant to penicillin therapy, [N. de C. Barbosa] Rev. brasil. med. 7:305-307, May, '50

50K2: in salmonellosis, [V. Márquez Biscayk, L. Fernández Urtiaga and J. Garcia Otero] Rev. méd. cubana 60:849-853, Dec. '49

50L1:  Lanza Castelli, R.A., and Elkeles, G., Bacteriology and bacteriotherapy in otorhinolaryngology, ANNALES D'OTO-LARYNGOLOGIE 67:2-3 (Feb.-Mar. 1950) p. 152-60 [16290]

50L2:  Barbosa, N. de C., Autogenous vaccine in cases resistant to penicillin, REVISTA BRASILEIRA DE MEDICINA 7:5 May 1950, p. 305-7. [32044]

51K1: autogenous, in penicillin resistant staphylococcic infections, [N. de C. Barbosa] Rev. brasil. med. 8:363-365, May, '51

51L1:  Zumsteeg, H., On focal infections, diagnostic and therapeutic considerations. AERZTLICHE WOCHENSCHRIFT 5:43 3 Nov. 1950, p. 841-6. [20244]

52J1: autogenous, clinical observations on use of autogenous vaccine made from cultures of coagulase positive hemolytic Staphylococcus aureus, [R. L. Goodale and A. B. Mangiaracine] Laryngoscope 62:299-310, March, '52

52J2: in acne vulgaris; record of 42 cases, [M. El-Zawahry] J. Roy. Egyptian M. A. 34:761-773, '51

52J3: treatment of chronic infections by new method, [F. Meyer] Quart. Bull. Sea View Hosp. 12:118-123, July-Oct. '51

52K1: autogenous, application of osmovaccines in general and in dermatology, [M. Héry] Bull. Soc. franç. dermat. et syph.

59:287-288, May-June, '52 F

52L1:  Bocage, A., Therapy of staphylococcus infections, GAZ. MÉD. FRANCE (GAZETTE MÉDICALE DE FRANCE ET DE PAYS DE LANGUE FRANCAISE, PARIS) 58:21 (November 1951), p. 1253 [18263]

52M1:  Liskova, K, Autovaccination in practice, PRAKT. LÉK., PRAHA (PRAKTICKY LÉKAR., PRAHA) 32:5 (5 March 52) [15767]

52M2:  Surjan, ZL., The specific treatment of ozaena; autovaccine in atrophic rhinitis, MAGYAR SEBÉSZET (BUDAPEST) 5;1 (March 1952), p. 61-5 [33553]

53J1: autogenous, [R. Cunha] Hospital, Rio de Janeiro 43:457-459, April '53 P

53J2: autogenous, analysis of series of asthma cases treated with autovaccine, [G. Bergquist] Acta med. scandinav. 144:101-106, '52

53J3: autovaccine in cholangitis, [H. Kipping and T. Schackow] Deutsches med. J. 4:81, Feb. 15, '53 G

53J4: therapy of pulmonary abscess by means of combination of antibiotics followed by endobronchial instillations of autovaccine, [J. Grenier, P. Collin and F. Lutier] Semaine hôp. Paris 29:1673-1679, May 20, '53 F

53L1:  Bergquist, G., Analysis

of a series of asthma [extrinsic and intrinsic] cases treated with autovaccine. ACTA. MED. SCAND. 144:2 (1052), p. 101-6 [32133]

53L2:   Albanese, P., Autovaccine therapy of diseases of peridontium, OSTERREICHISCHE ZEITSCHRIFT FUER STOMATOLOGIE (Wien)
49:9 (Sept. 1952), p. 497-9 [38418]

53M1:   Cunha, R., Autogenous vaccine, considerations, Hospital (Rio de Janeiro) 43:4 (April 1953) ,p. 457-9.   [39670]

53M2:   autovacc., ther. of cholangitis Kipping, H., Schackow, T., Autovaccines in cholangitis, DEUTSCHES MEDIZINISCHES JOURNAL (Berlin) 4:3-4 (15 Feb. 1953), p. 81 [30810]

54J1: autogenous, results of use of total autovaccine in chronic progressive polyarthritis, [A.R. Prévot] Bull. Acad. nat. méd. 138:120-123, Feb. 23-March 2, '54 F

54K1: autogenous, review of cases, [M. M. Wilson] J. J. Australia 2:509-511, Sept. 25, '54

54L1:   Kucera, K., Experience with therapeutic and preventive use
of autovaccines, LÉKARSKÉ LISTYY (Brno) 8:23 (1 Dec. 1953) p. 544-50   [52128]

54M1:   Serradell Capdevila, J.,

Simplification of the technic for preparing autovaccines, LABORATORIO (Granada) 17 (Feb. 1954) p. 111-4. [26994]

54M2:   Silcox, L.E., "Treatment of hyperplastic sinusitis.", TR. AM. LAR. RHIN. OTOL. SOC. 56TH MEETING, 1952, p. 60-72  [19675]

54M3:   Goodale, R.L., Mangiaracine, A.B., "Clinical observations on the use of autogenous vaccine made from cultures of coagulase
positive hemolytic Staphylococcus aureus.", TR. AM. LAR. RHIN. OTOL. SOC. 56TH MEETING, 1952, p. 22-37. [19672]

54M4:   Prévot, A.R., Results of treatment of rheumatoid arthritis with total autovaccinotherapy, BULL. ACAD. NAT. MÉD., PAR. 138:7-8 (23 Feb.-2 Mar. 1954), p. 120-3. [23284]

55J1: autogenous, bacterial autovaccines; immunitary, specific and allergic desensitizing effect, [R. F. Carron and G. R. Villarquide] Semana méd. 106:524-526, April 28, '55 S

55J2: myth of autogenous vaccines, [K. A. Baird] Am. Pract. and Digest Treat. 6:211-213, Feb. '55

55J3: very serious staphylococcic infection with pleuropulmonary manifestations; cure by erythromycin, autovaccine and transfusions, [P. and J. Michon] Presse méd.

62:1790, Dec. 25, '54 F

[58403]

55K1: autogenous, bacterial vaccines in treatment of asthma, [A.W. Frankland, W.H. Hughes and R. H. Gorrill] Brit. M. J. 2:941-944, Oct. 15, '55

55L1: Wilson, M.M., "Autogenous vaccine therapy; infections: a review of cases.", MED. J. AUSTRALIA 41, Vol 2 (12) 18 Sept.
1954, p. 507-9. [25164]

55L2: Wagner, V., Maratka, Z., Changes in skin tests following treatment of ulcerative colitis with autovaccines, SBORNIK LÉKARSKÝ 56 (4), April 1954, p. 94-8. [50069]

55L3: Michon, P., and J. Michon, Very grave staphylococcal infections with pleuropulmonary manifestations, autovaccine with erythromycin and blood transfusion, PRESSE MÉDICALE (Paris) 62 (86), 25 Dec. 1954, p. 1790. [49282]

55M1: Carron, R.F., Villarquide, G.R., Bacterial autovaccines; their immunization action and specific and allergic desensitization, SEM. MÉD, B. AIR. 106 (17), 28 Apr. 1955, p. 524-6. [37053]

55M2: Morales Villazín, N., Giovannetti, D.E., Studies of the citreus variety of the staphylococcal genus in antibiotic-resistant skin infections, SEM. MÉD, B. AIR. 107(1), 7 July, 1955, p. 45-8.

56J1: autogenous, resistant urinary tract infections; combined autogenous vaccine and drug therapy, [J.H. Winer] California Med. 84:204-205, March, '56

56K1: autogenous, autovaccine in urologic diseases, [L. Rebaudi, L. M. Veiga and A. S. Rebaudi] Rev. argent. urol. 24:667-668, Oct.-Dec. '55 S

56M1: Lahiri, D.C., Chatterji, S.N., Mukherjee, A.M., Neogy, K.N., Basu, S.N., "Use of autovaccine made out of selective
pathogen culture for the treatment of chronic bowel [intestinal]
diseases of unknown aetiology.", J. IND. M. ASS. 26(9), 1 May 1956, p. 333-8. [28084]

56M2: Winer, J.H., "Resistant urinary tract infections; combined autogenous vaccine and drug therapy.", CALIFORNIA MEDICINE (San Francisco) 84(3), March 1956, p. 204-5. [12885]

57M1: Uldrich, J., Chronic inflammation of male adnexa/chronic prostatitis, autovaccines with antibiotics, ZEITSCHR. UROL. 50(6), 1957, p. 343-8. [55310]

57M2: Gross, H., Autovaccines and autonosodes, MEDIZINISCHE (Stuttgart) No. 20 (17 May 1957), p. 756-7. [38723]

57M3:  Rebaudi, L., Veiga, L.M., and Rebaudi, A.S., Autovaccines in urological diseases, REV. ARGENT. UROL. 24(10-12), Oct.-Dec. 1955, p. 667-8. [18653]

58L1:  Barbosa, N. De C., New technic for the preparation of autogenous vaccines, p. 387-8. [8955]
[1958 d]

58M1:  Benoist, F., Héraud, G., Leliévre, A., Labrousse, C., Supprative air cysts of lung with renal amylosis; remarkable action of vaccinotherapy, BULL. SOC. MÉD. HOP. PARIS 74(17-18), 16-23 May 1958, 407-10.  [39618]

58M2:  Wegmann, T., Schindler-Baumann, I., Critical remarks on
vaccine therapy. in focal infection, PRAXIS, Bern 47(12), 20
March 1958, p. 296-8.  [34986]

59L1:  Thiers, H., Coudert, J., Colomb, D., Fayolle, J., and Moulin, G., Autovaccine therapy of fungal diseases; technic, indications and complications, BULL. SOC. FR. DERM. SYPH. 65(2) Apr.-May 1958, p. 185-6.  [2410]

59M1:  Hackl, H., Auto-vaccines in modern medicine, MEDIZIN-ISCHE (Stuttgart), No. 6, 7 Feb. 1959, p. 247-50.  [17328]

59M2:  Ritchie, J.M., "Control of the common cold by autogenous vaccine or by antibiotics.",

ANTIBIOTICS ANNUAL (New York) 1958-1959, p. 174-7.  [11619]

59M3:  Febbraro, E.E., Rheumatism, periodontosis and autovaccinotherapy, DIA MÉDICO (Buenos Aires) 30(94), 25 Dec. 1958, p. 3266.  [3979]

59M4:  Hodek, B., Autovaccine therapy in allergic diseases of the
upper respiratory tract, ALLERGIE & ASTHMA, LPZ. 5(1), Feb. 1959,
p. 39-44.  [23442]

59M5:  Banchieri, G.C., and Milillo, V.A., Autovaccine therapy
of broncopneumopathy in aged, GIORNALE DI GERONT. 7(4), Apr. 1959, p. 283-7.  [38114]

60P1:  Kollarova K, Sonak R: Treatment of allergic diseases with autovaccines.  Bratisl Lek Listy 42:36-43, 15 Jan 62  (Cz)

60P2:  Kim HS: Autovaccine-induced alteration of drug resistance of nongonorrheal urethritis.  J. Korea Med. Ass. 5:1774-7, 30 Apr 62  (Kor)

61P1:  Chachaj W, Suchnicka R: Oral administration of autovaccine in bronchial asthma of bacterial origin.  Pol Tyg Lek 15:1263-6, 15 Aug 60 (Pol)

61P2:  Soeltz-Szoets J: Autoinoculation and local vaccination in recurrent herpes simplex.  Derm Wschr 143:343-5,

1 Apr 61 (Ger)

61P3: Thiers H, Coudert J, Colomb D, Fayolle J, Moulin G: Reflexions on autovaccine therapy of candidiases. Bull Soc Franc Derm Syph 67:710-1, Aug-Oct 60 (Fr)

62P1: Ambroso GA, Zinicola M: On the utility of autovaccinotherapy in migrating phlebitis. Minerva Chir 15:38-40, 15 Jan 60 (It)

62P2: Gernand K, Haehnel H: Auto vaccine therapy in chronic recurrent infections. Deutsch Gesundh. 15:10-3, 7 Jan 60 (Ger)

62P3: Hammer JM, MacGregor JR: An autoclaved vaccine in the treatment of chronic staphylococcic infections. J. Michigan Med. Soc. 59:292, Feb 60

62P4: McCoy KL, Kennedy ER: Autogenous vaccine therapy in staphylococcic infections. JAMA 174:35-8, 3 Sept 60

63P1: Bube FW: Long-term autovacine-furadantin treatment in chronic pyelonephritis. Med Welt 9:480-1, 2 Mar 63 (Ger)

63P2: Gorgiev TB, Ketkov GF, Zaslavskaia ES: Autovaccine therapy in treatment of septicopyemia in children. Khirurgiia (Moskva) 38:57-9, Dec 62 (Rus)

63P3: Glaser-Tuerk M: Follow-up treatment of patients treated for focal infection with dentin autovaccines. Med. Welt 44:2356-9, 3 Nov. 62 (Ge)

63P4: Prevot, AR: Curability of anaerobic corynebacteriosis by autovacinotherapy. Ann Inst Pasteur (Paris) 104:697-8, May 63 (Fr)

64P1: Autovaccine therapy in chronic bacillary dysentery. Tyagi MN. Indian Med J 57:215, Aug 63

64P2: Use of staphylococcus toxoid and autogenous vaccine in the treatment of boils. Paulson G, etal. North Carolina Med. J. 24:385-6, Sept. 1963

64P3: Treatment of urinary infections with autovaccine. Karapandov M. Khirurgiia (Sofiia) 16:627-31, 1963 (Bul)

64P4: Attempted treatment of chronic supprative otitis media in children with the aid of autovaccines. Lewandowski H. Otolaryng Pol 17:63-8, 1963 (Pol)

64P5: Use of an auto-vaccine in allergic diseases in children. Preliminary communication. Lewandowska J, et al. Pediat Pol 38:897-903, Oct 63 (Pol)

64P6: Asthma and autogenous vaccine. Arico SA, Sem Med (B Air) 122:1394-8, 13 Jun 63 (Sp)

65P1: Leg ulcer due to moraxella. Intense allergic reaction and success of autovaccine. Thiers H, et al. Bull Soc Franc Derm Syph 71:343-4, May-Jun 64 (Fr)

67P1:  Evaluation of an autogenous laryngeal papilloma vaccine. Shipkowitz NL, et al. Laryngoscope 77:1047-66, Jun 67

67P2:  Experiences with auto-vaccine treatment in childhood diseases.  Szakáll S. Kinderaerztl Prax 34:485-90, Nov. 66  (Ger)

68P1:  Autovaccine therapy. Morozova VT, et al.  Ter Arkh 38:98-101, Feb. 66  (Rus)

68P2:  Experience with auto-vaccine therapy under hospital conditions.  Kuzhushko LN. Brach Delo 1:136-7, Jan 68 (Rus)

69P1:  Analysis of an autogenous vaccine in the treatment of juvenile papillomatosis of the larynx.  Strome M.  Laryngoscope 79:272-9, Feb 69

69P2:  Preliminary experiences with the combined autovaccine and polyvalent vaccine.  Roglová J, et al.  Sborn Ved Prac Lek Fak Karlov Univ 11:659-64, 1968 (Ger)

69P3:  Autovaccine therapy of chronic atrophic rhinitis in children.  Paunescu C, et al. Otorinolaringologie (Bucur) 13:269-73, Jul-Sep 68  (Rum)

69P4:  Autovaccine therapy of ulcerous blepharitis in combination with modern methods

of therapy.  Filippovich Ba, et al. Oftal Zh 23:192-4, 1968 (Rus)

70P1:  Autogenous vaccines in theory and in practice. Personal experience.  Smith DT. Arch Intern Med (Chicago) 125:344-50, Feb 70

70P2:  Pseudomyxoma peritonei treated with autogenous vaccine Graham JB, et al.  Clin Obstet Gynec 12:955-7, Dec 69

71P1:  Use of autovaccines in the treatment of various chronic diseases. Lipkin ME, et al.  Zh Mikrobiol Epidemiol Immunobiol 46:71-3, Oct 69  (Rus)

72P1:  Is autovaccine therapy still of importance in the era of chemotherapy? Schmid W., Med Welt 23:889-92, 10 Jun 72 (Ger)

72P2:  Treatment with autovaccine prepared from sputum in intrinsic bronchial asthma. Popescu IG, et al.  Stud Cercet Med Interna 12: 259-63, 1971 (Eng. Abstr.)

72P3:  Treatment of chronic nonspecific inflammatory diseases of the lungs and bronchi using autovacine. Masuev AM, et al.  Klin Med (Mosk) 49:36-8, May 71 (Eng. Abstr.)  (Rus)

72P4:  Effect of an autovaccine on the development of staphylococcal infection of experimentally injured eyes inoculated with a culture insensitive to antibiotics.

Filippovich BA, et al. Vestn Oftalmol 3:72-3, 1971 (Eng. Abstr.) (Rus)

72P5: Desensitizing effect of autovaccino- and anatoxin therapy in staphylococcal infections. Proskurov VA. Zh Mikrobiol Epidemiol Immunobiol 48:46-8, Sep 71 (Eng. Abstr.)

73P1: Surgery of rheumatoid arthritis. The role of synovectomy and use of autologous vaccine. Cobey MC. Clin Orthop 88:110-2, 1972

73P2: Experience in the therapy of allergic respiratory diseases using complex autovaccines. Hlasivcova V, et al. Cesk Otolaryngol 22:93-9, Apr 73 (Eng Abstr) Cze)

73P3: Case of acne rosacea cured with autovaccine. Podkowi_ska I, et. al. Wiad Lek 26:573-4, 15 Mar. 73 Oeng. Abstr.) (Pol)

73P4: Occurrence of antibodies in bovine mastitis following intradermal and subcutaneous injection of polyvalent autovaccine. I. Antibodies in serum. Kurek C. Pol Arch Weter 15:431-43, 1972 (Eng.Abstr.) (Pol)

73P5: Occurrence of antibodies in bovine mastitis and after intradermal and subcutaneous injection of polyvalent auto-vaccine. II. Antibodies in milk. Kurek C. Pol Arch Weter 15:445-62, 1972 (Eng. Abstr.) (Pol)

74P1: Proceedings: Clinical trial of autogenous tumor vaccine for treatment of osteogenic sarcoma. Southam CM, Et al. Proc Natl Cancer Conf 7:91-100, 1973

74P2: Our experience with combined autovaccine and heterovaccine therapy in chronic bronchitis with asthma (author's transl). Roglová J, etal. Cas Lek Cesk 114: 491-3, 19 Apr 74 (Eng.Abstr.) (Cze)

75P1: A clinical trial of autogenous vaccines in the treatment of osteogenic sarcoma. Marcove RC. Beitr Pathol 153 (1):65-72, Oct 74

75P2: Condylomata acuminata: treatment by autogenous vaccine. Ablin RJ, et al. Ill Med J 147(4):343-4, 346, Apr 75

75P3: Autovaccination in cases of nonspecific parotitis. Polenichkin VK. Stomatologiia (Mosk) 53(4):29-31, Jul-Aug (Eng.Abstr.) (Rus)

76P1: Chronic posttraumatic osteomyelitis. Attempt at oral autovaccine therapy. Ring J, et al. Fortschr Med 94(5):264-5, 268, 12 Feb 76 (Eng Abstr.) (Ger)

76P2: Importance of individual method of vaccine therapy in brucellosis. Otaraev IB, et al. Sov Med (8):153-4, Aug 75 (Rus)

77P1:  Intralymphatic infusion
of autochthonous tumor cells in
canine lymphoma.  Julliard GJ et
al., Int J Radiat Oncol Biol
Phys 1(5-6):497-503, March-Apr.
1976


77P2:  Autovaccine treatment of
rhiniologic diseases of allergic
pharynx.  Mitrovic K, et al.  J
Fr. Otorhinolaryngol. 25(1):45-
7, Jan '76


78P1:  Effect of autovaccine on
various immunologic indices in
chronic staphylococcal
infections.  Giedrys-Galant S.
Ann Acad Med Stetin 23:279-303,
1977 (Eng Abstr)  (Pol)


78P2:  Bacterial autovaccine
therapy in children with
respiratory allergy in early
childhood.  Dolezalova K, et al.
 Sb Ved Lek Fak Univ Karlovy
[Suppl]19(5):599-601, 1976 (Eng
Abst)  (Cze)


79P1:  Preparation of immuno-
therapeutic autologous tumor
cell vaccines from solid tumors
 Peters LC, et al.  Cancer Res.
39(4):1353-60, Apr 79


80P1:  Use of an autovaccine and
proteolytic enzymes in the
overall treatment of chronic
osteomyelitis.  Zebzeev EF, et
al.  Klin Khir 1980;(1):38-40
(Engl Abstr)  (Rus)


83P - - ["VACCINE THERAPY"
disappears w/out reference
elsewhere]

# APPENDIX E:   SUPPLEMENTAL BIBLIOGRAPHY

Ager, L.C., NYMJ, Sept. 16, 1916, [I.M. reinjection of 0.5 to 3 cc spinal fluid in polio

Allen, R.W., Vaccine Therapy and Opsonic Method of Treatment, 1908

Arrhenius, Svante A., Immunology, MacMillan Co. 1907

Bagley 1987 [homeopathy]

Bazell R, in The New Republic, 203, 9-10+ (Dec. 31, 1990), "Topic of Cancer"

Berger, Leslie, Los Angeles Times, August 24, 1994 [coining]

Boetcher, 1964 [oral autotherapy for dog bite]

Brain, Peter, Galen, on Bloodletting, Cambridge U. Press, 1986

Buchsel PC and Kelleher J [Nursing Clinics of N. America 24, Dec. 1989, 907-938]

Burke, D. S., Vaccine 11 (1993), p. 883-94

Chao NJ and Blume KG, West. J. Med 152 (Jan. 1990)

Chase, Allan, Magic Shots, William Morrow, 1982, p. 50

Chou NJ, etal, West J. Med. 151 (Dec. 1989) 638-43

CLARK, W.R., Experimental Foundations of Modern Immuniz. (1986), 416.

Clendening, L., Methods of Treatment, 1943, p. 65

Cohen, J., Science 265 (1994)

Colebrook, L., Almroth Wright, Provocative Doctor and Thinker, 1954

Copeland, N.G., etal., Science, Oct. 1, 1993, "Genome Maps IV"

Cushing, JE and DH Campbell, Principles of Immunology, McGraw-Hill, New York, 1957.

Cuyugan, San Francisco, USA, Jan.,1988 (personal communications)

Dowling, HF, Fighting Infection, 1977, Harvard U. Press

Duncan, NYMJ, November 4, 1916, p. 901 [poison ivy]

Editorial, The London Times (Aug. 30, 1942) [on penicillin]

Encyclopedia Britannica, 1991, 12 p. 228 [bacterial vaccines]

Encyclopedia Britannica 1972, "Vaccine Therapy"

FAUCI, A.S., Science 239 (5

Feb. 1988), 620.

Ferreira OC and Barcinski MA, Cellular Immunology 101 (1986), 259-265, "Autologous Induction of the Human T-Cell-Dependent Monocyte Procoagulent Activity: A Possible Link between Immunoregulatory Phenomena and Blood Coagulation"

Fleming, A, and G. F. Petrie of the Lister Institute wrote Recent Advances in Vaccine and Serum Therapy for "The Recent Advances Series" [P. Blakiston's Son & Co., Inc., Philadelphia 1934]

Fleming, A., "Serum and vaccine therapy in combination with sulfanilimide ...", Proc. Roy. Soc. Med. 32:911-920, June 1939. [on vaccinetherapy]

Florey H., and Chain, British J. of Exper. Pathology, 1940

Freeman, John, "Skin reactions in asthma", protein idiopathies. The Practitioner 116:73-8, January 1926..

Freeman,J.,"Toxic Idiopathies", Lancet, July 31, 1920, 229-35.

French, J. M., NYMJ, Sept. 23, 1916, 608 [oral autotherapy for poison ivy]

Goldman, J, Bone Marrow Transplantation (July) 1994, 14:1, "'Blood and marrow transplantation': a message from the editor"

Gorin NC, Comptes Rendus des Seances de la Societe de Biologie et de Sesfilialie, 1993, 187 (4), 452-86

Greger, etal, 1987, p. 4057 [on transplants]

HEKTOEN 1929

Hippocrates, Adams 1886, p. 261
Hippocrates, Translated by WHS Jones, Wm Heinemann Ltd., London, 1923, Vol. 1

Hippocrates, Vol. 2, Transl by WHS Jones, 1923

Hippocrates, Jones 1931, 1967, Harvard U. Press, Vol. 4

Hughes, H. in D. Wilson, 1976 [on Fleming]

Landsteiner, Karl, THE SPECIFICITY OF SEROLOGICAL REACTIONS (Harvard U. Press, Cambridge 1945)

Lederberg, J, JAMA 260 (Aug. 5, 1988), p. 684-5, on wonder drugs and tissue-culture advances

Lederberg, J., JAMA 260, 685, Aug.5, 1988

Lehrer, Steven, EXPLORERS OF THE BODY, Doubleday, 1979.

Levins, R., etal. (Harvard Working Group on New and Resurgent Diseases), American Scientist 82 (Jan.-Feb. 1994), 52-60, "The Emergence of New Diseases", p. 60

Lewis GP, Mangham BA, J. Pathology 1979 Jan., 127 (1):39-49, "Blood flow and permeability changes in the immune lymphocyte transfer reaction"

Lohr, 1988, p. A11 [on leeches]

Maddox, J., Nature 362, 105 (1993) [on Francis Crick]

Mann, 1973, p. 5, Chapter 1, "General Considerations, Neural Theory of the Action of Acupuncture"

Marks, G., and W.K. Beatty, EPIDEMICS.

Marks 1976, p. 221-2 [on Colebrook and puerperal sepsis]

Marx J, in Science 252, 27-8 (Apr. 5, 1991) [oral antigen]

Mayer, A, Munchener Med. Woch., 27 Dec. 1910: 2757-9, "Ein Versuch, Schwangerschaftstoxikosen durch Einspritzungen von Schwangerschaftserum zu heilen".

Mayer and Linser, 1910

McManus, J .F. A., Fundamental Ideas of Medicine - A Brief History of Medicine, Charles C. Thomas, Springfield, Ill. 1963

MEDICAL TIMES 854 (Aug. 1968) [on Pasteur]

Merigan, T., Science 264, 22 Apr. 94.

Osler, per W. H. Welch in McManus, J .F. A., The Fundamental Ideas of Medicine - A Brief History of Medicine, Charles C. Thomas, Springfield, Ill. 1963, p.6

Ossenkoppele GJ etal, Bone Marrow Transpl. 13 (Jan) 1994

Parham, P., Nature 368, 495-6 (7 Apr. 94)

Parish, HJ, History of Immunization 1965 [on Leishman]

Pasteur - Medical Times, 854, August 1968

Pauling, Linus, "The Future of Orthomolecular Medicine", pp. 249-253, in R. P. Huemer, ed., Roots of Molecular Medicine, W.H. Freeman, N.Y., 1986.

Pauling, Linus, and Ewan Cameron, CANCER AND VITAMIN C, Linus Pauling Institute of Science and Medicine 1979, 114

Pauling, L., Science 160 (19 Apr. 1968), 265-271

Pauling, L., Vitamin C and the Common Cold, W. H. Freeman & Co., San Francisco 1970

Pauling, Linus, "Molecular Structure and Intermolecular Forces" in Karl Landsteiner, THE SPECIFICITY OF SEROLOGICAL REACTIONS (Harvard U. Press, Cambridge 1945)

Physicians of the Mayo Clinic

and the Mayo Foundation, U.
Minn. Press, Minneapolis, 1937

Pierce, EA [15H1]: abstr.:
JAMA April 18, 1915

Poller, L., Recent Advances in
Blood Coagulation 2 (1977)

Rennie, John, in Scientific
American 264, 120 (June 1991)
[autolymphocyte therapy]

Roitt, Ivan M., Essential
Immunology, Third Ed.,
Blackwell Scientific
Publications, Oxford 1977

Romer, A.S., THE VERTEBRATE
BODY (1962)

Russell, P.E., MAN'S MASTERY OF
MALARIA (1955)

Sabin, Florence, J. EXPER. MED.
70, 67-82, "Cellular Reactions
to a Dye-Protein with a Concept
of the Mechanism of Antibody
Formation", 1939

Sandler, S. G., & A. J.
Silvergleid, Eds., AUTOLOGOUS
TRANSFUSION, 1983, Arlington,
VA: American Association of
Blood Banks

Schrup 1910

Shryock, R.H., The Development
of Modern Medicine, New York:
Alfred A. Knopf, 1947, p. 277,
283  [on Koch]

Smith, Kent, Homeopathy
Medicine for Today's Living,
Glendale, CA 1982

Stephenson 1960 [homeopathy]

Stern, Heinrich, JAMA LV (Nov.
19, 1910) 1781-5 [history of
bloodletting in children]

Unger, Lester J, "Blood
Transfusion", Canad. Pract. &
Rev., Oct. 1916 per NYMJ 4 Nov.
1916, 914

Wegman, M., JAMA 271 (8), 632,
Feb. 23, '94  [on Koch]

Wien p. 1629; Encyclopedia
Britannica, 1986; Bier 1901

Williams, T.I., Howard Florey,
Oxford U. Press, 1984, 65, 209

Wilson, D., 1978 [on Wright and
Freeman]

Wright, Almroth E., "Immunity"
in Encyclopedia Brit. 1929.

Wright, Almroth E., Studies on
Immunization, A Constable and
Co. Ltd., London 1909, 311]

Wright - Encyclopedia Brit.,
1972, "Vaccine Therapy"

Yang etal [Am J. Neph. 1994,
14(1):72-5 [on transplants]

Zamichow N, Los Angeles Times
Dec. 19, 1991, A40

# INDEX